CONTENTS

Introduction

Slow cookers are a simple way to make home-cooked comfort foods. This small electric appliance, a staple of many homes for more than 30 years, is based on the principles of slow cooking. The concept of slow cooking is simple: Put food into some sort of container or contained area and let it cook slowly. It's a method used in barbecue pits and pig roasts, where low temperatures and a lot of time allow meat to become tender. Slow cooking can be done via dry heat, as in an oven or roaster, or it can be moist, by involving liquid during the cooking process. Slow cookers use moisture in a unique way because they remain sealed during the cooking process. As food cooks and lets off steam, the condensation collects inside the device.

The slow cooking method has been around for centuries, and the electrical slow cooker first became popular in the 1970s kitchen -- the original slow cookers came in chic colors of the day, such as avocado and goldenrod. But when microwaves came into vogue a few years later, the slow cooker was left behind as people started zapping their food. However, the tide has turned back to slow cooking and new cookbooks that provide a variety of tasty recipes for this one-pot wonder. Manufacturers developed newer, more stylish versions of the device, which led to its resurgence over the last decade as a must-have appliance for time-strapped cooks. In the next section, we'll look at how a pot for preparing beans revolutionized cooking.

How it works

A slow cooker has three main components:
An outer casing
An inner container
A lid
The outer casing is metal and contains low-wattage heating coils, the component responsible for cooking the food, and these heating coils are completely encapsulated by the outer casing. The inner container, which is also called a crock, is made of glazed ceramic and fits inside the metal heating element. In some models, you can remove this cooking crock from the outer shell. The third piece of the appliance is a domed lid that fits tightly onto the crock.

The appliance cooks based on a combination of wattage and time. When turned on, the electrical coils heat up and transfer heat indirectly from the outer casing to the space between the base wall and the stoneware container. This indirect heat warms the crock to between 180 and 300 degrees Fahrenheit (82 to 149 degrees Celsius). This method of heat transfer simmers the ingredients inside the crock at a low temperature for several hours, until the food is thoroughly cooked.

As the food cooks, it releases steam, which the lid traps. The condensation creates a vacuum seal between the lid and the rim of the crock, which adds moisture to the food while helping the cooking process -- the lid is integral to the cooking process. The slow cooker typically has three settings: low, high and off. In programmable slow cookers, the device will switch to a warm setting after it has cooked the food to keep the meal at a proper temperature.

Benefits of using a slow cooker

Using a slow cooker is a great way to save time and still prepare a nutritious meal. Assemble the meal in the morning, put it in the slow cooker, and at the end of the day, dinner is ready -- without much mess or many dishes to clean. The device requires only a small amount of electricity only to do its work -- compared with a standard oven, a slow cooker uses a lot less energy, so it won't heat up an entire kitchen the way an oven does. Cooking with a slow cooker can also be an economically smart choice, because you can use cheaper cuts of meat. Condensation acts as a self-baster, so traditionally tougher cuts of meat become tender in a slow cooker. And just because you're saving time and money doesn't mean you're sacrificing taste. Vegetables cooked in a slow cooker can absorb stocks and spices, giving them fuller flavors.

The high and low settings on the device allow you to adjust the temperature for the length of time you want the meal to cook. Although cooking on low is completely safe, if you're home during the process, cooking on high for an hour first to ensure the food is thoroughly cooked.

What to cook in a slow cooker

Meats are one of the most popular items to make in a slow cooker, but they need to be thawed beforehand or they'll take too long to cook. When cooking meat, it's important to heat the meat to 140 degrees Fahrenheit (60 degrees Celsius) as quickly as possible to kill any bacteria. Always make sure the internal temperature of the meat is within recommended guidelines before serving. When cooking poultry, use poultry with the skin still attached -- this will help keep the meat moist throughout the cooking process.

Prepping vegetables for slow cooking may take longer to prepare than the meat -- it's important to cut them uniformly so they'll cook evenly. Vegetables may also take longer to cook than meat, so when preparing stews or meat-and-vegetable dishes, layer the vegetables on the bottom of the pot.

Some of the best slow cooker meals are soups and stews because the slow cooker is designed to simmer on the low setting for long periods of time. Cover soup ingredients with water, and if you need to add more liquid during cooking, bring it to a boil first, so it doesn't lower the soup's cooking temperature.

Dips and spreads are another category where slow cookers shine. The low heat keeps a cheese-based dip warm without burning the ingredients, and maintaining a dip at a low heat prevents ingredients from congealing during a party.

Grains are sometimes a surprising way to use a slow cooker. Oatmeal, cracked wheat and rice porridge can be cooked overnight to provide a hot, nutritious breakfast. Bread and bread-based dishes like stuffing can also be baked in a slow cooker -- the low heat setting also helps bread dough rise. Another surprising slow-cooking category is desserts. While rice and tapioca puddings may seem like a no-brainer, you can also use slow cookers to make hot fruit desserts and even cakes.

Some recipes call for adding ingredients near the end of the cooking time because of the nature of the ingredients and their tolerance for the slow-cooking process. Spices and herbs may become too concentrated during cooking, so be sure to adjust their levels at the end of the process. Likewise, some vegetables, dairy products and seafood will lose their flavor and texture if simmered for too long, so if the recipe calls for including them near the end of the process, be sure to follow the directions carefully.

Breakfast Recipes

1.   Mushroom Quiche

Servings: 2   Cooking Time: 6 Hours
Ingredients:

- 2 cups baby Bella mushrooms, chopped
- ½ cup cheddar cheese, shredded
- 4 eggs, whisked
- ½ cup heavy cream
- 1 tablespoon basil, chopped
- 2 tablespoons chives, chopped
- A pinch of salt and black pepper
- ½ cup almond flour
- ¼ teaspoons baking soda
- Cooking spray

Directions:
In a bowl, mix the eggs with the cream, flour and the other ingredients except the cooking spray and stir well.   Grease the Crock Pot with the cooking spray, pour the quiche mix, spread well, put the lid on and cook on High for 6 hours.   Slice the quiche, divide between plates and serve for breakfast.
Nutrition Info: calories 211, fat 6, fiber 6, carbs 6, protein 10

2.   "baked" Creamy Brussels Sprouts

Servings: 2 (serving Size Is ½ Of Recipe—6.3 Ounces)   Cooking Time: 2 Hours And 25 Minutes
Ingredients:

- 14 Brussels sprouts
- ¼ cup Parmesan cheese, grated
- 2 garlic cloves
- 2 tablespoons extra virgin olive oil
- ½ cup cream cheese
- 1 teaspoon balsamic vinegar
- Salt and pepper to taste

Directions:
Rinse the Brussels sprouts in cold water to remove dirt and dust.   Discard the first leaves.   Pour oil into Crock-Pot and add Brussels sprouts.   Add in the remaining ingredients and stir.   Cover and cook for 3-4 hours on low or 2 hours on HIGH.   Before serving, sprinkle with Parmesan or feta cheese.   Let cheese melt for 2 or 3 minutes.
Nutrition Info: Calories: 228.7, Total Fat: 15.85 g, Saturated Fat: 8.95 g, Cholesterol: 49.28 mg, Sodium: 332.45 mg, Potassium: 522.11 mg, Total Carbohydrates: 8.57 g, Sugar: 4.16 g, Protein: 10.93 g

3.   Eggs With Brussel Sprouts

Servings: 4   Cooking Time: 6 Hours
Ingredients:

- 1 cup Brussel sprouts, halved
- ½ cup Mozzarella, shredded
- 5 eggs, beaten
- 1 teaspoon chili powder
- 1 teaspoon olive oil

Directions:
Pour olive oil in the Crock Pot.   Then add the layer of the Brussel sprouts.   Sprinkle the vegetables with chili powder and eggs.   Then add mozzarella and close the lid.   Cook the meal on Low for 6 hours.
Nutrition Info: Per Serving: 110 calories, 8.8g protein, 2.9g carbohydrates, 7.5g fat, 1.1g fiber, 206mg cholesterol, 110mg sodium, 172mg potassium

4.   Egg Bake

Servings: 8   Cooking Time: 8 Hours
Ingredients:

- 20 ounces tater tots
- 2 yellow onions, chopped
- 6 ounces bacon, chopped
- 2 cups cheddar cheese, shredded
- 12 eggs
- ¼ cup parmesan, grated
- 1 cup milk
- Salt and black pepper to the taste
- 4 tablespoons white flour
- Cooking spray

Directions:
Grease your Crock Pot with cooking spray and layer half of the tater tots, onions, bacon, cheddar and parmesan.   Continue layering the rest of the tater tots, bacon, onions, parmesan and cheddar.   In a bowl, mix the eggs with milk, salt, pepper and flour and whisk well.   Pour this into the Crock Pot, cover and cook on Low for 8 hours.   Slice, divide between plates and serve for breakfast.
Nutrition Info: calories 290, fat 9, fiber 1, carbs 9, protein 22

5.   Quinoa And Chia Pudding

Servings: 2   Cooking Time: 6 Hours
Ingredients:

- 1 cup coconut cream
- 2 tablespoons chia seeds
- ½ cup almond milk
- 1 tablespoon sugar
- ½ cup quinoa, rinsed
- ½ teaspoon vanilla extract

Directions:
In your Crock Pot, mix the cream with the chia seeds and the other ingredients, toss, put the lid on and cook on Low for 6 hours.   Divide into bowls and serve for breakfast.
Nutrition Info: calories 120, fat 2, fiber 1, carbs 6, protein 4

6.   Apple Breakfast Rice

Servings: 4   Cooking Time: 7 Hours
Ingredients:

- 4 apples, cored, peeled and chopped
- 2 teaspoons cinnamon powder
- 1 and ½ cups brown rice
- 2 tablespoons butter
- ½ teaspoon vanilla extract
- A pinch of nutmeg, ground
- 5 cups milk

Directions:

13

Put the butter in your Crock Pot, add apples, cinnamon, rice, vanilla, nutmeg and milk, cover, cook on Low for 7 hours, stir, divide into bowls and serve for breakfast.
Nutrition Info:calories 214, fat 4, fiber 5, carbs 7, protein 4

7. Greek Mushrooms Casserole

Servings: 4   Cooking Time: 4 Hrs
Ingredients:

12 eggs, whisked	½ cup sun-dried
Salt and black pepper	tomatoes
to the taste	1 tsp garlic, minced
½ cup milk	2 cups spinach
1 red onion, chopped	½ cup feta cheese,
1 cup baby bell	crumbled
mushrooms, sliced	

Directions:
Beat eggs with milk, salt, and black pepper in a suitable bowl.   Toss mushrooms, spinach, onion, garlic, and tomatoes in your Crock Pot.   Pour the egg mixture on top and drizzle the cheese over it. Put the cooker's lid on and set the cooking time to hours on Low settings.   Slice and serve.
Nutrition Info: Per Serving: Calories 325, Total Fat 7g, Fiber 7g, Total Carbs 27g, Protein 18g

8. Pumpkin And Quinoa Mix

Servings: 2   Cooking Time: 8 Hours
Ingredients:

Cooking spray	½ teaspoon vanilla
½ cup quinoa	extract
1 cup almond milk	¼ teaspoon
1 tablespoon honey	cinnamon powder
¼ cup pumpkin	
puree	

Directions:
Grease your Crock Pot with the cooking spray, add the quinoa, milk, honey and the other ingredients, stir, put the lid on and cook on Low for 7 hours. Divide the mix into bowls and serve for breakfast.
Nutrition Info:calories 242, fat 3, fiber 8, carbs 20, protein 7

9. Creamy Strawberries Oatmeal

Servings: 8   Cooking Time: 8 Hours
Ingredients:

6 cups water	1 cup Greek yogurt
2 cups milk	2 cups strawberries,
2 cups steel cut oats	halved
1 teaspoon cinnamon	1 teaspoon vanilla
powder	extract

Directions:
In your Crock Pot, mix water with milk, oats, yogurt, cinnamon, strawberries and vanilla, toss, cover and cook on Low for 8 hours.   Divide into bowls and serve for breakfast.
Nutrition Info:calories 200, fat 4, fiber 6, carbs 8, protein 4

10. Apple And Chia Mix

Servings: 2   Cooking Time: 8 Hours
Ingredients:

¼ cup chia seeds	1 teaspoon vanilla
2 apples, cored and	extract
roughly cubed	½ tablespoon
1 cup almond milk	cinnamon powder
2 tablespoons maple	Cooking spray
syrup	

Directions:
Grease your Crock Pot with the cooking spray, add the chia seeds, milk and the other ingredients, toss, put the lid on and cook on Low for 8 hours. Divide the mix into bowls and serve for breakfast.
Nutrition Info:calories 453, fat 29.3, fiber 8, carbs 51.1, protein 3.4

11. Vanilla Maple Oats

Servings: 4   Cooking Time: 8 Hrs
Ingredients:

1 cup steel-cut oats	2 tsp cinnamon
2 tsp vanilla extract	powder
2 cups vanilla almond	2 cups of water
milk	2 tsp flaxseed
2 tbsp maple syrup	Cooking spray
	2 tbsp blackberries

Directions:
Coat the base of your Crock Pot with cooking spray. Stir in oats, almond milk, vanilla extract, cinnamon, maple syrup, flaxseeds, and water. Put the cooker's lid on and set the cooking time to 8 hours on Low settings.   Stir well and serve with blackberries on top.   Devour.
Nutrition Info: Per Serving: Calories 200, Total Fat 3g, Fiber 6g, Total Carbs 9g, Protein 3g

12. Scrambled Spinach Eggs

Servings: 9   Cooking Time: 2 Hrs
Ingredients:

8 eggs	3 tbsp butter
½ cup spinach	1 tsp minced garlic
½ cup cherry	5 oz. Cheddar cheese
tomatoes	½ cup milk
1 tsp dried oregano	
1 tsp salt	

Directions:
First, beat the eggs with cheddar cheese, milk, oregano, garlic, salt, cherry tomatoes, and spinach in a large bowl.   Coat the base of your Crock Pot with butter.   Pour the egg-tomato mixture into the Crock Pot.   Put the cooker's lid on and set the cooking time to 2 hours on High settings.   Serve.
Nutrition Info: Per Serving: Calories 187, Total Fat 14.3g, Fiber 0g, Total Carbs 3.55g, Protein 11g

13. Breakfast Spinach Pie

Servings: 4   Cooking Time: 2 Hours
Ingredients:

5 flour tortillas
2 eggs, beaten
3 cups spinach, chopped
¼ cup milk
½ cup mozzarella, shredded
Cooking spray

Directions:
Spray the Crock Pot with cooking spray. Then put 3 flour tortilla in the bottom of the Crock Pot. Mix milk with eggs. Sprinkle the small amount of the milk mixture over the flour tortilla. Add chopped spinach and mozzarella. Cover the mixture with remaining tortillas and add milk mixture. Close the lid and cook the pie on High for 2 hours.

Nutrition Info: Per Serving: 120 calories, 6.6g protein, 15.3g carbohydrates, 4.1g fat, 2.4g fiber, 85mg cholesterol, 91mg sodium, 220mg potassium

14. Chicken Frittata

Servings: 2   Cooking Time: 3 Hours
Ingredients:
½ cup chicken, cooked and shredded
1 teaspoon mustard
1 tablespoon mayonnaise
2 bacon slices, cooked and crumbled
1 tomato, chopped
4 eggs
1 small avocado, pitted, peeled and chopped
Salt and black pepper to the taste

Directions:
In a bowl, mix the eggs with salt, pepper, chicken, avocado, tomato, bacon, mayo and mustard, toss, transfer to your Crock Pot, cover and cook on Low for 3 hours. Divide between plates and serve for breakfast

Nutrition Info:calories 300, fat 32, fiber 6, carbs 15, protein 25

15. Peach, Vanilla And Oats Mix

Servings: 2   Cooking Time: 8 Hours
Ingredients:
½ cup steel cut oats
2 cups almond milk
½ cup peaches, pitted and roughly chopped
½ teaspoon vanilla extract
1 teaspoon cinnamon powder

Directions:
In your Crock Pot, mix the oats with the almond milk, peaches and the other ingredients, toss, put the lid on and cook on Low for 8 hours. Divide into bowls and serve for breakfast right away.

Nutrition Info:calories 261, fat 5, fiber 8, carbs 18, protein 6

16. Eggplant Pate

Servings: 15   Cooking Time: 6 Hrs
Ingredients:
5 medium eggplants, peeled and chopped
2 sweet green pepper, chopped
1 cup bread crumbs
2 yellow onion, chopped
1 tbsp minced garlic
¼ chili pepper,

1 tsp salt
1 tbsp sugar
½ cup tomato paste
chopped
1 tsp olive oil
1 tsp kosher salt
1 tbsp mayonnaise

Directions:
Place the eggplants in a colander and drizzle salt on top. Leave them for 10 minutes at room temperature. Whisk tomatoes paste with sugar, salt, mayonnaise, and garlic in a bowl. Grease the base of your Crock Pot with olive oil. Spread chopped onion and eggplant in the cooker. Pour the tomato sauce over the veggies. Top the sauce with green peppers and chili pepper. Put the cooker's lid on and set the cooking time to 6 hours on Low settings. Blend the cooked eggplant mixture with an immersion blender until smooth. Top the eggplant pate with breadcrumbs. Serve.

Nutrition Info: Per Serving: Calories 83, Total Fat 0.8g, Fiber 7g, Total Carbs 18.15g, Protein 3g

17. Baguette Boats

Servings: 4   Cooking Time: 3 Hours
Ingredients:
6 oz baguette (2 baguettes)
4 ham slices
1 teaspoon minced garlic
½ cup Mozzarella, shredded
1 teaspoon olive oil
1 egg, beaten

Directions:
Cut the baguettes into the halves and remove the flesh from the bread. Chop the ham and mix it with egg, Mozzarella, and minced garlic. Fill the baguettes with ham mixture. Then brush the Crock Pot bowl with olive oil from inside. Put the baguette boats in the Crock Pot and close the lid. Cook them for 3 hours on High.

Nutrition Info: Per Serving: 205 calories, 12.1g protein, 25.5g carbohydrates, 6.1g fat, 1.4g fiber, 59mg cholesterol, 678mg sodium, 152mg potassium.

18. Squash Bowls

Servings: 2   Cooking Time: 6 Hours
Ingredients:
2 tablespoons walnuts, chopped
2 cups squash, peeled and cubed
½ cup coconut cream
½ teaspoon cinnamon powder
½ tablespoon sugar

Directions:
In your Crock Pot, mix the squash with the nuts and the other ingredients, toss, put the lid on and cook on Low for 6 hours. Divide into bowls and serve.

Nutrition Info:calories 140, fat 1, fiber 2, carbs 2, protein 5

19. Jalapeno Muffins

Servings: 4   Cooking Time: 3 Hours

Ingredients:

4 tablespoons flour	2 tablespoons cream
4 jalapeno pepper, diced	cheese
2 eggs, beaten	1 oz Parmesan, grated
	1 teaspoon olive oil

Directions:
Brush the silicone muffin molds with olive oil. Then mix all remaining ingredients in the mixing bowl. In the end, you will get a smooth batter. Transfer the batter in the prepared muffin molds. Then put the molds in the Crock Pot and close the lid. Cook the muffins on High for 3 hours.
Nutrition Info: Per Serving: 114 calories, 6.4g protein, 7.3g carbohydrates, 6.8g fat, 0.6g fiber, 92mg cholesterol, 112mg sodium, 74mg potassium

20. Cheesy Eggs

Servings: 2   Cooking Time: 3 Hours
Ingredients:

4 eggs, whisked	2 ounces feta cheese,
¼ cup spring onions, chopped	crumbled
	A pinch of salt and
1 tablespoon oregano, chopped	black pepper
	Cooking spray
1 cup milk	

Directions:
In a bowl, combine the eggs with the spring onions and the other ingredients except the cooking spray and whisk.   Grease your Crock Pot with cooking spray, add eggs mix, stir , put the lid on and cook on Low for 3 hours.   Divide between plates and serve for breakfast.
Nutrition Info: calories 214, fat 4, fiber 7, carbs 18, protein 5

21. Ham Stuffed Pockets

Servings: 6   Cooking Time: 1.5 Minutes
Ingredients:

6 pita bread, sliced	7 oz. ham, sliced
7 oz. mozzarella, sliced	1 big tomato, sliced
	1 tbsp mayo
1 tsp minced garlic	1 tbsp heavy cream

Directions:
First, heat your Crock Pot for 30 minutes on High setting.   Meanwhile, whisk the mayonnaise with garlic and cream.   Layer inside each half of the pita bread with mayo-garlic mixture.   Now add a slice of tomato, ham, and mozzarella to the bread. Wrap the bread pieces with a foil sheet.   Place the packed pita bread in the Crock Pot.   Put the cooker's lid on and set the cooking time to 1 hour 30 minutes on Low settings.   Remove the bread from the foil.   Serve.
Nutrition Info: Per Serving: Calories 273, Total Fat 3.3g, Fiber 2g, Total Carbs 38.01g, Protein 22g

22. Morning Banana Bread

Servings: 4   Cooking Time: 4 Hrs
Ingredients:

2 eggs	1 tsp baking powder
1 cup of sugar	3 bananas, mashed
2 cups flour	½ tsp baking soda
½ cup butter	

Directions:
Crack eggs in a bowl and beat until well mixed. Stir in eggs, sugar, baking powder, baking soda, bananas, and flour.   Continue mixing the eggs-flour mixture until it forms a smooth batter. Pour the egg-flour mixture in a loaf pan.   Place this loaf pan in the Crock Pot.   Put the cooker's lid on and set the cooking time to 4 hours on Low settings.   Slice the bread.   Serve.
Nutrition Info: Per Serving: Calories 261, Total Fat 9g, Fiber 6g, Total Carbs 20g, Protein 16g

23. Herbed Egg Scramble

Servings: 2   Cooking Time: 6 Hours
Ingredients:

4 eggs, whisked	¼ cup heavy cream
¼ cup mozzarella, shredded	1 tablespoon rosemary, chopped
1 tablespoon chives, chopped	A pinch of salt and black pepper
1 tablespoon oregano, chopped	Cooking spray

Directions:
Grease your Crock Pot with the cooking spray, and mix the eggs with the cream, herbs and the other ingredients inside.   Stir well, put the lid on, cook for 6 hours on Low, stir once again, divide between plates and serve.
Nutrition Info: calories 203, fat 15.7, fiber 1.7, carbs 3.8, protein 12.8

24. Creamy Asparagus Chicken

Servings: 7   Cooking Time: 8 Hrs
Ingredients:

1 cup cream	1 tsp oregano
2 lb. chicken breast, skinned, boneless, sliced	1 tsp ground white pepper
	1 tsp sriracha
1 tsp chili powder	6 oz. asparagus
3 tbsp flour	1 tsp sage

Directions:
Whisk chili powder, oregano, sage, white pepper, and flour in a shallow tray.   Add the chicken slices to this spice mixture and coat them well. Now add cream, chopped veggies, and Sriracha to the Crock Pot.   Place the coated chicken slices in the cooker.   Put the cooker's lid on and set the cooking time to 8 hours on Low settings.   Serve warm.
Nutrition Info: Per Serving: Calories 311, Total Fat 18.8g, Fiber 1g, Total Carbs 5.71g, Protein 29g

25. Sausage Pie(1)

Servings: 5   Cooking Time: 3 Hours
Ingredients:

7 oz potato, cooked, mashed	1 teaspoon Italian seasonings

3 eggs, beaten
4 oz sausages, chopped

2 oz Mozzarella, shredded
1 teaspoon olive oil

Directions:
Mix eggs with mashed potato and Italian seasonings.   Then brush the Crock Pot bottom with olive oil.   Put the mashed potato mixture inside and flatten it.   Then add sausages and Mozzarella.   Close the lid and cook the pie on High for 3 hours.

Nutrition Info: Per Serving: 188 calories, 11.7g protein, 7.6g carbohydrates, 12.3g fat, 0.9g fiber, 124mg cholesterol, 278mg sodium, 270mg potassium

26. Butternut Squash Pate

Servings: 7   Cooking Time: 4 Hours

Ingredients:

8 oz butternut squash puree
1 tablespoon honey
¼ teaspoon ground clove

1 teaspoon cinnamon
1 tablespoon lemon juice
2 tablespoons coconut oil

Directions:
Put all ingredients in the Crock Pot, gently stir, and cook on Low for 4 hours.

Nutrition Info: Per Serving: 63 calories, 0g protein, 6.9g carbohydrates, 3.9g fat, 0.8g fiber, 0mg cholesterol, 3mg sodium, 7mg potassium.

27. Breakfast Banana Bread

Servings: 4   Cooking Time: 4 Hours

Ingredients:

2 eggs
1 cup sugar
2 cups flour
1 teaspoon baking powder

½ cup butter
3 bananas, mashed
½ teaspoon baking soda

Directions:
In a bowl, mix butter with sugar and eggs and whisk well.   Add baking soda, baking powder, flour and bananas, stir really well and pour into a bread pan that fits your Crock Pot.   Put the pan into your Crock Pot, cover and cook on Low for 4 hours.   Slice and serve for breakfast.

Nutrition Info:calories 261, fat 9, fiber 6, carbs 20, protein 16

28. Beans Salad

Servings: 2   Cooking Time: 6 Hours

Ingredients:

1 cup canned black beans, drained
1 cup canned red kidney beans, drained
1 cup baby spinach
2 spring onions, chopped
½ red bell pepper, chopped

½ teaspoon garam masala
¼ cup veggie stock
A pinch of cumin, ground
A pinch of chili powder
A pinch of salt and

¼ teaspoon turmeric powder

black pepper
½ cup salsa

Directions:
In your Crock Pot, mix the beans with the spinach, onions and the other ingredients, toss, put the lid on and cook on High for 6 hours.   Divide the mix into bowls and serve for breakfast.

Nutrition Info:calories 130, fat 4, fiber 2, carbs 5, protein 4

29. Chocolate Quinoa

Servings: 4   Cooking Time: 6 Hours

Ingredients:

1 cup quinoa
1 cup coconut milk
1 cup milk
2 tablespoons cocoa powder

3 tablespoons maple syrup
4 dark chocolate squares, chopped

Directions:
In your Crock Pot, mix quinoa with coconut milk, milk, cocoa powder, maple syrup and chocolate, stir, cover and cook on Low for 6 hours.   Stir quinoa mix again, divide into bowls and serve.

Nutrition Info:calories 215, fat 5, fiber 8, carbs 17, protein 4

30. Italian Style Scrambled Eggs

Servings: 4   Cooking Time: 4 Hours

Ingredients:

4 eggs, beaten
3 oz Mozzarella, shredded
1 teaspoon Italian seasonings

¼ cup milk
¼ teaspoon salt
1 teaspoon butter, melted

Directions:
Mix eggs with milk, Italian seasonings, and salt. Pour butter and milk mixture in the Crock Pot and close the lid.   Cook the meal on high for 1 hour. Then open the lid and scramble the eggs.   After this, top the meal with cheese and cook the eggs on low for 3 hours more.

Nutrition Info: Per Serving: 143 calories, 12.1g protein, 2g carbohydrates, 9.7g fat, 0g fiber, 180mg cholesterol, 351mg sodium, 69mg potassium.

31. Cheesy Cauliflower Hash

Servings: 5   Cooking Time: 8 Hrs

Ingredients:

7 eggs
¼ cup milk
1 tsp salt
1 tsp ground black pepper
10 oz. cauliflower, shredded

½ tsp ground mustard
¼ tsp chili flakes
5 oz. breakfast sausages, chopped
½ onion, chopped
5 oz. Cheddar cheese, shredded

Directions:
First, beat the eggs with milk, mustard, black pepper, salt, onion, and chili flakes in a bowl.

Spread the cauliflower shreds in the Crock Pot. Pour the egg-milk mixture over the cauliflower shreds. Drizzle cheese and chopped sausages on top. Put the cooker's lid on and set the cooking time to 8 hours on Low settings. Slice and serve.
Nutrition Info: Per Serving: Calories 329, Total Fat 21.8g, Fiber 2g, Total Carbs 10.31g, Protein 23g

32. Cinnamon Berries Oatmeal

Servings: 2   Cooking Time: 6 Hours
Ingredients:

1 cup old fashioned oats	½ teaspoon cinnamon powder
3 cups almond milk	½ teaspoon vanilla extract
1 cup blackberries	
½ cup Greek yogurt	

Directions:
In your Crock Pot, mix the oats with the milk, berries and the other ingredients, toss, put the lid on and cook on Low for 6 hours. Divide into bowls and serve for breakfast.
Nutrition Info:calories 932, fat 43, fiber 16.7, carbs 82.2, protein 24.3

33. Salmon Frittata

Servings: 3   Cooking Time: 3 Hours And 40 Minutes
Ingredients:

4 eggs, whisked	Salt and black pepper to the taste
½ teaspoon olive oil	4 ounces smoked salmon, chopped
2 tablespoons green onions, chopped	

Directions:
Drizzle the oil in your Crock Pot, add eggs, salt and pepper, whisk, cover and cook on Low for 3 hours. Add salmon and green onions, toss a bit, cover, cook on Low for 40 minutes more and divide between plates. Serve right away for breakfast.
Nutrition Info:calories 220, fat 10, fiber 2, carbs 15, protein 7

34. Mexican Egg Bake

Servings: 8   Cooking Time: 2 Hours And 15 Minutes
Ingredients:

Cooking spray	½ tsp chili powder
10 eggs	A pinch of salt and black pepper
12 oz. Monterey Jack, shredded	10 oz. taco sauce
1 cup half and half	4 oz. canned green chilies, chopped
1 garlic clove, minced	8 corn tortillas

Directions:
Beat eggs with 8 oz. cheese, half and half, black pepper, salt, green chilies, chili powder, and garlic in a bowl. Coat the base of your Crock Pot with cooking spray. Pour the egg-cheese mixture into the cooker. Put the cooker's lid on and set the cooking time to 2 hours on Low settings. Now top the egg with remaining cheese and taco sauce.

Cover again and cook for 15 minutes on the low setting. Serve warm with a tortilla.
Nutrition Info: Per Serving: Calories 312, Total Fat 4g, Fiber 8g, Total Carbs 12g, Protein 5g

35. Breakfast Meat Rolls

Servings: 12   Cooking Time: 4.5 Hours
Ingredients:

1-pound puff pastry	1 egg, beaten
1 cup ground pork	1 tablespoon sesame oil
1 tablespoon garlic, diced	

Directions:
Roll up the puff pastry. Then mix ground pork with garlic and egg. Then spread the puff pastry with ground meat mixture and roll. Cut the puff pastry rolls on small rolls. Then sprinkle the rolls with sesame oil. Arrange the meat rolls in the Crock Pot and close the lid. Cook breakfast on High for 4.5 hours.
Nutrition Info: Per Serving: 244 calories, 4.9g protein, 17.3g carbohydrates, 17.2g fat, 0.6g fiber, 20mg cholesterol, 106mg sodium, 31mg potassium.

36. Peppers Rice Mix

Servings: 2   Cooking Time: 3 Hours
Ingredients:

½ cup brown rice	1 cup chicken stock
2 spring onions, chopped	½ cup canned black beans, drained
½ orange bell pepper, chopped	½ cup mild salsa
½ red bell pepper, chopped	½ teaspoon sweet paprika
½ green bell pepper, chopped	½ teaspoon lime zest, grated
2 ounces canned green chilies, chopped	A pinch of salt and black pepper

Directions:
In your Crock Pot, mix the rice with the stock, spring onions and the other ingredients, toss, put the lid on and cook on High for 3 hours. Divide the mix into bowls and serve for breakfast.
Nutrition Info:calories 140, fat 2, fiber 2, carbs 5, protein 5

37. Sweet Pepper Eggs

Servings: 2   Cooking Time: 2.5 Hours
Ingredients:

1 sweet pepper	4 eggs
¼ teaspoon ground black pepper	1 teaspoon butter, melted

Directions:
Slice the sweet pepper into 4 rounds. Then brush the Crock Pot with butter from inside. Put the sweet pepper rounds in the Crock Pot in one layer. Then crack the eggs in the sweet pepper rounds. Sprinkle the eggs with ground black pepper and close the lid. Cook the meal on High for 2.5 hours.

Nutrition Info: Per Serving: 162 calories, 11.7g protein, 5.4g carbohydrates, 10.8g fat, 0.9g fiber, 332mg cholesterol, 138mg sodium, 234mg potassium.

38. Honey Pumpkin

Servings: 4   Cooking Time: 7 Hours

Ingredients:

1 tablespoon ground cinnamon	2 tablespoons honey
1 tablespoon ground cardamom	1-pound pumpkin, cubed
	¼ cup of water

Directions:
Put pumpkin in the Crock Pot.   Add honey, ground cinnamon, cardamom, and water. Mix the ingredients and close the lid.   Cook the pumpkin on Low for 7 hours.
Nutrition Info: Per Serving: 79 calories, 1.5g protein, 20.2g carbohydrates, 0.4g fat, 4.6g fiber, 0mg cholesterol, 7mg sodium, 263mg potassium.

39. Worcestershire Asparagus Casserole

Servings: 4   Cooking Time: 5 Hours

Ingredients:

2 pounds asparagus spears, cut into 1-inch pieces	Salt and black pepper to the taste
	2 cups coconut milk
1 cup mushrooms, sliced	1 teaspoon Worcestershire sauce
1 teaspoon olive oil	5 eggs, whisked

Directions:
Grease your Crock Pot with the oil and spread asparagus and mushrooms on the bottom.   In a bowl, mix the eggs with milk, salt, pepper and Worcestershire sauce, whisk, pour into the Crock Pot, toss everything, cover and cook on Low for 6 hours.   Divide between plates and serve right away for breakfast.
Nutrition Info:calories 211, fat 4, fiber 4, carbs 8, protein 5

40. Raspberry Vanilla Oatmeal

Servings: 4   Cooking Time: 8 Hrs

Ingredients:

2 cups of water	½ tsp vanilla extract
1 tbsp coconut oil	1 cup raspberries
1 cup steel-cut oats	4 tbsp walnuts, chopped
1 tbsp sugar	
1 cup milk	

Directions:
Add oil, oats, water, milk, vanilla, raspberries, and sugar to the Crock Pot.   Put the cooker's lid on and set the cooking time to 8 hours on Low settings.   Give the oatmeal a gentle stir then divide it into the serving bowls.   Garnish with walnuts.   Serve.
Nutrition Info: Per Serving: Calories 200, Total Fat 10g, Fiber 4g, Total Carbs 20g, Protein 4g

41. Apricots Bread Pudding

Servings: 9   Cooking Time: 5 Hrs

Ingredients:

10 oz. French bread	1 tsp vanilla sugar
6 tbsp dried apricots	½ tsp ground nutmeg
10 oz. milk	
3 eggs, beaten	½ tsp ground cardamom
4 tbsp butter	
½ tsp salt	¼ cup whipped cream
	4 tbsp brown sugar

Directions:
Melt butter by heating in a saucepan then add milk. Cook until warm, then stir in vanilla sugar, salt, ground cardamom, ground nutmeg, and brown sugar.   Continue mixing the milk mixture until sugar is fully dissolved.   Spread French bread and dried apricots in the Crock Pot.   Beat eggs in a bowl and add to the milk mixture.   Stir in cream and mix well until fully incorporated. Pour this milk-cream mixture over the bread and apricots in the Crock Pot.   Put the cooker's lid on and set the cooking time to 5 hours on Low settings.   Serve.
Nutrition Info: Per Serving: Calories 229, Total Fat 11.5g, Fiber 1g, Total Carbs 24.3g, Protein 8g

42. Broccoli Omelet

Servings: 4   Cooking Time: 2 Hours

Ingredients:

1 tablespoon cream cheese	5 eggs, beaten
	1 tomato, chopped
3 oz broccoli, chopped	1 teaspoon avocado oil

Directions:
Mix eggs with cream cheese and transfer in the Crock Pot.   Add avocado oil, broccoli, and tomato.   Close the lid and cook the omelet on High for 2 hours.
Nutrition Info: Per Serving: 99 calories, 7.9g protein, 2.6g carbohydrates, 6.6g fat, 0.8g fiber, 207mg cholesterol, 92mg sodium, 184mg potassium.

43. Chai Breakfast Quinoa

Servings: 2   Cooking Time: 6 Hours

Ingredients:

1 cup quinoa	2 cups milk
1 egg white	¼ teaspoon cinnamon powder
¼ teaspoon vanilla extract	
1 and ½ tablespoons brown sugar	¼ teaspoon vanilla extract
¼ teaspoon cardamom, ground	¼ teaspoon nutmeg, ground
¼ teaspoon ginger, grated	1 tablespoons coconut flakes

Directions:

In your Crock Pot, mix quinoa with egg white, milk, vanilla, sugar, cardamom, ginger, cinnamon, vanilla and nutmeg, stir a bit, cover and cook on Low for 6 hours.   Stir, divide into bowls and serve for breakfast with coconut flakes on top.
Nutrition Info:calories 211, fat 4, fiber 6, carbs 10, protein 4

44. Broccoli Omelette

Servings: 4   Cooking Time: 2 Hrs
Ingredients:

½ cup milk	1 cup broccoli florets
6 eggs	1 yellow onion, chopped
Salt and black pepper to the taste	1 garlic clove, minced
A pinch of chili powder	1 tbsp cheddar cheese, shredded
A pinch of garlic powder	Cooking spray
1 red bell pepper, chopped	

Directions:
Start by cracking eggs in a large bowl and beat them well.   Stir in all the veggies, cheese, and spices then mix well.   Pour the eggs-veggie mixture into the Crock Pot.   Put the cooker's lid on and set the cooking time to 2 hours on High settings.   Slice and serve warm.
Nutrition Info: Per Serving: Calories 142, Total Fat 7g, Fiber 1g, Total Carbs 8g, Protein 10g

45. Nutty Sweet Potatoes

Servings: 8   Cooking Time: 6 Hrs
Ingredients:

2 tbsp peanut butter	2 tbsp lemon juice
¼ cup peanuts	1 cup onion, chopped
1 lb. sweet potato, peeled and cut in strips.	½ cup chicken stock
1 garlic clove, peeled and sliced	1 tsp salt
	1 tsp paprika
	1 tsp ground black pepper

Directions:
Toss the sweet potato with lemon juice, paprika, salt, black pepper, and peanut butter in a large bowl.   Place the sweet potatoes in the Crock Pot. Add onions and garlic clove on top of the potatoes. Put the cooker's lid on and set the cooking time to 6 hours on Low settings.   Serve with crushed peanuts on top.   Devour.
Nutrition Info: Per Serving: Calories 376, Total Fat 22.4g, Fiber 6g, Total Carbs 39.36g, Protein 5g

46. Banana And Coconut Oatmeal

Servings: 6   Cooking Time: 7 Hours
Ingredients:

Cooking spray	¼ teaspoon nutmeg, ground
2 bananas, sliced	
1 cup steel cut oats	½ teaspoon cinnamon powder
28 ounces canned coconut milk	

½ cup water
1 tablespoon butter
2 tablespoons brown sugar
½ teaspoon vanilla extract
1 tablespoon flaxseed, ground

Directions:
Grease your Crock Pot with cooking spray, add banana slices, oats, coconut milk, water, butter, sugar, cinnamon, butter, vanilla and flaxseed, toss a bit, cover and cook on Low for 7 hours.   Divide into bowls and serve for breakfast.
Nutrition Info:calories 251, fat 6, fiber 8, carbs 16, protein 6

47. Chia Oatmeal

Servings: 2   Cooking Time: 8 Hours
Ingredients:

2 cups almond milk	½ teaspoon almond extract
1 cup steel cut oats	
2 tablespoons butter, soft	2 tablespoons chia seeds

Directions:
In your Crock Pot, mix the oats with the chia seeds and the other ingredients, toss, put the lid on and cook on Low for 8 hours.   Stir the oatmeal one more time, divide into bowls and serve.
Nutrition Info:calories 812, fat 71.4, fiber 9.4, carbs 41.1, protein 11

48. Breakfast Rice Pudding

Servings: 4   Cooking Time: 4 Hours
Ingredients:

1 cup coconut milk	2 tablespoons flaxseed
2 cups water	
1 cup almond milk	1 teaspoon cinnamon powder
½ cup raisins	
1 cup brown rice	2 tablespoons coconut sugar
2 teaspoons vanilla extract	Cooking spray

Directions:
Grease your Crock Pot with the cooking spray, add coconut milk, water, almond milk, raisins, rice, vanilla, flaxseed and cinnamon, cover, cook on Low for 4 hours, stir, divide into bowls, sprinkle coconut sugar all over and serve.
Nutrition Info:calories 213, fat 3, fiber 6, carbs 10, protein 4

49. Cinnamon French Toast

Servings: 2   Cooking Time: 4 Hours
Ingredients:

½ French baguette, sliced	1 egg, whisked
2 ounces cream cheese	2 tablespoons honey
1 tablespoon brown sugar	½ teaspoon cinnamon powder
3 tablespoons almond milk	1 tablespoon butter, melted
	Cooking spray

Directions:

Spread the cream cheese on all bread slices, grease your Crock Pot with the cooking spray and arrange the slices in the pot.   In a bowl, mix the egg with the cinnamon, almond milk and the remaining ingredients, whisk and pour over the bread slices. Put the lid on, cook on High for 4 hours, divide the mix between plates and serve for breakfast.

Nutrition Info:calories 316, fat 23.5, fiber 0.5, carbs 23.9, protein 5.6

50. Walnut And Cheese Balls

Servings: 5   Cooking Time: 1.5 Hours

Ingredients:

1 cup walnuts, grinded	¼ cup breadcrumbs
2 eggs, beaten	2 tablespoons coconut oil, melted
3 oz Parmesan, grated	

Directions:
Mix grinded walnuts and breadcrumbs.   Then add eggs and Parmesan.   Carefully mix the mixture and make the medium size balls from them.   Then pour melted coconut oil in the Crock Pot.   Add walnuts balls. Arrange them in one layer and close the lid.   Cook the balls on high for 1 hour.   Then flip them on another side and cook for 30 minutes more.

Nutrition Info: Per Serving: 303 calories, 14.4g protein, 7.1g carbohydrates, 25.9g fat, 1.9g fiber, 78mg cholesterol, 223mg sodium, 165mg potassium

51. Peppers And Eggs Mix

Servings: 2   Cooking Time: 4 Hours

Ingredients:

4 eggs, whisked	1 yellow bell pepper, cut into strips
½ teaspoon coriander, ground	¼ cup heavy cream
½ teaspoon rosemary, dried	½ teaspoon garlic powder
2 spring onions, chopped	A pinch of salt and black pepper
1 red bell pepper, cut into strips	1 teaspoon sweet paprika
1 green bell pepper, cut into strips	Cooking spray

Directions:
Grease your Crock Pot with the cooking spray, and mix the eggs with the coriander, rosemary and the other ingredients into the pot.   Put the lid on, cook on Low for 4 hours, divide between plates and serve for breakfast.

Nutrition Info:calories 172, fat 6, fiber 3, carbs 6, protein 7

52. Granola Bowls

Servings: 2   Cooking Time: 4 Hours

Ingredients:

½ cup granola	¼ cup coconut cream
2 tablespoons brown sugar	

2 tablespoons cashew butter	1 teaspoon cinnamon powder
	½ teaspoon nutmeg, ground

Directions:
In your Crock Pot, mix the granola with the cream, sugar and the other ingredients, toss, put the lid on and cook on Low for 4 hours.   Divide into bowls and serve for breakfast.

Nutrition Info:calories 218, fat 6, fiber 9, carbs 17, protein 6

53. Breakfast Potatoes

Servings: 8   Cooking Time: 4 Hours

Ingredients:

3 potatoes, peeled and cubed	12 ounces smoked chicken sausage, sliced
1 green bell pepper, chopped	½ cup sour cream
1 red bell pepper, chopped	¼ teaspoon basil, dried
1 yellow onion, chopped	10 ounces cream of chicken soup
1 and ½ cups cheddar cheese, shredded	2 tablespoons parsley, chopped
¼ teaspoon oregano, dried	Salt and black pepper to the taste

Directions:
In your Crock Pot, mix potatoes with red bell pepper, green bell pepper, sausage, onion, oregano, basil, cheese, salt, pepper and cream of chicken, cover and cook on Low for 4 hours.   Add parsley, divide between plates and serve for breakfast.

Nutrition Info:calories 320, fat 5, fiber 7, carbs 10, protein 5

54. Baby Carrots In Syrup

Servings: 5   Cooking Time: 7 Hours

Ingredients:

3 cups baby carrots	1 cup apple juice
2 tablespoons brown sugar	1 teaspoon vanilla extract

Directions:
Mix apple juice, brown sugar, and vanilla extract. Pour the liquid in the Crock Pot.   Add baby carrots and close the lid.   Cook the meal on Low for 7 hours.

Nutrition Info: Per Serving: 81 calories, 0g protein, 18.8g carbohydrates, 0.1g fat, 3.7g fiber, 0mg cholesterol, 363mg sodium, 56mg potassium.

55. Spinach Frittata

Servings: 6   Cooking Time: 2 Hours

Ingredients:

2 cups spinach, chopped	7 eggs, beaten
1 teaspoon smoked paprika	2 tablespoons coconut oil
1 teaspoon sesame oil	¼ cup heavy cream

Directions:
Mix eggs with heavy cream.   Then grease the Crock Pot with coconut oil and pour the egg mixture inside.   Add smoked paprika, sesame oil, and spinach.   Carefully mix the ingredients and close the lid.   Cook the frittata on High for 2 hours.

Nutrition Info: Per Serving: 140 calories, 6.9g protein, 1.1g carbohydrates, 12.3g fat, 0.4g fiber, 198mg cholesterol, 82mg sodium, 137mg potassium.

56. Shrimp Omelet

Servings: 4   Cooking Time: 3.5 Hours
Ingredients:

4 eggs, beaten	½ teaspoon ground paprika
4 oz shrimps, peeled	
½ teaspoon ground turmeric	¼ teaspoon salt
	Cooking spray

Directions:
Mix eggs with shrimps, turmeric, salt, and paprika. Then spray the Crock Pot bowl with cooking spray. After this, pour the egg mixture inside. Flatten the shrimps and close the lid.   Cook the omelet for 3.5 hours on High.

Nutrition Info: Per Serving: 98 calories, 12.1g protein, 1.1g carbohydrates, 4.9g fat, 0.2g fiber, 223mg cholesterol, 278mg sodium, 120mg potassium.

57. Milk Oatmeal

Servings: 4   Cooking Time: 2 Hours
Ingredients:

2 cups oatmeal	1 cup milk
1 cup of water	1 tablespoon coconut oil
1 tablespoon liquid honey	
1 teaspoon vanilla extract	¼ teaspoon ground cinnamon

Directions:
Put all ingredients except liquid honey in the Crock Pot and mix.   Close the lid and cook the meal on High for hours.   Then stir the cooked oatmeal and transfer in the serving bowls.   Top the meal with a small amount of liquid honey.

Nutrition Info: Per Serving: 234 calories, 7.4g protein, 35.3g carbohydrates, 7.3g fat, 4.2g fiber, 5mg cholesterol, 33mg sodium, 189mg potassium.

58. Asparagus Egg Casserole

Servings: 4   Cooking Time: 2.5 Hours
Ingredients:

7 eggs, beaten	1 oz Parmesan, grated
4 oz asparagus, chopped, boiled	1 teaspoon sesame oil
	1 teaspoon dried dill

Directions:
Pour the sesame oil in the Crock Pot.   Then mix dried dill with parmesan, asparagus, and eggs. Pour the egg mixture in the Crock Pot and close the lid.   Cook the casserole on high for 2.5 hours.

Nutrition Info: Per Serving: 149 calories, 12.6g protein, 2.1g carbohydrates, 10.3g fat, 0.6g fiber, 292mg cholesterol, 175mg sodium, 169mg potassium

59. Green Buttered Eggs

Servings: 2   Cooking Time: 3 Hours
Ingredients:

2 tablespoons organic grass-fed butter	1 teaspoon thyme leaves
1 tablespoon coconut oil	4 organic eggs, beaten
2 cloves of garlic, chopped	¼ teaspoon cayenne pepper
½ cup cilantro, chopped	Salt and pepper to taste

Directions:
Place butter and coconut oil in a skillet heated over medium flame.   Add in the garlic and sauté until fragrant.   Add in the cilantro and thyme leaves. Continue stirring until crisp.   Pour into the CrockPot and add in the beaten eggs.   Season with cayenne pepper, salt and black pepper to taste. Close the lid and cook on high for 2 hours and on low for 3 hours.

Nutrition Info: Calories per serving:311; Carbohydrates: 2.5g; Protein: 14.6g; Fat: g27.5 Sugar:0 g; Sodium: 362mg; Fiber: 1g

60. Bacon And Egg Casserole

Servings: 8   Cooking Time: 5 Hours
Ingredients:

20 ounces hash browns	Cooking spray
8 ounces cheddar cheese, shredded	½ cup milk
8 bacon slices, cooked and chopped	12 eggs
6 green onions, chopped	Salt and black pepper to the taste
	Salsa for serving

Directions:
Grease your Crock Pot with cooking spray, spread hash browns, cheese, bacon and green onions and toss.   In a bowl, mix the eggs with salt, pepper and milk and whisk really well.   Pour this over hash browns, cover and cook on Low for 5 hours. Divide between plates and serve with salsa on top.

Nutrition Info:calories 300, fat 5, fiber 5, carbs 9, protein 5

61. Zucchini Quinoa

Servings: 3   Cooking Time: 3 Hours
Ingredients:

½ zucchini, grated	1 teaspoon salt
1 teaspoon coconut oil	1 tablespoon cream cheese
1 cup quinoa	1 oz goat cheese, crumbled
2 cup chicken stock	

Directions:

Mix grated zucchini with coconut oil, quinoa, and chicken stock and transfer in the Crock Pot. Then add cream cheese and salt.   Cook the meal on High for hours.   Then stir the cooked quinoa well and transfer in the serving plates.   Top the meal with crumbled goat cheese.
Nutrition Info: Per Serving: 288 calories, 12g protein, 38.3g carbohydrates, 9.9g fat, 4.3g fiber, 14mg cholesterol, 1333mg sodium, 423mg potassium.

62. Potato Muffins

Servings: 4   Cooking Time: 2 Hours
Ingredients:

4 teaspoons flax meal	1 teaspoon ground paprika
1 bell pepper, diced	
1 cup potato, cooked, mashed	2 oz Mozzarella, shredded
2 eggs, beaten	

Directions:
Mix flax meal with potato and eggs.   Then add ground paprika and bell pepper. Stir the mixture with the help of the spoon until homogenous. After this, transfer the potato mixture in the muffin molds. Top the muffins with Mozzarella and transfer in the Crock Pot.   Close the lid and cook the muffins on High for 2 hours.
Nutrition Info: Per Serving: 107 calories, 8g protein, 7.2g carbohydrates, 5.7g fat, 1.7g fiber, 89mg cholesterol, 118mg sodium, 196mg potassium

63. Apple Cinnamon Granola

Servings: 6   Cooking Time: 4 Hrs
Ingredients:

2 green apples, peeled, cored and sliced	¼ cup apple juice
	1/8 cup maple syrup
½ cup granola	1 tsp cinnamon powder
½ cup bran flakes	2 tbsp soft butter
	½ tsp nutmeg, ground

Directions:
Toss the apples with granola, bran flakes, maple syrup, apple juice, butter, cinnamon, nutmeg, and butter in a large bowl.   Spread this apple crumble into the base of your Crock Pot.   Put the cooker's lid on and set the cooking time to 4 hours on Low settings.   Serve and devour.
Nutrition Info: Per Serving: Calories 363, Total Fat 5g, Fiber 6g, Total Carbs 20g, Protein 6g

64. Creamy Yogurt

Servings: 8   Cooking Time: 10 Hours
Ingredients:

3 teaspoons gelatin	
½ gallon milk	1 and ½ tablespoons vanilla extract
7 ounces plain yogurt	
	½ cup maple syrup

Directions:

Put the milk in your Crock Pot, cover and cook on Low for 3 hours.   In a bowl, mix 1 cup of hot milk from the Crock Pot with the gelatin, whisk well, pour into the Crock Pot, cover and leave aside for hours.   Combine 1 cup of milk with the yogurt, whisk really well and pour into the pot.   Also add vanilla and maple syrup, stir, cover and cook on Low for 7 more hours.   Leave yogurt aside to cool down and serve it for breakfast.
Nutrition Info:calories 200, fat 4, fiber 5, carbs 10, protein 5

65. Cauliflower Rice Pudding

Servings: 2   Cooking Time: 2 Hours
Ingredients:

¼ cup maple syrup	3 cups almond milk
1 cup cauliflower rice	2 tablespoons vanilla extract

Directions:
Put cauliflower rice in your Crock Pot, add maple syrup, almond milk and vanilla extract, stir, cover and cook on High for 2 hours.   Stir your pudding again, divide into bowls and serve for breakfast.
Nutrition Info:calories 240, fat 2, fiber 2, carbs 15, protein 5

66. French Toast

Servings: 2   Cooking Time: 3.5 Hours
Ingredients:

1 teaspoon cream cheese	2 white bread slices
	1 egg, beaten
1 teaspoon white sugar	¼ cup milk
	1 tablespoon butter

Directions:
Put butter in the Crock Pot.   Add cream cheese, white sugar, egg, and milk. Stir the mixture. Then put the bread slices in the Crock Pot and close the lid.   Cook the toasts for 3.5 hours on High.
Nutrition Info: Per Serving: 135 calories, 4.7g protein, 8.3g carbohydrates, 9.5g fat, 0.2g fiber, 101mg cholesterol, 152mg sodium, 60mg potassium.

67. Cranberry Quinoa

Servings: 4   Cooking Time: 2 Hours
Ingredients:

3 cups coconut water	3 teaspoons honey
1 teaspoon vanilla extract	1/8 cup coconut flakes
1 cup quinoa	¼ cup cranberries, dried
1/8 cup almonds, sliced	

Directions:
In your Crock Pot, mix coconut water with vanilla, quinoa, honey, almonds, coconut flakes and cranberries, toss, cover and cook on High for 2 hours.   Divide quinoa mix into bowls and serve.
Nutrition Info:calories 261, fat 7, fiber 8, carbs 18, protein

68. Bacon Tater

Servings: 4   Cooking Time: 8 Hours 10 Minutes

Ingredients:

½ pound Canadian bacon, diced
¼ cup Parmesan cheese, grated
½ cup whole milk
1 pound package frozen tater tot potatoes
Salt and black pepper, to taste
2 onions, chopped
1½ cups Cheddar cheese, shredded
6 eggs
2 tablespoons flour

Directions:

Grease a crockpot and layer 3 of the tater tots, bacon, onions, and cheeses.   Repeat the layers twice, ending with cheeses.   Mix together eggs, milk, flour, salt and black pepper in a medium mixing bowl.   Drizzle this mixture over the layers in the crock pot and cover the lid.   Cook on LOW about for 8 hours and dish out to serve.

Nutrition Info: Calories:614 Fat:36g Carbohydrates:36.6g

69. Crock-pot Veggie Omelet

Servings: 4   Cooking Time: 2 Hours

Ingredients:

6 large eggs
4 cups spinach, fresh, chopped
1 ½ cups white mushrooms, sliced
2 cloves garlic, crushed
1 cup feta cheese, crumbled
2 tablespoons of coconut oil
Salt and pepper to taste

Directions:

Heat the coconut oil in Crock-Pot.   Set aside.   In a mixing bowl, combine garlic, eggs, salt, and pepper.   Add mushrooms and spinach to the mix.   Cover and cook for about 2 hours, or until omelet is set.   Check it at about hour and 15 minutes into cooking time.   When the omelet is cooked, add the feta and fold in half.   Transfer to serving plate.

Nutrition Info: Calories: 659, Total Fat: 55.5 g, Saturated Fat: 30.3 g, Net Carbs: 7.7 g, Dietary Fiber: 2.8 g, Protein: 30.9 g

70. Chicken- Pork Meatballs

Servings: 8   Cooking Time: 7 Hrs

Ingredients:

1 cup bread crumbs
2 tbsp sour cream
9 oz. ground chicken
7 oz. ground pork
1 tsp onion powder
1 onion, chopped
1 tsp ketchup
¼ tsp olive oil

Directions:

Thoroughly mix ground chicken, onion powder, sour cream, ground pork, ketchup, and onion in a large bowl.   Add breadcrumbs to bind this mixture well.   Make small meatballs out of this mixture and roll them in extra breadcrumbs. Brush the base of your Crock Pot with olive oil. Gently place the chicken-pork meatballs in the Crock Pot.   Put the cooker's lid on and set the cooking time to 7 hours on Low settings.   Serve warm.

Nutrition Info: Per Serving: Calories 116, Total Fat 5g, Fiber 0g, Total Carbs 4.08g, Protein 14g

71. Potato And Ham Mix

Servings: 2   Cooking Time: 6 Hours

Ingredients:

Cooking spray
4 eggs, whisked
½ cup red potatoes, peeled and grated
¼ cup heavy cream
¼ cup ham, chopped
1 tablespoon cilantro, chopped
½ teaspoon turmeric powder
Salt and black pepper to the taste

Directions:

Grease your Crock Pot with cooking spray, add the eggs, potatoes and the other ingredients, whisk, put the lid on and cook on High for 6 hours.   Divide between plates and serve for breakfast.

Nutrition Info:calories 200, fat 4, fiber 6, carbs 12, protein 6

72. Tomato And Zucchini Eggs Mix

Servings: 2   Cooking Time: 3 Hours

Ingredients:

Cooking spray
4 eggs, whisked
2 spring onions, chopped
1 tablespoon basil, chopped
½ teaspoon turmeric powder
½ cup tomatoes, cubed
1 zucchini, grated
¼ teaspoon sweet paprika
A pinch of salt and black pepper
1 tablespoon parsley, chopped
2 tablespoons parmesan, grated

Directions:

Grease your Crock Pot with cooking spray, add the eggs mixed with the zucchini, tomatoes and the other ingredients except the cheese and stir well. Sprinkle the cheese, put the lid on and cook on High for 3 hours.   Divide between plates and serve for breakfast right away.

Nutrition Info:calories 261, fat 5, fiber 7, carbs 19, protein 6

73. Basil Sausages

Servings: 5   Cooking Time: 4 Hours

Ingredients:

1-pound Italian sausages, chopped
1 teaspoon dried basil
¼ cup of water
1 tablespoon olive oil
1 teaspoon ground coriander

Directions:

Sprinkle the chopped sausages with ground coriander and dried basil and transfer in the Crock Pot.   Add olive oil and water.   Close the lid and cook the sausages on high for 4 hours.

Nutrition Info: Per Serving: 338 calories, 12.9g protein, 0.6g carbohydrates, 31.2g fat, 0g fiber,

69mg cholesterol, 664mg sodium, 231mg potassium.

74. Almond And Quinoa Bowls

Servings: 2   Cooking Time: 5 Hours
Ingredients:

- 1 cup quinoa
- 2 cups almond milk
- 2 tablespoons butter, melted
- 2 tablespoons brown sugar
- A pinch of cinnamon powder
- A pinch of nutmeg, ground
- ¼ cup almonds, sliced
- Cooking spray

Directions:
Grease your Crock Pot with the cooking spray, add the quinoa, milk, melted butter and the other ingredients, toss, put the lid on and cook on Low for 5 hours.   Divide the mix into bowls and serve for breakfast.
Nutrition Info:calories 211, fat 3, fiber 6, carbs 12, protein 5

75. Sweet Toasts

Servings: 4   Cooking Time: 5 Hours
Ingredients:

- 4 slices of white bread
- 3 eggs, beaten
- 1 tablespoon sugar
- 1 teaspoon olive oil
- 1 teaspoon vanilla extract

Directions:
Mix eggs with sugar and vanilla extract.   Then pour the mixture in the Crock Pot.   Add olive oil and bread slices.   Close the lid and cook the meal on Low for 5 hours.
Nutrition Info: Per Serving: 95 calories, 4.8g protein, 7.9g carbohydrates, 4.8g fat, 0.2g fiber, 123mg cholesterol, 108mg sodium, 55mg potassium

76. Egg Scramble

Servings: 4   Cooking Time: 2.5 Hours
Ingredients:

- 4 eggs, beaten
- 1 tablespoon butter, melted
- 2 oz Cheddar cheese, shredded
- ¼ teaspoon cayenne pepper
- 1 teaspoon ground paprika

Directions:
Mix eggs with butter, cheese, cayenne pepper, and ground paprika.   Then pour the mixture in the Crock Pot and close the lid.   Cook it on high for 2 hours.   Then open the lid and scramble the eggs. Close the lid and cook the meal on high for 30 minutes.
Nutrition Info: Per Serving: 147 calories, 9.2g protein, 0.9g carbohydrates, 12g fat, 0.2g fiber, 186mg cholesterol, 170mg sodium, 88mg potassium.

77. Chia Seeds And Chicken Breakfast

Servings: 4   Cooking Time: 3 Hours
Ingredients:

- 1 pound chicken breasts, skinless, boneless and cubed
- ½ teaspoon basil, dried
- ¾ cup flaxseed, ground
- ¼ cup parmesan, grated
- ¼ cup chia seeds
- ½ teaspoon oregano, chopped
- Salt and black pepper to the taste
- 2 eggs
- 2 garlic cloves, minced

Directions:
In a bowl, mix flaxseed with chia seeds, parmesan, salt, pepper, oregano, garlic and basil and stir. Put the eggs in a second bowl and whisk them well. Dip chicken in eggs mix, then in chia seeds mix, put them in your Crock Pot after you've greased it with cooking spray, cover and cook on High for hours. Serve them right away for a Sunday breakfast.
Nutrition Info:calories 212, fat 3, fiber 4, carbs 17, protein 4

78. Bacon Eggs

Servings: 2   Cooking Time: 2 Hours
Ingredients:

- 2 eggs, hard-boiled, peeled
- ¼ teaspoon ground black pepper
- 2 bacon slices
- 1 teaspoon olive oil
- ½ teaspoon dried thyme

Directions:
Sprinkle the bacon with ground black pepper and dried thyme.   Then wrap the eggs in the bacon and sprinkle with olive oil.   Put the eggs in the Crock Pot and cook on High for 2 hours.
Nutrition Info: Per Serving: 187 calories, 12.6g protein, 0.9g carbohydrates, 14.7g fat, 0.2g fiber, 185mg cholesterol, 501mg sodium, 172mg potassium.

79. Corn Casserole

Servings: 6   Cooking Time: 8 Hours
Ingredients:

- 1 cup sweet corn kernels
- 1 chili pepper, chopped
- 1 tomato, chopped
- 1 cup Mozzarella, shredded
- 2 tablespoons cream cheese
- 5 oz ham, chopped
- 1 teaspoon garlic powder
- 2 eggs, beaten

Directions:
Mix sweet corn kernels, with chili pepper, tomato, and ham.   Add minced garlic and stir the ingredients.   Transfer it in the Crock Pot and flatten gently.   Top the casserole with eggs, cream cheese, and Mozzarella.   Cook the casserole on LOW for 8 hours.

Nutrition Info: Per Serving: 110 calories, 8.3g protein, 7.2g carbohydrates, 5.8g fat, 1g fiber, 74mg cholesterol, 449mg sodium, 159mg potassium.

80. Strawberry Yogurt

Servings: 7   Cooking Time: 3 Hours
Ingredients:

4 cup milk	1 cup Greek yogurt
1 cup strawberries, sliced	1 teaspoon coconut shred

Directions:
Pour the milk into the Crock Pot and cook it on HIGH for 3 hours.   Cool the milk till it reaches the temperature of 100F.   Add Greek yogurt, mix the liquid carefully, and cover with a towel. Leave the yogurt for 10 hours in a warm place. Pour the thick yogurt mixture in the colander or cheese mold and leave for hours to avoid the extra liquid.   Transfer the cooked yogurt in the ramekins and top with sliced strawberries and coconut shred.
Nutrition Info: Per Serving: 105 calories,7.6g protein, 9.9g carbohydrates, 4.2g fat, 0.6g fiber, 13mg cholesterol, 76mg sodium, 152mg potassium.

81. Ginger Raisins Oatmeal

Servings: 2   Cooking Time: 8 Hours
Ingredients:

1 cup almond milk	¼ cup raisins
½ cup steel cut oats	1 tablespoon orange juice
½ teaspoon ginger, ground	
1 tablespoon orange zest, grated	½ teaspoon vanilla extract
	½ tablespoon honey

Directions:
In your Crock Pot, combine the milk with the oats, raisins and the other ingredients, toss, put the lid on and cook on Low for 8 hours.   Divide into bowls and serve for breakfast.
Nutrition Info:calories 435, fat 30.1, fiber 5.8, carbs 41.2, protein 6.2

82. Vanilla Quinoa

Servings: 2   Cooking Time: 4 Hours
Ingredients:

½ cup quinoa	2 cups of milk
1 teaspoon vanilla extract	1 tablespoon butter

Directions:
Put quinoa, milk, and vanilla extract in the Crock Pot.   Cook it for 4 hours on Low.   Then add butter and stir the quinoa carefully.
Nutrition Info: Per Serving: 335 calories, 14.1g protein, 39.5g carbohydrates, 13.3g fat, 3g fiber, 35mg cholesterol, 158mg sodium, 384mg potassium.

83. Cranberry Almond Quinoa

Servings: 4   Cooking Time: 2 Hrs

Ingredients:

3 cups of coconut water	3 tsp honey
1 tsp vanilla extract	1/8 cup coconut flakes
1 cup quinoa	¼ cup cranberries, dried
1/8 cup almonds, sliced	

Directions:
Add coconut water, honey, vanilla, quinoa, almonds, cranberries, and coconut flakes to the Crock Pot.   Put the cooker's lid on and set the cooking time to hours on High settings.   Dish out and serve.
Nutrition Info: Per Serving: Calories 261, Total Fat 7g, Fiber 8g, Total Carbs 18g, Protein 4g

84. Oats Craisins Granola

Servings: 8   Cooking Time: 2 Hrs
Ingredients:

5 cups old-fashioned rolled oats	½ cup peanut butter
1/3 cup coconut oil	1 tbsp vanilla
2/3 cup honey	2 tsp cinnamon powder
½ cup almonds, chopped	1 cup craisins
	Cooking spray

Directions:
Toss oats with honey, oil, craisins, cinnamon, vanilla, peanut butter, and almonds in the Crock Pot.   Put the cooker's lid on and set the cooking time to hours on High settings.   Serve.
Nutrition Info: Per Serving: Calories 200, Total Fat 3g, Fiber 6g, Total Carbs 9g, Protein 4g

85. Peas And Rice Bowls

Servings: 2   Cooking Time: 6 Hours
Ingredients:

¼ cup peas	¼ cup heavy cream
1 cup wild rice	
2 cups veggie stock	½ teaspoon allspice, ground
1 tablespoon dill, chopped	A pinch of salt and black pepper
3 spring onions, chopped	
½ teaspoon coriander, ground	¼ cup cheddar cheese, shredded
	1 teaspoon olive oil

Directions:
Grease the Crock Pot with the oil, add the rice, peas, stock and the other ingredients except the dill and heavy cream, stir, put the lid on and cook on Low for 3 hours.   Add the remaining ingredients, stir the mix, put the lid back on, cook on Low for 3 more hours, divide into bowls and serve for breakfast.
Nutrition Info:calories 442, fat 13.6, fiber 6.8, carbs 66, protein 17.4

86. Chocolate Toast

Servings: 4   Cooking Time: 40 Minutes
Ingredients:

4 white bread slices
1 tablespoon vanilla extract
2 tablespoons Nutella
1 banana, mashed
1 tablespoon coconut oil
¼ cup full-fat milk

Directions:
Mix vanilla extract, Nutella, mashed banana, coconut oil, and milk.   Pour the mixture in the Crock Pot and cook on High for 40 minutes. Make a quick pressure release and cool the chocolate mixture.   Spread the toasts with cooked mixture.

Nutrition Info: Per Serving: 148 calories, 2g protein, 18.2g carbohydrates, 7.1g fat, 1.5g fiber, 2mg cholesterol, 73mg sodium, 182mg potassium.

87. Chicken Cabbage Medley

Servings: 5   Cooking Time: 4.5 Hrs

Ingredients:
6 oz. ground chicken
10 oz. cabbage, chopped
1 white onion, sliced
½ cup tomato juice
1 tsp sugar
½ tsp salt
1 tsp ground black pepper
4 tbsp chicken stock
2 garlic cloves

Directions:
Whisk tomato juice with black pepper, salt, sugar, and chicken stock in a bowl.   Spread the onion slices, chicken, and cabbage in the Crock Pot. Pour the tomato-stock mixture over the veggies and top with garlic cloves.   Put the cooker's lid on and set the cooking time to hours 30 minutes on High settings.   Serve.

Nutrition Info: Per Serving: Calories 91, Total Fat 3.1g, Fiber 2g, Total Carbs 9.25g, Protein 8g

88. Breakfast Casserole

Servings: 5   Cooking Time: 7 Hours

Ingredients:
1 cup Cheddar cheese, shredded
1 potato, peeled, diced
½ cup carrot, grated
1 teaspoon ground turmeric
½ teaspoon cayenne pepper
5 eggs, beaten
5 oz ham, chopped
½ cup bell pepper, chopped

Directions:
Make the layer from potato in the Crock Pot mold. Then put the layer of carrot over the potatoes. Sprinkle the vegetables with ground turmeric and cayenne pepper.   Then add ham and bell pepper. Pour the beaten eggs over the casserole and top with shredded cheese.   Cook the meal on LOW for 7 hours.

Nutrition Info: Per Serving: 237 calories, 16.8g protein, 10g carbohydrates, 14.4g fat, 1.7g fiber, 204mg cholesterol, 582mg sodium, 378mg potassium.

89. Lentils And Quinoa Mix

Servings: 6   Cooking Time: 8 Hours

Ingredients:
3 garlic cloves, minced
1 yellow onion, chopped
1 celery stalk, chopped
2 red bell peppers, chopped
12 ounces canned tomatoes, chopped
4 cups veggie stock
1 cup lentils
14 ounces pinto beans
2 tablespoons chili powder
½ cup quinoa
1 tablespoons oregano, chopped
2 teaspoon cumin, ground

Directions:
In your Crock Pot, mix garlic with the onion, celery, bell peppers, tomatoes, stock, lentils, pinto beans, chili powder, quinoa, oregano and cumin, stir, cover, cook on Low for 8 hours, divide between plates and serve for breakfast

Nutrition Info: calories 231, fat 4, fiber 5, carbs 16, protein 4

90. Chili Eggs Mix

Servings: 2   Cooking Time: 3 Hours

Ingredients:
3 spring onions, chopped
2 tablespoons sun dried tomatoes, chopped
1 ounce canned and roasted green chili pepper, chopped
½ teaspoon rosemary, dried
Cooking spray
Salt and black pepper to the taste
3 ounces cheddar cheese, shredded
4 eggs, whisked
¼ cup heavy cream
1 tablespoon chives, chopped

Directions:
Grease your Crock Pot with cooking spray and mix the eggs with the chili peppers and the other ingredients except the cheese.   Toss everything into the pot, sprinkle the cheese on top, put the lid on and cook on High for 3 hours.   Divide between plates and serve.

Nutrition Info: calories 224, fat 4, fiber 7, carbs 18, protein 11

91. Crock-pot Breakfast Casserole

Servings: 8   Cooking Time: 10-12 Hours

Ingredients:
1 lb. ground sausage, cooked, drained
12-ounce package bacon slices, crumbled, cooked, drained
1 dozen eggs
1 cup heavy white cream
½ cup feta cheese, chopped
1 teaspoon black pepper
1 teaspoon sea salt
2 cups Monterrey Jack cheese, shredded
1 ½ cups spinach, fresh
1 ½ cups mushrooms, fresh, sliced
1 green bell pepper, diced
1 medium sweet yellow onion, diced

4 cups daikon radish hashed browns

Directions:
Place a layer of hashed browns on bottom of Crock-Pot. Follow with a layer of sausage and bacon, then add onions, spinach, green pepper, mushrooms and cheese. In a mixing bowl, beat the eggs, cream, salt, and pepper together. Pour over mixture in Crock-Pot. Cover and cook on LOW for -12 hours.
Nutrition Info: Calories: 443.6, Carbohydrates: 8 g, Fiber: 1.95 g, Net Carbohydrates: 6.05 g, Protein: 18.1 g, Fat: 38.25 g

92. Egg Sandwich

Servings: 4   Cooking Time: 2.5 Hours
Ingredients:

4 bread slices	4 ham slices
4 eggs, beaten	½ teaspoon minced
1 teaspoon smoked paprika	garlic
½ teaspoon ground turmeric	1 tablespoon coconut oil

Directions:
In the bowl mix eggs, smoked paprika, ground turmeric, and minced garlic. Then dip every bread slice in the egg mixture. Put the coconut oil in the Crock Pot. Arrange the bread slices in the Crock Pot in one layer and top with ham. Close the lid and cook the meal on HIGH for 2.hours.
Nutrition Info: Per Serving: 165 calories, 11g protein, 6.6g carbohydrates, 10.6g fat, 0.9g fiber, 180mg cholesterol, 488mg sodium, 169mg potassium.

93. Mushrooms Casserole

Servings: 4   Cooking Time: 4 Hours
Ingredients:

1 teaspoon lemon zest, grated	10 ounces spinach, torn
10 ounces goat cheese, cubed	½ cup yellow onion, chopped
1 tablespoon lemon juice	½ teaspoon basil, dried
1 tablespoon apple cider vinegar	8 ounces mushrooms, sliced
1 tablespoon olive oil	Salt and black pepper to the taste
2 garlic cloves, minced	Cooking spray

Directions:
Spray your Crock Pot with cooking spray, arrange cheese cubes on the bottom and add lemon zest, lemon juice, vinegar, olive oil, garlic, spinach, onion, basil, mushrooms, salt and pepper. Toss well, cover, cook on Low for 4 hours, divide between plates and serve for breakfast right away.
Nutrition Info:calories 276, fat 6, fiber 5, carbs 7, protein 4

94. Coconut Oatmeal

Servings: 6   Cooking Time: 5 Hours
Ingredients:

2 cups oatmeal	2 tablespoons
2 cups of coconut milk	coconut shred
1 cup of water	1 tablespoon maple syrup

Directions:
Put all ingredients in the Crock Pot and carefully mix. Then close the lid and cook the oatmeal on low for 5 hours.
Nutrition Info: Per Serving: 313 calories, 5.4g protein, 25.8g carbohydrates, 22.5g fat, 4.8g fiber, 0mg cholesterol, 16mg sodium, 316mg potassium

95. Tomato Hot Eggs

Servings: 3   Cooking Time: 2.5 Hours
Ingredients:

3 eggs, beaten	1 bell pepper, diced
2 tomatoes, chopped	1 tablespoon hot sauce
1 teaspoon coconut oil	

Directions:
Grease the Crock Pot with coconut oil from inside. Then mix hot sauce with beaten eggs. Add chopped tomatoes and bell pepper. Pour the mixture in the Crock Pot and close the lid. Cook the meal on high for 2.hours.
Nutrition Info: Per Serving: 104 calories, 6.7g protein, 6.6g carbohydrates, 6.2g fat, 1.5g fiber, 164mg cholesterol, 193mg sodium, 335mg potassium.

96. Cranberry Maple Oatmeal

Servings: 2   Cooking Time: 6 Hours
Ingredients:

1 cup almond milk	½ cup cranberries
½ cup steel cut oats	1 tablespoon maple syrup
½ teaspoon vanilla extract	1 tablespoon sugar

Directions:
In your Crock Pot, mix the oats with the berries, milk and the other ingredients, toss, put the lid on and cook on Low for 6 hours. Divide into bowls and serve for breakfast.
Nutrition Info:calories 200, fat 5, fiber 7, carbs 14, protein 4

97. Berry-berry Jam

Servings: 6   Cooking Time: 4 Hrs
Ingredients:

1 cup white sugar	1 tbsp lemon zest
1 cup strawberries	1 tsp lemon juice
1 tbsp gelatin	½ cup blueberries
3 tbsp water	

Directions:
Take a blender jug and add berries, sugar, lemon juice, and lemon zest to puree. Blend this blueberry-strawberry mixture for 3 minutes until smooth. Pour this berry mixture into the base of

your Crock Pot.   Put the cooker's lid on and set the cooking time to 1 hour on High settings.   Mix gelatin with 3 tbsp water in a bowl and pour it into the berry mixture.   Again, put the cooker's lid on and set the cooking time to 3 hours on High settings.   Allow the jam to cool down.   Serve.
Nutrition Info: Per Serving: Calories 163, Total Fat 8.3g, Fiber 2g, Total Carbs 20.48g, Protein 3g

98. Nutmeg Squash Oatmeal

Servings: 6   Cooking Time: 8 Hrs
Ingredients:

½ cup almonds, soaked for 12 hours in water and drained
½ cup walnuts, chopped
2 apples, peeled, cored and cubed
1 butternut squash, peeled and cubed
½ tsp nutmeg, ground
1 tsp cinnamon powder
1 tbsp sugar
1 cup milk

Directions:
Toss almond with apples, walnuts, nutmeg, sugar, squash, and cinnamon in the base of your Crock Pot.   Pour in milk and give it a gentle stir.   Put

the cooker's lid on and set the cooking time to 8 hours on Low settings.   Serve.
Nutrition Info: Per Serving: Calories 178, Total Fat 7g, Fiber 7g, Total Carbs 9g, Protein 4g

99. Chocolate Vanilla Toast

Servings: 4   Cooking Time: 4 Hrs
Ingredients:

Cooking spray
1 loaf of bread, cubed
¾ cup brown sugar
3 eggs
1 and ½ cups of milk
1 tsp vanilla extract
¾ cup of chocolate chips
1 tsp cinnamon powder

Directions:
Cover the base of your Crock Pot with cooking spray.   Spread the bread pieces in the cooker. Beat eggs with vanilla, milk, sugar, chocolate chips, and cinnamon in a bowl.   Pour this egg-chocolate mixture over the bread pieces.   Put the cooker's lid on and set the cooking time to 4 hours on Low settings.   Serve.
Nutrition Info: Per Serving: Calories 261, Total Fat 6g, Fiber 5g, Total Carbs 19g, Protein 6g

Lunch & Dinner Recipes

100.   Bbq Tofu

Servings: 4   Cooking Time: 2 1/4 Hours

Ingredients:

4 thick slices firm tofu	1 cup BBQ sauce
1 shallot, sliced	1/4 teaspoon cumin powder
2 garlic cloves, minced	1 pinch cayenne pepper
1 teaspoon Worcestershire sauce	1 thyme sprig

Directions:

Combine the shallot, garlic, BBQ sauce, Worcestershire sauce, cumin powder, cayenne pepper and thyme in your Crock Pot.   Add the tofu and coat it well.   Cover the pot with its lid and cook on high settings for 2 hours.   Serve the tofu warm with your favorite side dish.

101.Beans Bourginon

Servings: 10   Cooking Time: 8 1/4 Hours

Ingredients:

2 tablespoons olive oil	2 leeks, sliced
2 large onions, chopped	2 cups sliced mushrooms
4 garlic cloves, chopped	2 carrots, sliced
1 teaspoon dried thyme	1/2 cup dry red wine
2 cups kidney beans, rinsed	4 cups vegetable stock or water
	2 bay leaves
	Salt and pepper to taste

Directions:

Heat the oil in a skillet and add the onions, leeks and garlic. cook for   minutes until softened then transfer in your Crock Pot.   Add the remaining ingredients and cook on low settings for 8 hours. The dish is best served warm.

102.   Dinner Millet Bowl

Servings: 5   Cooking Time: 8 Hours

Ingredients:

2 cups whole-grain millet	1 teaspoon salt
2 cups chicken stock	1/4 cup pomegranate seeds
3 cups of water	1 cup sauerkraut
1 teaspoon butter	

Directions:

Mix water with chicken stock and pour the liquid in the Crock Pot.   Add salt and millet and cook the ingredients on low for 8 hours.   Then mix the cooked millet with butter and pomegranate seeds. Transfer the millet in the bowls and top with sauerkraut.

Nutrition Info: Per Serving: 323 calories, 9.4g protein, 61g carbohydrates, 4.4g fat, 7.7g fiber, 2mg cholesterol, 972mg sodium, 212mg potassium.

103.   Beef Broccoli Sauté

Servings: 4   Cooking Time: 2 1/4 Hours

Ingredients:

2 flank steaks, cut into thin strips	2 tablespoons soy sauce
1 tablespoon peanut oil	1/4 cup beef stock
1 pound broccoli florets	1 teaspoon hot sauce
1/4 cup peanuts, chopped	1/2 teaspoon sesame oil
1 tablespoon tomato paste	1 tablespoon sesame seeds
	Salt and pepper to taste

Directions:

Combine all the ingredients in your crock pot. Add salt and pepper to taste and cook on high settings for hours.   Serve the sauté warm.

104.   Buffalo Chicken Drumsticks

Servings: 8   Cooking Time: 7 1/4 Hours

Ingredients:

4 pounds chicken drumsticks	2 cups hot BBQ sauce
2 tablespoons tomato sauce	1 teaspoon Worcestershire sauce
1 tablespoon cider vinegar	1 cup cream cheese
	Salt and pepper to taste

Directions:

Combine the chicken and the remaining ingredients in your crock pot.   Add salt and pepper to taste and cook on low settings for 7 hours.   Serve the chicken warm and fresh.

105.   Quinoa Tofu Veggie Stew

Servings: 6   Cooking Time: 6 1/4 Hours

Ingredients:

6 oz. firm tofu, cubed	1/2 cup green peas
1/2 cup quinoa, rinsed	1 cup broccoli florets
1 celery stalk, sliced	1 tablespoon Pesto sauce
1 parsnip, diced	2 tablespoons green lentils
1 carrot, diced	1 cup vegetable stock
1 cup cauliflower florets	Salt and pepper to taste

Directions:

Combine all the ingredients in your crock pot. Add salt and pepper to taste and cook on low settings for 6 hours.   Serve the stew warm and fresh.

106.   Black Bean Pork Stew

Servings: 10   Cooking Time: 9 1/4 Hours

Ingredients:

2 red onions, chopped	2 cups chicken stock
4 garlic cloves,	1 teaspoon dried basil
	1 teaspoon cumin

chopped
1 pound dried black beans
1 can fire roasted tomatoes
2 chipotle peppers, chopped
1 teaspoon dried oregano

powder
1 teaspoon chili powder
3 pounds pork roast, cubed
Salt and pepper to taste

Directions:
Combine the onions, garlic, black beans, tomatoes, stock, chipotle peppers, oregano, basil, cumin powder, chili powder and pork roast in a Crock Pot. Add salt and pepper to taste and cook on low settings for 9 hours.   Serve the stew warm and fresh or chilled.

107.   Chicken Shrimp Jambalaya

Servings: 8   Cooking Time: 8 1/4 Hours
Ingredients:

2 tablespoons olive oil
1 1/2 pounds skinless chicken breasts, cubed
2 large onions, chopped
2 red bell peppers, cored and diced
1 celery stalk, sliced
2 garlic cloves, chopped

1/2 teaspoon dried oregano
1 cup diced tomato
1 1/2 cups chicken stock
Salt and pepper to taste
1 pound fresh shrimps, peeled and cleaned
Cooked white rice for serving

Directions:
Heat the oil in a skillet and add the chicken. Cook for 5 minutes until golden then transfer in your crock pot.   Add the onions, bell peppers, celery, garlic, oregano, tomato and stock.   Add salt and pepper to taste and cook on low settings for 6 hours.   At this point, add the shrimps and cook for 2 more hours.   Serve the jambalaya warm and fresh.

108.   Spinach Bean Casserole

Servings: 8   Cooking Time: 6 1/2 Hours
Ingredients:

2 bacon slices, chopped
2 sweet onions, chopped
1 carrot, diced
1 celery stalk, sliced
4 garlic cloves, chopped
2 tablespoons tomato paste
1/2 cup tomato sauce

1/2 teaspoon dried sage
1 1/2 cups dried black beans, rinsed
2 cups vegetable stock
2 cups water
4 cups fresh spinach, shredded
1 bay leaf
Salt and pepper to taste

Directions:
Heat a skillet over medium flame and add the bacon. Cook until crisp then stir in the onions and garlic. cook for 2 minutes until softened.

Transfer in your Crock Pot and add the remaining ingredients.   Season with salt and pepper to taste and cook on low settings for 6 hours.   Serve the stew warm and fresh.

109.   Mustard Pork Chops And Carrots

Servings: 2   Cooking Time: 4 Hours
Ingredients:

1 tablespoon butter
1 pound pork chops, bone in
2 carrots, sliced
1 cup beef stock

½ tablespoon honey
½ tablespoon lime juice
1 tablespoon lime zest, grated

Directions:
In your Crock Pot, mix the pork chops with the butter and the other ingredients, toss, put the lid on and cook on High for 4 hours.   Divide between plate sand serve.
Nutrition Info: calories 300, fat 8, fiber 10, carbs 16, protein 16

110. Boston Baked Beans

Servings: 8   Cooking Time: 6 1/4 Hours
Ingredients:

1 pound dried kidney beans
2 tablespoons molasses
1 teaspoon mustard seeds
1 teaspoon Worcestershire sauce
2 tablespoons brown sugar
1 cup water

1 large onion, chopped
2 cups vegetable stock
1/2 teaspoon celery seeds
1/2 teaspoon cumin seeds
1 bay leaf
Salt and pepper to taste

Directions:
Combine the kidney beans, molasses, mustard seeds, Worcestershire sauce, brown sugar, onion and stock in your Crock Pot.   Season with salt and pepper and add the celery seeds, cumin seeds, water and bay leaf.   Cook on low settings for 6 hours.   Serve the beans warm and fresh.

111. Chickpea Tikka Masala

Servings: 6   Cooking Time: 6 1/2 Hours
Ingredients:

2 tablespoons olive oil
1 large onion, chopped
4 garlic cloves, chopped
1 teaspoon grated ginger
1 teaspoon garam masala
1 can diced tomatoes

1/2 teaspoon turmeric powder
1/2 teaspoon red chili, sliced
2 cans (15 oz. each) chickpeas, drained
1 cup coconut milk
Salt and pepper to taste
Chopped cilantro for serving

Directions:

Heat the oil in a skillet and stir in the onion and garlic. Cook for 2 minutes until softened and translucent then transfer in your crock pot. Add the remaining ingredients and season well with salt and pepper. Cover and cook on low settings for 6 hours. The chickpea tikka masala is best served warm.

Grease the Crock Pot with the cooking spray and mix the bell peppers with the onion, garlic and the other ingredients into the pot. Put the lid on, cook on Low for 8 hours, divide into bowls and serve.

Nutrition Info:calories 272, fat 4, fiber 7, carbs 19, protein 7

112. Intense Mustard Pork Chops

Servings: 4   Cooking Time: 5 1/4 Hours
Ingredients:

4 pork chops	1 tablespoon honey
2 tablespoons Dijon mustard	4 garlic cloves, minced
2 tablespoons olive oil	1 cup chicken stock
1 shallot, finely chopped	Salt and pepper to taste

Directions:
Season the pork chops with salt and pepper and place them in your crock pot. Add the rest of the ingredients and adjust the taste with salt and pepper. Cover with a lid and cook on low settings for 5 hours. Serve the pork chops and the sauce formed in the pan warm with your favorite side dish.

113. Creamy Salsa Verde Chicken

Servings: 6   Cooking Time: 4 1/4 Hours
Ingredients:

2 pounds chicken breast, cubed	1/4 cup chicken stock
1 jar salsa verde	Salt and pepper to taste
1 cup cream cheese	1 ripe avocado for serving
2 tablespoons chopped cilantro	1 lime for serving

Directions:
Combine the chicken, salsa verde, cream cheese, cilantro, stock, salt and pepper in a crock pot. Cover with a lid and cook on low settings for 4 hours. Serve the chicken warm, topped with sliced or cubed avocado and a drizzle of lime juice.

114. Beans And Mushroom Stew

Servings: 2   Cooking Time: 8 Hours
Ingredients:

Cooking spray	1 cup white mushrooms, sliced
½ green bell pepper, chopped	1 cup canned kidney beans, drained
½ red bell pepper, chopped	
½ red onion, chopped	½ teaspoon turmeric powder
2 garlic cloves, minced	½ teaspoon coriander, ground
1 cup tomatoes, cubed	1 tablespoon parsley, chopped
1 cup veggie stock	
Salt and black pepper to the taste	½ tablespoon Cajun seasoning

Directions:

115. Asiago Chickpea Stew

Servings: 4   Cooking Time: 2 1/4 Hours
Ingredients:

2 cans (15 oz. each) chickpeas, drained	Salt and pepper to taste
2 ripe tomatoes, peeled and diced	1/2 teaspoon dried oregano
1/2 cup vegetable stock	1 cup grated Asiago cheese
1/2 cup light cream	

Directions:
Combine the chickpeas, tomatoes, stock, cream, salt, pepper and oregano in your crock pot. Top with grated cheese and cook on high settings for hours. Serve the stew warm and fresh.

116. African Sweet Potato Stew

Servings: 6   Cooking Time: 6 1/2 Hours
Ingredients:

1 onion, chopped	1 cup vegetable stock
2 garlic cloves, chopped	1 teaspoon grated ginger
1 1/2 pounds sweet potatoes, peeled and cubed	1 pinch chili powder
	4 cups fresh spinach
1 can diced tomatoes	Salt and pepper to taste
2 tablespoons peanut butter	Chopped peanuts for serving

Directions:
Mix the onion, garlic, potatoes, tomatoes, stock and peanut butter in your crock pot. Add the remaining ingredients and season with salt and pepper as needed. Cook on low settings for 6 hours. The stew is best served warm, topped with chopped peanuts.

117. Garlic Roasted Pork Belly

Servings: 8   Cooking Time: 8 1/4 Hours
Ingredients:

4 pounds pork belly	1 teaspoon cayenne pepper
8 garlic cloves	
1 teaspoon cumin powder	Salt and pepper to taste
1 teaspoon garlic powder	1 cup dry white wine

Directions:
Make a few holes in the pork meat and stuff them with garlic cloves. Season the piece of meat with cumin, garlic powder, cayenne pepper, salt and pepper. Place the pork belly in your Crock Pot and add the wine. Cook on low settings for 8 hours. Serve the pork belly warm and fresh.

118. White Bean Chard Stew

Servings: 6   Cooking Time: 6 1/4 Hours

Ingredients:

2 cans (15 oz. each) white beans, drained	1 fennel bulb, sliced
1 bunch green chard, shredded	1/2 cup vegetable stock
1 shallot, chopped	1 cup diced tomatoes
2 garlic cloves, minced	1/2 teaspoon dried oregano
1 leek, sliced	1/2 teaspoon dried basil
1 red bell pepper, cored and sliced	Salt and pepper to taste

Directions:
Combine the white beans and the remaining ingredients in your crock pot.   Add enough salt and pepper and cook on low settings for 6 hours. Serve the stew warm and fresh or freeze it in individual portions for as long as needed.

119. Roasted Bell Pepper Cannellini Stew

Servings: 6   Cooking Time: 6 1/4 Hours

Ingredients:

1 can (15 oz.) cannellini beans, drained	1/2 cup tomato sauce
4 roasted red bell peppers, chopped	1 cup vegetable stock
2 garlic cloves, chopped	1/2 teaspoon dried basil
1 shallot, chopped	Salt and pepper to taste
2 ripe tomatoes, peeled and diced	1 pinch cumin powder
	2 tablespoons chopped parsley

Directions:
Combine the beans, bell peppers, garlic, shallot, tomatoes, tomato sauce, stock, basil and cumin in your Crock Pot.   Add salt and pepper to taste and cook on low settings for 6 hours.   When done, stir in the parsley and serve the stew warm or chilled.

120. Cuban Beans

Servings: 6   Cooking Time: 8 1/4 Hours

Ingredients:

1 cup dried black beans, rinsed	1/2 teaspoon cumin seeds
2 cups vegetable stock	1/2 teaspoon ground coriander
2 cups water	1 teaspoon sherry wine vinegar
1 cup chopped onion	1 can fire roasted tomatoes
2 red bell peppers, cored and diced	1 green chile, chopped
1 green bell pepper, cored and diced	Salt and pepper to taste
1 teaspoon fennel seeds	

Directions:
Combine the beans and the remaining ingredients in your Crock Pot.   Add salt and pepper as needed and cook on low settings for 8 hours. Serve the beans warm in tortillas or over cooked rice.

121. Spicy Swiss Steak

Servings: 4   Cooking Time: 8 Hours 20 Minutes

Ingredients:

¼ teaspoon kosher salt	¼ cup carrots, sliced
½ tablespoon liquid smoke mesquite flavor	½ (14½ oz.) can Rotel tomatoes (tomatoes with a hint of chili to give them some heat)
½ cup celery, sliced	
1 garlic clove, peeled and minced	¾ cup beef broth
½ teaspoon black pepper	¼ cup onions, sliced
1¼ pounds boneless round steak	¼ cup red bell peppers

Directions:
Put all the ingredients in a crock pot and mix well. Cover and cook on LOW for about 8 hours.   Dish out and serve hot.

Nutrition Info: Calories:332 Fat:12.9g Carbohydrates:4.5g

122.   Farro Pilaf

Servings: 4   Cooking Time: 7 Hours

Ingredients:

¼ onion, diced	3 cups of water
1 tablespoon olive oil	1 teaspoon dried sage
1 cup farro	4 oz beef sirloin, chopped

Directions:
Heat olive oil in the skillet.   Add beef sirloin and roast it on medium heat for 3 minutes per side. Then transfer the meat in the Crock Pot.   Add water, farro, sage, and onion.   Close the lid and cook the pilaf on Low for 7 hours.

Nutrition Info: Per Serving: 246 calories,15.7g protein, 33.7g carbohydrates, 5.3g fat, 3.2g fiber, 25mg cholesterol, 54mg sodium, 128mg potassium.

123.   Veggie Soup

Servings: 2   Cooking Time: 4 Hours

Ingredients:

½ pound gold potatoes, peeled and roughly cubed	4 cups veggie stock
1 carrot, sliced	3 tablespoons tomato paste
1 zucchini, cubed	1 sweet onion, chopped
1 eggplant, cubed	1 tablespoon lemon juice
1 cup tomatoes, cubed	1 tablespoon chives, chopped
A pinch of salt and black pepper	

Directions:
In your Crock Pot, mix the potatoes with the carrot, zucchini and the other ingredients, toss, put the lid

on and cook on Low for 4 hours. Divide the soup into bowls and serve.
Nutrition Info:calories 392, fat 7, fiber 8, carbs 12, protein 28

124. Herbed Broccoli Soufflé

Servings: 6   Cooking Time: 2 1/4 Hours

Ingredients:

1 1/2 pounds fresh or frozen broccoli	1 cup mayonnaise
1 can cream of celery soup	2 eggs, beaten
	1 cup grated Cheddar
1/2 teaspoon onion powder	Salt and pepper to taste
1/2 teaspoon garlic powder	1 cup crushed crackers

Directions:
Cook the broccoli in a pot of hot water for minutes. Drain and place in a food processor. Pulse until ground. Stir in the celery soup, mayonnaise, onion powder, garlic powder and eggs. Pour the mixture in your greased crock pot. Top with crackers and cheese and cook on high settings for 2 hours. Serve the soufflé right away.

125. Honey Sesame Glazed Chicken

Servings: 4   Cooking Time: 6 1/4 Hours

Ingredients:

4 chicken breasts	2 tablespoons soy sauce
3 tablespoons honey	
1/2 teaspoon red pepper flakes	1/4 cup ketchup
	1/4 cup chicken stock
2 garlic cloves, minced	2 tablespoons sesame seeds
1 teaspoon grated ginger	1 teaspoon sesame oil

Directions:
Combine the chicken and the remaining ingredients in your crock pot. Cover with a lid and cook on low settings for 6 hours. Serve the chicken warm with your favorite side dish.

126. Red Chile Pulled Pork

Servings: 8   Cooking Time: 7 1/4 Hours

Ingredients:

4 pounds pork roast	1 cup tomato sauce
2 red chilis, seeded and chopped	1 cup red salsa
	Salt and pepper to taste
1 large onion, chopped	

Directions:
Combine all the ingredients in your Crock Pot. Add salt and pepper to fit your taste and cook under the lid on low settings for 7 hours. When done, shred the pork into fine threads using two forks. Serve the pork warm and fresh or re-heat it later.

127. Summer Squash Lasagna

Servings: 8   Cooking Time: 6 1/2 Hours

Ingredients:

2 summer squashes, cut into thin strips	1/2 cup chopped parsley
4 tablespoons Italian pesto	1 lemon, juiced
	1/2 teaspoon dried thyme
4 ripe tomatoes, pureed	1 pinch chili flakes
1 can chickpeas, drained	Salt and pepper to taste
1/2 cup red lentils	1 1/2 cups shredded mozzarella
1 shallot, chopped	

Directions:
Mix the chickpeas, lentils, parsley, lemon juice, thyme and chili flakes in a bowl. Add salt and pepper to taste and mix well. Place a few squash slices in your Crock Pot. Brush with pesto and top with part of the chickpea mix. Pour a few spoonfuls of tomato puree and continue layering squash slices, pesto, chickpea mix and tomato puree. End with a layer of mozzarella and cook on low settings for 6 hours. Serve the lasagna warm.

128. Spicy Sweet Potato Chili

Servings: 8   Cooking Time: 5 1/2 Hours

Ingredients:

2 tablespoons olive oil	1 carrot, diced
2 shallots, chopped	1 can (15 oz.) black beans, drained
1 garlic clove, chopped	1/2 teaspoon chili powder
1/4 teaspoon cumin powder	2 cups vegetable stock
1/2 teaspoon curry powder	2 tablespoons tomato paste
1 1/2 pounds sweet potatoes, peeled and cubed	Salt and pepper to taste

Directions:
Heat the oil in a skillet and add the shallots and garlic. Sauté for 2 minutes then transfer in your Crock Pot. Add the remaining ingredients and season with salt and pepper. Cook the chili on low settings for 5 hours. Serve the chili warm.

129. Onion Pork Tenderloin

Servings: 6   Cooking Time: 8 1/4 Hours

Ingredients:

3 large sweet onions, sliced	6 bacon slices
	1 thyme sprig
2 tablespoons canola oil	1/2 cup white wine
	1/2 cup chicken stock
2 pounds pork tenderloin	Salt and pepper to taste

Directions:
Heat the oil in a skillet and add the onions. Cook for minutes on all sides until softened and slightly caramelized. Transfer the onions in your crock pot and add the rest of the ingredients. Season with salt and pepper and cook on low settings for 8 hours.

130. Zucchini Bean Stew

Servings: 6   Cooking Time: 2 1/4 Hours

Ingredients:

1 can (15 oz.) white beans, drained	1 can diced tomatoes
1 red bell pepper, cored and diced	1 teaspoon dried Italian herbs
1 zucchini, cubed	Salt and pepper to taste
1 celery stalk, diced	1 cup vegetable stock
2 garlic cloves, chopped	1 bay leaf

Directions:
Combine the beans, bell pepper and zucchini in your Crock Pot.   Add the remaining ingredients and adjust the taste with salt and pepper.   Cook on high settings for 2 hours.   The stew is best served warm.

131. Green Bean Casserole

Servings: 6   Cooking Time: 6 1/4 Hours

Ingredients:

1 pound green beans, trimmed and chopped	1 cup whole milk
	4 eggs, beaten
1/2 pound fresh spinach, shredded	1/2 cup breadcrumbs
	Salt and pepper to taste
1/2 cup cream cheese	
1 shallot, chopped	

Directions:
Combine all the ingredients in your Crock Pot. Add salt and pepper to taste and cook on low settings for 6 hours.   Serve the casserole warm or chilled.

132. Buttered Broccoli

Servings: 4   Cooking Time: 1 1/2 Hours

Ingredients:

2 heads broccoli, cut into florets	1 shallot, sliced
	4 tablespoons butter
2 garlic cloves, chopped	Salt and pepper to taste

Directions:
Combine all the ingredients in your Crock Pot. Add enough salt and pepper and cook the broccoli on high settings for 1 1/4 hours.   Serve the broccoli warm and fresh.

133. Leek Potato Stew

Servings: 6   Cooking Time: 4 1/2 Hours

Ingredients:

2 tablespoons olive oil	2 tablespoons tomato paste
2 leeks, sliced	1/2 cup diced tomatoes
2 celery stalks, sliced	
2 carrots, diced	1 bay leaf
1 1/2 pounds potatoes, peeled and cubed	1 thyme sprig
	Salt and pepper to taste

Directions:

Heat the oil in your Crock Pot and add the leeks. Cook for 5 minutes until softened then transfer the mix in your Crock Pot.   Add the remaining ingredients and season with salt and pepper. Cook on low settings for 4 hours.   The stew is best served warm.

134. Wild Rice Medley

Servings: 4   Cooking Time: 6 Hours

Ingredients:

1/3 cup wild rice	1 teaspoon butter
1 cup carrot, chopped	1.5 cup vegetable stock
1 onion, chopped	
1 oz pine nuts	

Directions:
Mix wild rice with vegetable stock and transfer in the Crock Pot.   Add carrot and onion.   Cook the mixture on low for 6 hours.   Then add butter and stir the medley.   Top it with pine nuts.
Nutrition Info: Per Serving: 128 calories, 3.6g protein, 16.5g carbohydrates, 6g fat, 2.6g fiber, 3mg cholesterol, 47mg sodium, 228mg potassium.

135. Chicken And Peppers Mix

Servings: 6   Cooking Time: 4 Hours

Ingredients:

24 ounces tomato sauce	Salt and black pepper to the taste
1/4 cup parmesan, grated	6 chicken breast halves, skinless and boneless
1 yellow onion, chopped	
2 garlic cloves, minced	1/2 green bell pepper, chopped
1 teaspoon basil, dried	1/2 yellow bell pepper, chopped
1 teaspoon oregano, dried	1/2 red bell pepper, chopped

Directions:
In your Crock Pot, mix tomato sauce with parmesan, onion, garlic, basil, oregano, salt, pepper, chicken, green bell pepper, yellow bell pepper and red bell pepper, toss, cover and cook on Low for 4 hours.   Divide between plates and serve for lunch.
Nutrition Info: calories 221, fat 6, fiber 3, carbs 16, protein 26

136. Tomato Bulgur

Servings: 6   Cooking Time: 6 Hours

Ingredients:

1 cup bulgur	1/4 cup onion, diced
2 cups of water	
1 tablespoon tomato paste	1 teaspoon cayenne pepper
1/4 cup bell pepper, diced	1 tablespoon sesame oil

Directions:
Heat sesame oil in the skillet.   Add onion and bell pepper and roast them for 5 minutes on medium

heat.   Then transfer the roasted vegetables in the Crock Pot.   Add water and tomato paste. Stir the ingredients.   Then add bulgur and cayenne pepper.   Close the lid and cook the meal on Low for hours.

Nutrition Info: Per Serving: 107 calories, 3.1g protein, 19.2g carbohydrates, 2.7g fat, 4.6g fiber, 0mg cholesterol, 9mg sodium, 146mg potassium.

137. Spinach Potato Stew

Servings: 6   Cooking Time: 4 1/4 Hours

Ingredients:

2 pounds potatoes, peeled and cubed	1/4 teaspoon coriander powder
2 tablespoons olive oil	1/4 teaspoon fennel seeds
1 shallot, chopped	4 cups spinach
2 garlic cloves, chopped	1 cup vegetable stock
1/4 teaspoon cumin powder	Salt and pepper to taste

Directions:

Heat the oil in a skillet and add the shallot and garlic. Cook for 2 minutes until softened then add the spices and sauté just for 30 seconds to release flavors.   Transfer in your Crock Pot and add the remaining ingredients.   Season with salt and pepper and cook on low settings for 4 hours. Serve the stew warm.

138. Beef Bolognese Sauce

Servings: 6   Cooking Time: 6 1/4 Hours

Ingredients:

2 tablespoons canola oil	1/2 teaspoon dried oregano
2 pounds ground beef	1/2 teaspoon dried basil
1 carrot, grated	1/4 cup red wine
1 celery stalk, finely chopped	1/2 cup beef stock
4 garlic cloves, minced	Salt and pepper to taste
1 can (15 oz.) diced tomatoes	Grated Parmesan cheese for serving
2 tablespoons tomato paste	Cooked pasta of your choice for serving

Directions:

Heat the oil in a frying pan and add the ground beef. Cook for a few minutes then transfer in your Crock Pot.   Add the rest of the ingredients and adjust the taste with salt and pepper.   Cook on low settings for 6 hours.   Serve the sauce warm, over cooked past, topped with grated cheese or freeze the sauce into individual portions for later serving.

139. Asian Eggplant Stew

Servings: 4   Cooking Time: 2 1/4 Hours

Ingredients:

1 large eggplant, peeled and cubed	1/2 cup coconut milk
3 tablespoons	1 teaspoon rice vinegar

coconut oil
1/4 cup hoisin sauce
1 tablespoon soy sauce

1/2 teaspoon grated ginger
1 pinch cayenne pepper

Directions:

Heat the oil in a skillet and add the eggplant. Cook on all sides until golden then transfer in your Crock Pot.   Add the remaining ingredients and cook on high settings for 4 hours.   Serve the stew chilled.

140. Beans Chili

Servings: 2   Cooking Time: 3 Hours

Ingredients:

½ red bell pepper, chopped	1 cup canned red kidney beans, drained
½ green bell pepper, chopped	1 cup canned white beans, drained
1 garlic clove, minced	1 cup canned black beans, drained
½ cup yellow onion, chopped	Salt and black pepper to the taste
½ cup roasted tomatoes, crushed	1 tablespoon chili powder
½ cup corn	1 cup veggie stock

Directions:

In your Crock Pot, mix the peppers with the beans and the other ingredients, toss, put the lid on and cook on High for 3 hours.   Divide into bowls and serve right away.

Nutrition Info: calories 400, fat 14, fiber 5, carbs 29, protein 22

141. Vegetarian Coconut Curry

Servings: 8   Cooking Time: 7 1/2 Hours

Ingredients:

1 1/2 pounds potatoes, peeled and cubed	1 cup green peas
2 carrots, sliced	2 red bell peppers, cored and diced
1 teaspoon curry powder	1 1/2 cups coconut milk
1/2 teaspoon chili powder	1/2 cup vegetable stock
1/2 teaspoon red pepper flakes	Salt and pepper to taste

Directions:

Combine the potatoes, carrots, green peas, curry powder, chili powder, red pepper flakes, bell peppers, coconut milk and stock in your Crock Pot. Add salt and pepper to taste and cook on low settings for 7 hours.   Serve the curry warm.

142. Broccoli With Peanuts

Servings: 6   Cooking Time: 2 1/4 Hours

Ingredients:

2 heads broccoli, cut into florets	2 tablespoons olive oil
1 cup raw peanuts, chopped	1 lemon, juiced
4 garlic cloves,	1 tablespoons soy sauce

chopped
1 shallot, sliced

Salt and pepper to taste

Directions:
Combine the broccoli, peanuts, garlic, shallot, olive oil, lemon juice and soy sauce in your Crock Pot. Add salt and pepper to taste and cook the dish on high settings for hours.   Serve the dish warm and fresh.

143.	**Bacon Millet**

Servings: 6   Cooking Time: 6 Hours
Ingredients:

2 cups millet
4 cups of water
2 tablespoons butter

½ teaspoon salt
2 oz bacon, chopped, cooked

Directions:
Put millet and salt in the Crock Pot.   Add water and cook the meal on low for 6 hours.   When the millet is cooked, carefully mix it with butter and transfer in the plates.   Add bacon.
Nutrition Info: Per Serving: 337 calories, 10.9g protein, 48.7g carbohydrates, 10.6g fat, 5.7g fiber, 21mg cholesterol, 447mg sodium, 186mg potassium.

144.	**Creamy Chicken And Mushroom Pot Pie**

Servings: 6   Cooking Time: 6 1/4 Hours
Ingredients:

4 cups sliced cremini mushrooms
4 carrots, sliced
2 chicken breasts, cubed
1 large onion, chopped

1 cup frozen peas
1 cup vegetable stock
Salt and pepper to taste
1/2 teaspoon dried thyme
1 sheet puff pastry

Directions:
Combine the mushrooms, carrots, chicken, onion, peas, stock and thyme in your crock pot.   Add salt and pepper to taste then top with the puff pastry.   Cover with a lid and cook on low settings for 6 hours.   Serve the pot pie warm and fresh.

145.	**Marinated Mushrooms**

Servings: 8   Cooking Time: 8 1/4 Hours
Ingredients:

24 oz. fresh mushrooms, sliced
1/2 cup butter
1 cup water
1 cup soy sauce

1/4 teaspoon chili powder
1 teaspoon rice vinegar

Directions:
Combine all the ingredients in your Crock Pot. Cook on low settings for 8 hours.   Serve the mushrooms warm or chilled.

146.	**Chicken Dip**

Servings: 4   Cooking Time: 3.5 Hours
Ingredients:

½ cup white beans, canned, drained
½ cup ground chicken
1 teaspoon dried parsley

¼ cup BBQ sauce
1 teaspoon cayenne pepper
½ cup of water

Directions:
Blend the canned beans and transfer them in the Crock Pot.   Add ground chicken, dried parsley, BBQ sauce, cayenne pepper, and water.   Stir the ingredients and close the lid.   Cook the dip on High for 3.5 hours.
Nutrition Info: Per Serving: 142 calories, 11g protein, 21.2g carbohydrates, 1.6g fat, 4.1g fiber, 16mg cholesterol, 195mg sodium, 539mg potassium.

147.	**Miso Braised Pork**

Servings: 8   Cooking Time: 7 1/4 Hours
Ingredients:

4 pounds pork shoulder
6 garlic cloves, minced
1 tablespoon grated ginger
1 cup vegetable stock

2 tablespoons canola oil
2 tablespoons miso paste
1 lemongrass stalk, crushed

Directions:
Mix the garlic, ginger, canola oil, miso paste, stock and lemongrass in your crock pot.   Place the pork shoulder in the pot as well and cover with a lid. Cook on low settings for 7 hours.   Serve the pork warm with your favorite side dish.

148.	**Hungarian Beef Goulash**

Servings: 6   Cooking Time: 7 1/4 Hours
Ingredients:

2 pounds beef steak, cubed
2 tablespoons canola oil
2 red bell peppers, cored and diced
1 carrot, sliced
2 garlic cloves, chopped
1 red onion, chopped
1 can fire roasted tomatoes
2 tablespoons tomato paste

2 pounds potatoes, peeled and cubed
1 teaspoon smoked paprika
1 teaspoon cumin seeds
2 bay leaves
1 cup tomato sauce
1 cup beef stock
Salt and pepper to taste
Sour cream for serving

Directions:
Heat the canola oil in a frying pan and add the beef steak. Cook on all sides for a few minutes then transfer in your crock pot.   Add the rest of the ingredients and adjust the taste with salt and pepper.   Cover with a lid and cook on low settings for 7 hours.   Serve the goulash warm and fresh, topped with sour cream.

149. Cauliflower Mashed Potatoes

Servings: 4   Cooking Time: 4 1/2 Hours

Ingredients:

1 pound potatoes, peeled and cubed	2 tablespoons coconut oil
2 cups cauliflower florets	1/4 cup coconut milk
1/4 cup vegetable stock	Salt and pepper to taste

Directions:

Combine the potatoes, cauliflower, stock, coconut oil and coconut milk in your Crock Pot.   Add salt and pepper to taste and cook on low settings for 4 hours.   When done, mash with a potato masher and serve right away.

150. Beef Brisket

Servings: 6   Cooking Time: 8 Hours 15 Minutes

Ingredients:

½ teaspoon vinegar	2 pounds beef brisket, well-trimmed
1/3 cup water	2 bay leaves
½ teaspoon salt	
¼ teaspoon black pepper	¼ teaspoon thyme
¼ cup tomato sauce	2 cloves garlic

Directions:

Put all the ingredients in a bowl and mix well. Arrange beef in the crock pot and pour the above mixture over beef.   Cover and cook on LOW for about 8 hours.   Dish out in a platter and serve hot.

Nutrition Info: Calories:285 Fat:9.5g Carbohydrates:1g

151. Smoky Pork Chili

Servings: 8   Cooking Time: 6 1/4 Hours

Ingredients:

1 tablespoon canola oil	1 cup dark beer
6 bacon slices, chopped	1 teaspoon cumin powder
1 pound ground pork	1 pound dried black beans, rinsed
2 onions, chopped	2 1/2 cups vegetable stock
4 garlic cloves, chopped	1 cup diced tomatoes
2 tablespoon tomato paste	2 bay leaves
1 1/2 teaspoons smoked paprika	1 thyme sprig
	Salt and pepper to taste

Directions:

Heat the oil in a skillet and add the bacon. Cook until crisp then stir in the pork. Sauté for a few additional minutes then transfer in your Crock Pot. Add the rest of the ingredients and adjust the taste with salt and pepper.   Cook on low settings for 6 hours.   Serve the chili warm and fresh.

152. Chipotle Pork Chili

Servings: 8   Cooking Time: 8 1/2 Hours

Ingredients:

2 tablespoons canola oil	1 teaspoon cumin powder
2 pounds pork shoulder, cubed	1/2 teaspoon ground coriander
2 shallots, chopped	1 cup tomato sauce
4 garlic cloves, chopped	1 cup chicken stock
3 chipotle peppers, chopped	2 tablespoons tomato paste
2 cans (15 oz. each) black beans, drained	2 bay leaves
1 can fire roasted tomatoes	Salt and pepper to taste
	1 lime for serving

Directions:

Heat the oil in a skillet and add the pork shoulder. Cook on all sides until golden then transfer in your crock pot.   Add the rest of the ingredients, including salt and pepper.   Cook on low settings for 8 hours.   Serve the chili warm and fresh.

153. Tempeh Carnitas

Servings: 6   Cooking Time: 6 1/2 Hours

Ingredients:

1 pound tempeh, cut into thin strips	1/2 teaspoon dried oregano
2 tablespoons canola oil	1/2 teaspoon dried basil
4 garlic cloves, minced	1 cup vegetable stock
1 large onion, finely chopped	Salt and pepper to taste

Directions:

Heat the oil in a skillet and add the tempeh. Cook on all sides until golden then transfer in your Crock Pot.   Add the remaining ingredients and cook on low settings for 6 hours.   Serve the dish warm.

154. Chunky Beef Pasta Sauce

Servings: 8   Cooking Time: 6 1/2 Hours

Ingredients:

2 pounds beef sirloin, cut into thin strips	1 celery stalk, diced
1 carrot, diced	2 cups sliced mushrooms
2 garlic cloves, chopped	1/4 cup red wine
1 can (28 oz.) diced tomatoes	1 cup tomato sauce
	1 bay leaf
	Salt and pepper to taste

Directions:

Combine the beef sirloin, carrot, celery, garlic, tomatoes, mushrooms, red wine, tomato sauce and bay leaf in your Crock Pot.   Add enough salt and pepper and cover with its lid.   Cook on low settings for 6 hours.   Serve the sauce right away with cooked pasta or freeze it into individual portions to serve later.

155. Pasta Fritters

Servings: 4   Cooking Time: 5 Hours

Ingredients:

5 oz whole-grain pasta, cooked
1 egg, beaten
1 teaspoon ground turmeric

½ cup Cheddar cheese
1 tablespoon whole-grain flour
1 teaspoon sesame oil

Directions:
Chop the pasta into small pieces and mix with egg, ground turmeric, and flour.   Then shred the cheese and add it in the pasta mixture.   Make the small fritters from the mixture.   After this, brush the Crock Pot bowl with sesame oil.   Put the fritters inside and cook them on low for hours.
Nutrition Info: Per Serving: 144 calories, 7g protein, 12.4g carbohydrates, 7.4g fat, 1.6g fiber, 56mg cholesterol, 103mg sodium, 103g potassium.

156.   Quinoa Chili(1)

Servings: 6   Cooking Time: 6 Hours
Ingredients:

2 cups veggie stock
30 ounces canned black beans, drained
28 ounces canned tomatoes, chopped
1 green bell pepper, chopped
1 yellow onion, chopped
2 sweet potatoes, cubed

½ cup quinoa
1 tablespoon chili powder
2 tablespoons cocoa powder
2 teaspoons cumin, ground
Salt and black pepper to the taste
¼ teaspoon smoked paprika

Directions:
In your Crock Pot, mix stock with quinoa, black beans, tomatoes, bell pepper, onion, sweet potatoes, chili powder, cocoa, cumin, paprika, salt and pepper, stir, cover and cook on High for 6 hours.   Divide into bowls and serve for lunch.
Nutrition Info: calories 342, fat 6, fiber 7, carbs 18, protein 4

157. Noodle Stroganoff

Servings: 6   Cooking Time: 6 1/2 Hours
Ingredients:

2 large Portobello mushrooms, sliced
1 oz. dried wild mushrooms, chopped
1 teaspoon Worcestershire sauce
1 large onion, chopped
1 cup tofu cream

1 can condensed cream of mushroom soup
1 1/2 cup vegetable stock
1/2 cup short pasta of your choice
Salt and pepper to taste

Directions:
Combine the mushrooms, Worcestershire sauce, onion, mushroom soup, tofu cream, stock and short pasta in your crock pot.   Season with salt and pepper and cook on low settings for 6 hours. Serve the stroganoff warm or chilled.

158.   Texas Style Braised Beef

Servings: 8   Cooking Time: 8 1/4 Hours
Ingredients:

4 pounds beef sirloin roast
2 chipotle peppers, chopped
2 green chile peppers, chopped
1 shallot, chopped
1 cup BBQ sauce

2 tablespoons brown sugar
1/2 teaspoon garlic powder
1/2 teaspoon chili powder
Salt and pepper to taste

Directions:
Mix the chipotle peppers, green chile peppers, shallot, BBQ sauce, brown sugar, garlic powder, chili powder, salt and pepper to taste in your Crock Pot.   Add the beef and coat it well with this mix. Cover and cook on low settings for 8 hours. When done, slice and serve the beef warm with your favorite side dish.

159.   Crock Pot Steamed Rice

Servings: 8   Cooking Time: 4 Hours
Ingredients:

2 cups white rice
4 cups water
1 bay leaf

Salt and pepper to taste

Directions:
Combine all the ingredients in your crock pot. Add salt and pepper as needed and cook on low settings for 4 hours. If possible, stir once during the cooking process.   Serve the rice warm or chilled, as a side dish to your favorite veggie main dish.

160.   Mexican Shredded Chicken

Servings: 8   Cooking Time: 8 1/4 Hours
Ingredients:

4 chicken breasts
1 can fire roasted tomatoes
2 chipotle peppers, chopped
2 red bell peppers, cored and sliced

1 can (10 oz.) sweet corn, drained
1 teaspoon taco seasoning
1 cup chicken stock
Salt and pepper to taste

Directions:
Combine the chicken and the rest of the ingredients in your crock pot, adding enough salt and pepper. Cover and cook on low settings for 8 hours. When done, shred the chicken finely and serve it warm or chilled.

161. Green Lentils Salad

Servings: 2   Cooking Time: 4 Hours
Ingredients:

¼ cup green lentils
1 cup chicken stock
½ teaspoon ground cumin

2 cups lettuce, chopped
¼ cup Greek Yogurt

Directions:

Mix green lentils with chicken stock and transfer in the Crock Pot. Cook the ingredients on High for 4 hours. Then cool the lentils and transfer them in the salad bowl. Add ground cumin, lettuce, and Greek yogurt. Mix the salad carefully.
Nutrition Info: Per Serving: 118 calories, 9.4g protein, 17.7g carbohydrates, 1.3g fat, 7.7g fiber, 1mg cholesterol, 395mg sodium, 359mg potassium.

162. Greek Style Chicken Ragout
Servings: 8   Cooking Time: 8 1/4 Hours
Ingredients:

4 chicken breasts, halved	4 artichoke hearts, chopped
1 pound new potatoes, washed	1 lemon, juiced
1 pound baby carrots	1 teaspoon dried oregano
1 zucchini, cubed	Salt and pepper to taste
4 garlic cloves, chopped	1 1/2 cups chicken stock
1 sweet onion, sliced	

Directions:
Combine the chicken, potatoes, carrots, zucchini, garlic, onion, artichoke hearts, lemon juice, oregano and stock in your Crock Pot. Add salt and pepper to taste and cover with a lid. Cook on low settings for 8 hours. Serve the chicken and veggies warm.

163. Teriyaki Pork
Servings: 8   Cooking Time: 7 Hours
Ingredients:

2 tablespoons sugar	¾ cup apple juice
2 tablespoons soy sauce	¼ teaspoon garlic powder
1 teaspoon ginger powder	3 pounds pork loin roast, halved
1 tablespoon white vinegar	7 teaspoons cornstarch
Salt and black pepper to the taste	3 tablespoons water

Directions:
In your Crock Pot, mix apple juice with sugar, soy sauce, vinegar, ginger, garlic powder, salt, pepper and pork loin, toss well, cover and cook on Low for 7 hours. Transfer cooking juices to a small pan, heat up over medium-high heat, add cornstarch mixed with water, stir well, cook for minutes until it thickens and take off heat. Slice roast, divide between plates, drizzle sauce all over and serve for lunch.
Nutrition Info: calories 247, fat 8, fiber 1, carbs 9, protein 33

164. Turkey And Mushrooms
Servings: 2   Cooking Time: 7 Hours And 10 Minutes
Ingredients:

2 garlic cloves, minced	1 red onion, sliced
1 pound turkey	A pinch of red pepper flakes

breast, skinless, boneless and cubed
1 tablespoon olive oil
1 teaspoon oregano, dried
1 teaspoon basil, dried
1 cup mushrooms, sliced
¼ cup chicken stock
½ cup canned tomatoes, chopped
A pinch of salt and black pepper

Directions:
Heat up a pan with the oil over medium-high heat, add the onion , garlic and the meat, brown for minutes and transfer to the Crock Pot. Add the oregano, basil and the other ingredients, toss, put the lid on and cook on Low for 7 hours. Divide into bowls and serve for lunch.
Nutrition Info: calories 240, fat 4, fiber 6, carbs 18, protein 10

165. Bbq Pork Ribs
Servings: 8   Cooking Time: 11 1/4 Hours
Ingredients:

5 pounds pork short ribs	1 large onion, sliced
2 cups BBQ sauce	1 tablespoon brown sugar
1 celery stalk, sliced	4 garlic cloves, minced
1 tablespoon Dijon mustard	1/4 cup chicken stock
1 teaspoon chili powder	Salt and pepper to taste

Directions:
Combine the pork short ribs, BBQ sauce, onion, celery and mustard, as well as chili, sugar, garlic and stock in your Crock Pot. Season with salt and pepper and cook on low settings for 11 hours. Serve the pork ribs warm and fresh.

166. Bavarian Beef Roast
Servings: 6   Cooking Time: 10 1/4 Hours
Ingredients:

2 tablespoons all-purpose flour	2 pounds beef roast
2 tablespoons mustard seeds	1 cup apple juice
1 teaspoon prepared horseradish	1/2 cup beef stock
	Salt and pepper to taste

Directions:
Season the beef with salt and pepper and sprinkle with flour. Combine the beef roast and the rest of the ingredients in your crock pot. Add salt and pepper as needed and cook on low settings for 10 hours. Serve the roast while still warm.

167. Lime Cilantro Chicken
Servings: 4   Cooking Time: 6 1/4 Hours
Ingredients:

4 chicken breasts	1/2 cup chicken stock
1 bunch cilantro	Salt and pepper to taste
1 lime, zested and juiced	1/2 cup grated Parmesan
1 tablespoon Italian pesto	

Directions:
Combine the cilantro, lime zest and lime juice, as well as stock and pesto in a blender. Pulse until smooth. Mix the chicken with the cilantro mix in a crock pot. Top with grated cheese and cook on low settings for 6 hours. Serve the chicken warm with your favorite side dish.

168. Sweet Potato Pork Stew

Servings: 6   Cooking Time: 6 1/4 Hours

Ingredients:

1 1/2 pounds pork tenderloin, cubed	1 pinch nutmeg
3 large sweet potatoes, peeled and cubed	1 teaspoon Dijon mustard
2 shallots, chopped	2 tablespoons tomato paste
2 red apples, peeled and cubed	2 cups chicken stock
	Salt and pepper to taste

Directions:
Combine the pork, sweet potatoes, shallots, apples, nutmeg, mustard, tomato paste and stock in your Crock Pot. Add enough salt and pepper and cook on low settings for 6 hours. Serve the pork stew warm or re-heated.

169. Madras Lentils

Servings: 6   Cooking Time: 4 1/4 Hours

Ingredients:

1 cup dried red lentils, rinsed	3 garlic cloves, chopped
1/2 cup brown lentils, rinsed	1/2 teaspoon cumin powder
1 cup tomato sauce	1/2 teaspoon dried oregano
2 cups vegetable stock	Salt and pepper to taste
1 large potato, peeled and cubed	1/2 cup coconut milk
1 shallot, chopped	

Directions:
Mix the lentils, tomato sauce, stock, potato, shallot, garlic, cumin powder, oregano and coconut milk in your Crock Pot. Add salt and pepper to taste and cook over low settings for 4 hours. Serve the lentils warm or store them in an airtight container in the freezer until needed.

170. Turkey Lunch

Servings: 12   Cooking Time: 4 Hours And 20 Minutes

Ingredients:

½ teaspoon thyme, dried	1 cup grape juice
½ teaspoon garlic powder	2 cups raspberries
Salt and black pepper to the taste	2 apples, peeled and chopped
2 turkey breast halves, boneless	2 cups blueberries
1/3 cup water	A pinch of red pepper flakes, crushed
	¼ teaspoon ginger powder

Directions:
In your Crock Pot, mix water with salt, pepper, thyme and garlic powder and stir. Add turkey breast halves, toss, cover and cook on Low for 4 hours. Meanwhile, heat up a pan over medium-high heat, add grape juice, apples, raspberries, blueberries, pepper flakes and ginger, stir, bring to a simmer, cook for 20 minutes and take off heat. Divide turkey between plates, drizzle berry sauce all over and serve for lunch.

Nutrition Info: calories 215, fat 2, fiber 3, carbs 12, protein 26

171. Spinach Lentil Stew

Servings: 6   Cooking Time: 6 1/4 Hours

Ingredients:

4 garlic cloves, chopped	1 shallot, chopped
2 tablespoon tomato paste	1/4 teaspoon garam masala
1/2 teaspoon cumin powder	1 cup red lentils, rinsed
1/2 teaspoon coriander seeds	1 cup diced tomatoes
1/2 teaspoon turmeric powder	1 1/2 cups vegetable stock
1/4 teaspoon chili powder	1/2 cup coconut cream
	1 thyme sprig
	Salt and pepper to taste

Directions:
Combine the shallot, garlic, tomato paste, spices, lentils, tomatoes, stock, coconut cream and thyme in your Crock Pot. Add salt and pepper to taste and cook on low settings for 6 hours. The stew is best served warm.

172. Oregano Wild Rice

Servings: 6   Cooking Time: 4 Hours

Ingredients:

2 cups wild rice	5 cups chicken stock
1 teaspoon dried oregano	1 tablespoon butter
½ teaspoon dried marjoram	½ teaspoon ground black pepper

Directions:
Put the wild rice in the Crock Pot. Add chicken stock, dried oregano, dried marjoram, and ground black pepper. Close the lid and cook the rice on high for 4 hours. Then add butter and stir the rice well.

Nutrition Info: Per Serving: 281 calories, 13g protein, 47.3g carbohydrates, 4.9g fat, 3.5g fiber, 11mg cholesterol, 304mg sodium, 445mg potassium.

173. Layered Vegetable Stew

Servings: 8   Cooking Time: 7 1/2 Hours

Ingredients:

2 tablespoons olive oil	2 carrots, sliced
2 large onions, sliced	1 1/2 cups tomato sauce

1 zucchini, sliced
1 large eggplant, peeled and sliced
2 potatoes, peeled and sliced
4 ripe tomatoes, sliced

1/4 teaspoon garlic powder
1/2 teaspoon dried oregano
1/2 teaspoon dried marjoram
Salt and pepper to taste

Directions:
Drizzle the oil at the bottom of your Crock Pot. Add the onions and layer the remaining vegetables in the exact order as they appear on the list above. Mix the tomato sauce, garlic powder, oregano, marjoram, salt and pepper in a bowl. Season properly and pour over the vegetables.   Cook on low settings for 7 hours.   Serve the stew warm and fresh or chilled.

174. Hoisin Braised Tofu

Servings: 4   Cooking Time: 2 1/4 Hours
Ingredients:

4 slices firm tofu
1 tablespoon soy sauce
1 teaspoon grated ginger
1 teaspoon rice vinegar

1/2 cup hoisin sauce
1/2 teaspoon sesame oil
2 garlic cloves, minced
1 teaspoon molasses

Directions:
Mix the hoisin sauce, ginger, vinegar, sesame oil, garlic and molasses in your Crock Pot.   Add the tofu and coat it well then cover the pot with its lid and cook on high settings for hours.   Serve the tofu warm with your favorite side dish.

175. Tomato Crouton Stew

Servings: 6   Cooking Time: 6 1/4 Hours
Ingredients:

4 ripe heirloom tomatoes, peeled and cubed
2 sweet onions, chopped
2 tablespoons olive oil
2 garlic cloves, chopped
2 red bell peppers, cored and diced

2 tablespoons tomato paste
1 1/2 cups vegetable stock
4 cups bread croutons
Salt and pepper to taste
1/2 teaspoon dried thyme
1/2 teaspoon dried oregano

Directions:
Heat the oil in a skillet and add the onions and garlic. Cook on low settings for 2 minutes until softened then transfer in your Crock Pot.   Add the remaining ingredients and season with salt and pepper.   Cook on low settings for 6 hours. Serve the stew warm and fresh.

176. Spinach Casserole

Servings: 6   Cooking Time: 6 1/4 Hours
Ingredients:

16 oz. frozen spinach
1 cup green peas
2 cups cottage cheese
2 tablespoons butter
1/4 cup all-purpose flour

4 eggs
1/2 teaspoon baking powder
Salt and pepper to taste

Directions:
Combine all the ingredients in a bowl and season with salt and pepper. Mix well.   Pour the mixture in your crock pot and cook on low settings for 6 hours.   Serve the casserole warm.

177. Carne Guisada

Servings: 8   Cooking Time: 6 1/2 Hours
Ingredients:

3 pounds beef chuck roast, cut into small cubes
2 red bell peppers, cored and diced
3 garlic cloves, minced
4 medium size potatoes, peeled and cubed

2 shallots, chopped
1/4 teaspoon chili powder
1/2 teaspoon cumin powder
1 1/2 cups beef stock
1 cup tomato sauce
Salt and pepper to taste

Directions:
Combine the chuck roast, bell peppers, shallots, garlic, tomatoes, chili powder, cumin powder, stock and tomato sauce in your crock pot.   Season with salt and pepper as needed and cook on low settings for 6 hours.   The carne guisada is best served in burritos or tortillas.

178.   Ginger Slow Roasted Pork

Servings: 8   Cooking Time: 7 1/4 Hours
Ingredients:

4 pounds pork shoulder
2 teaspoons grated ginger
1 tablespoon soy sauce

1 tablespoon honey
1 1/2 cups vegetables stock
Salt and pepper to taste

Directions:
Season the pork with salt and pepper, as well as ginger, soy sauce and honey.   Place the pork in your Crock Pot and add the stock.   Cover and cook on low settings for 7 hours.   Serve the pork warm with your favorite side dish.

179. African Inspired Chicken Stew

Servings: 8   Cooking Time: 5 1/4 Hours
Ingredients:

1 1/2 cups red lentils
2 pounds skinless chicken drumsticks
1 tablespoon butter
2 large red onions, chopped
4 garlic cloves, minced

1/2 teaspoon chili powder
1 teaspoon coriander powder
1/4 teaspoon all-spice powder
1/4 teaspoon ground cloves

1 teaspoon grated ginger

1 cup coconut milk
1 cup vegetable stock

Directions:
Combine the lentils, chicken, butter, spices, coconut milk and stock in your Crock Pot. Add enough salt and pepper and cook on low settings for 5 hours. Serve the stew warm and fresh.

180. Root Vegetable Risotto

Servings: 6   Cooking Time: 6 1/4 Hours

Ingredients:

1 cup white rice	1 parsley root, diced
2 tablespoons olive oil	Salt and pepper to taste
1 parsnip, diced	1/4 cup white wine
1 carrot, diced	1 3/4 cups vegetable stock
1 sweet potato, peeled and diced	2 tablespoons grated Parmesan
1/2 teaspoon dried sage	

Directions:
Combine the rice, oil, parsnip, carrot, parsley root, potato, sage, white wine and stock in your Crock Pot. Season with salt and pepper as needed and cook on low settings for 6 hours. When done, stir in the grated cheese and serve the risotto warm and fresh.

181. Beef Stroganoff

Servings: 6   Cooking Time: 6 1/4 Hours

Ingredients:

1 1/2 pounds beef stew meat, cubed	1 tablespoon Worcestershire sauce
1 large onion, chopped	1 cup cream cheese
4 garlic cloves, minced	Salt and pepper to taste
1/2 cup water	Cooked pasta for serving

Directions:
Mix all the ingredients in a crock pot. Add salt and pepper to taste and cook on low settings for 6 hours. Serve the stroganoff warm and serve it with cooked pasta of your choice.

182. Curried Beef Short Ribs

Servings: 6   Cooking Time: 8 1/4 Hours

Ingredients:

4 pounds beef short ribs	1 cup tomato sauce
3 tablespoons red curry paste	2 shallots, chopped
1 teaspoon curry powder	1 teaspoon grated ginger
1/2 teaspoon garlic powder	1 lime, juiced
	Salt and pepper to taste

Directions:
Mix the curry paste, tomato sauce, curry powder, garlic powder, shallots, ginger and lime juice in a crock pot. Add salt and pepper then place the ribs in the pot as well. Coat the ribs well and

cover with a lid. Cook on low settings for 8 hours. Serve the ribs warm and fresh.

183. Refried Red Kidney Beans

Servings: 4   Cooking Time: 6 Hours

Ingredients:

2 cups red kidney beans, soaked	1 teaspoon onion powder
1 cayenne pepper, chopped	8 cups of water
½ teaspoon garlic powder	1 teaspoon coconut oil

Directions:
Put all ingredients in the Crock Pot. Cook the mixture for 6 hours on high. Then transfer the cooked bean mixture in the blender and pulse for 15 seconds. Transfer the meal in the bowls

Nutrition Info: Per Serving: 324 calories, 20.9g protein, 57.4g carbohydrates, 2.2g fat, 14.2g fiber, 0mg cholesterol, 26mg sodium, 1274mg potassium.

184. Sticky Glazed Pork Ribs

Servings: 8   Cooking Time: 8 1/4 Hours

Ingredients:

6 pounds short pork ribs	1/4 cup hoisin sauce
1/2 cup hot ketchup	1 cup crushed pineapple in juice
2 tablespoons maple syrup	2 shallots, chopped
1 teaspoon onion powder	1 teaspoon grated ginger
1 teaspoon garlic powder	2 tablespoons soy sauce

Directions:
Combine all the ingredients in your Crock Pot. Mix until the ribs are evenly coated then cover with a lid and cook on low settings for 8 hours. Serve the sticky ribs warm.

185. Mustard Short Ribs

Servings: 2   Cooking Time: 8 Hours

Ingredients:

2 beef short ribs, bone in and cut into individual ribs	½ cup BBQ sauce
Salt and black pepper to the taste	1 tablespoon mustard
	1 tablespoon green onions, chopped

Directions:
In your Crock Pot, mix the ribs with the sauce and the other ingredients, toss, put the lid on and cook on Low for 8 hours. Divide the mix between plates and serve.

Nutrition Info: calories 284, fat 7, 4, carbs 18, protein 20

186. Curried Coconut Chickpeas

Servings: 6   Cooking Time: 2 1/4 Hours

Ingredients:

2 cans (15 oz.can) chickpeas, drained	1 cup coconut milk
2 shallots, chopped	1 teaspoon curry powder

2 garlic cloves, chopped
1 can diced tomatoes
1/2 cup vegetable stock

Salt and pepper to taste
2 tablespoons chopped cilantro

Directions:
Combine the chickpeas, shallots, garlic, tomatoes, coconut milk, stock and curry powder in your Crock Pot.   Add salt and pepper to taste and cook on high settings for hours.   When done, stir in the chopped cilantro and serve the dish warm.

187.   Swiss Steaks

Servings: 4   Cooking Time: 8 1/4 Hours
Ingredients:

2 tablespoons all-purpose flour
2 tablespoons canola oil
2 red bell peppers, cored and sliced

4 beef steaks
1 shallot, sliced
1 can (15 oz.) diced tomatoes
Salt and pepper to taste

Directions:
Season the steaks with salt and pepper and sprinkle with flour.   Heat the oil in a frying pan and add the steaks in the hot oil. Fry on each side until golden then place the steaks in your Crock Pot. Add the remaining ingredients and add salt and pepper if needed.   Cover and cook on low settings for 8 hours.   Serve the steaks and sauce warm.

188.   Garlicky Lentil Stew

Servings: 6   Cooking Time: 4 1/4 Hours
Ingredients:

1 cup red lentils
6 garlic cloves, chopped
1 onion, chopped
1/2 teaspoon grated ginger
1/2 teaspoon garam masala
1 teaspoon brown sugar

2 tablespoons tomato paste
1 cup vegetable stock
1 cup diced tomatoes
1 cup coconut milk
1 bay leaf
1 thyme sprig
Salt and pepper to taste

Directions:
Combine the lentils, garlic, onion, garam masala and the remaining ingredients in your Crock Pot. Add salt and pepper to taste and cook on low settings for 4 hours.   The stew is best served warm and fresh.

189.   White Bean Chili Over Creamy Grits

Servings: 8   Cooking Time: 6 3/4 Hours
Ingredients:

2 cups dried white beans, rinsed
2 cups vegetable stock
2 cups water
1 onion, chopped
2 garlic cloves,

1 red chili, chopped
1 cup fire roasted tomatoes
1 bay leaf
2 cups spinach, shredded
Salt and pepper to

chopped
1 carrot, diced
1 celery stalk, diced
1/2 teaspoon cumin powder

taste
1 cup grits
2 cups whole milk
1 cup grated Cheddar

Directions:
Combine the beans, stock, water, onion, garlic, carrot, celery, red chili, tomatoes, cumin powder and bay leaf in your Crock Pot. Top with shredded spinach.   Add salt and pepper to taste and cook on low settings for 6 1/hours.   To make the creamy grits, pour the milk in a saucepan. Bring to a boil and add the grits. Cook on low heat until creamy then remove from heat and add the cheese. Spoon the grits into the serving bowls and top with white bean stew.

190.   Spicy Chickpea Stew

Servings: 6   Cooking Time: 8 1/4 Hours
Ingredients:

1 1/2 cups dried chickpeas, rinsed
2 shallots, chopped
1 can fire roasted tomatoes
1 teaspoon dried oregano
2 cups vegetable stock

1 celery stalk, diced
1 bay leaf
1/2 teaspoon garlic powder
1/4 teaspoon chili powder
Salt and pepper to taste

Directions:
Combine the chickpeas, shallots, celery, tomatoes, oregano, stock and spices in your crock pot.   Add salt and pepper as needed and cook on low settings for 7 hours.   Serve the chickpea chili warm and fresh or store it in individual containers in the freezer.

191. Spinach Chicken

Servings: 6   Cooking Time: 6 1/2 Hours
Ingredients:

6 chicken thighs, boneless
2 tablespoons canola oil
1/4 cup chopped cilantro
1/4 cup chopped parsley
3 cups fresh spinach, shredded
1 cup vegetable stock

2 potatoes, peeled and cubed
Salt and pepper to taste
1/4 teaspoon cumin powder
1/4 teaspoon chili powder
1/4 teaspoon all-spice powder

Directions:
Combine the chicken and canola oil in a skillet and fry the chicken on all sides until golden.   Transfer the chicken in your crock pot and add the remaining ingredients, including the spices, salt and pepper.   Cook on low settings for 6 hours. Serve the chicken warm and fresh, although it tastes great chilled as well.

192. Lime And Thyme Chicken

Servings: 2   Cooking Time: 6 Hours

Ingredients:

- 1 pound chicken thighs, boneless and skinless
- Juice of 1 lime
- 1 tablespoon lime zest, grated
- 2 teaspoons olive oil
- ½ cup tomato sauce
- 2 garlic cloves, minced
- 1 tablespoon thyme, chopped
- Salt and black pepper to the taste

Directions:

In your Crock Pot, mix the chicken with the lime juice, zest and the other ingredients, toss, put the lid on and cook on High for 6 hours.   Divide between plates and serve right away.

Nutrition Info: calories 324, fat 7, fiber 8, carbs 20, protein 17

193. Mustard Baked Potatoes

Servings: 6   Cooking Time: 4 1/4 Hours

Ingredients:

- 3 pounds potatoes, peeled and cubed
- 1 tablespoon Dijon mustard
- 1/4 cup vegetable stock
- 1/2 teaspoon cumin seeds
- 4 garlic cloves, minced
- 1/2 teaspoon salt

Directions:

Combine all the ingredients in your Crock Pot. Mix well until evenly coated.   Cover with a lid and cook on low settings for 4 hours.   Serve the potatoes warm.

194. Chili Bbq Ribs

Servings: 8   Cooking Time: 8 1/2 Hours

Ingredients:

- 6 pounds pork short ribs
- 1 1/2 teaspoons chili powder
- 1 teaspoon cumin powder
- 2 tablespoons brown sugar
- 2 cups BBQ sauce
- 2 tablespoons red wine vinegar
- 1 teaspoon Worcestershire sauce
- Salt and pepper to taste

Directions:

Mix the BBQ sauce, chili powder, sugar, vinegar, Worcestershire sauce, salt and pepper in a Crock Pot.   Add the short ribs and mix until well coated.   Cover with a lid and cook on low settings for 8 1/4 hours.   Serve the ribs warm and fresh.

195. Spring Mashed Potatoes

Servings: 4   Cooking Time: 2 1/2 Hours

Ingredients:

- 1 1/2 pounds potatoes, peeled and cubed
- 1 cup water
- Salt and pepper to taste
- 1/4 cup coconut milk
- 1 green onion, chopped
- 1 garlic clove, minced

Directions:

Combine the potatoes and water in your Crock Pot. Add salt and pepper and cook on high settings for 2 hours.   When done, puree the potatoes with a masher and stir in the coconut milk, onion and garlic.   Serve the mashed potatoes warm.

196. Chicken Noodle Soup

Servings: 4   Cooking Time: 6 Hours And 15 Minutes

Ingredients:

- 1 and ½ pound chicken breast, boneless, skinless and cubed
- 1 yellow onion, chopped
- 3 carrots, chopped
- 2 celery stalks, chopped
- 3 garlic cloves minced
- 2 bay leaves
- 1 cup water
- 6 cups chicken stock
- 1 teaspoon Italian seasoning
- 2 cup cheese tortellini
- 1 tablespoon parsley, chopped

Directions:

In your Crock Pot, mix chicken with onion, carrots, celery, garlic, bay leaves, water, stock and seasoning, stir, cover and cook on Low for 6 hours. Add tortellini, stir, cover, cook on Low for 15 minutes more, ladle into bowls and serve for lunch.

Nutrition Info: calories 231, fat 3, fiber 4, carbs 17, protein 22

197. Simple Potato Stew

Servings: 8   Cooking Time: 6 1/2 Hours

Ingredients:

- 1 large onion, chopped
- 2 garlic cloves, chopped
- 2 red bell peppers, cored and diced
- 1 celery root, peeled and cubed
- 2 pounds potatoes, peeled and cubed
- 2 carrots, sliced
- 2 ripe tomatoes, peeled and diced
- 2 cups vegetable stock
- Salt and pepper to taste
- 2 bay leaves
- 2 tablespoons chopped parsley for serving

Directions:

Combine all the ingredients in your crock pot. Add salt and pepper as needed and cook on low settings for 6 hours.   Serve the stew warm, topped with chopped parsley.

198. Provence Summer Veggie Stew

Servings: 8   Cooking Time: 6 1/2 Hours

Ingredients:

- 1 cup frozen pearl onions
- 3 large carrots, sliced
- 1 cup frozen corn
- 1 cup frozen green peas
- 1 cup vegetable stock
- 2 zucchinis, cubed
- 1 teaspoon herbs de Provence
- 1 can (15 oz.) chickpeas, drained
- Salt and pepper to taste

2 ripe tomatoes, peeled and cubed / Cooked white rice for serving

Directions:
Combine the onions, carrots, corn, green peas, stock, zucchinis, tomatoes, herbs, chickpeas, salt and pepper in your crock pot.   Add salt and pepper to taste and cook on low settings for 6 hours.   Serve the stew fresh over cooked white rice or simple.

---

199.   Oriental Beef Brisket

Servings: 8   Cooking Time: 8 1/4 Hours

Ingredients:

4 pounds beef brisket, cubed	1 teaspoon chili powder
1 tablespoon peanut oil	1 cup beef stock
1/4 cup hoisin sauce	1 bay leaf
1 cup red salsa	Salt and pepper to taste
1 teaspoon cumin seeds	Cooked rice for serving

Directions:
Combine all the ingredients in your crock pot, adding salt and pepper to taste   Cover and cook on low settings for 8 hours.   Serve the beef brisket warm over cooked rice.

---

200.   Three Bean Chili

Servings: 8   Cooking Time: 8 1/2 Hours

Ingredients:

1/2 cup dried white beans, rinsed	1 onion, chopped
1/2 cup cannellini beans, rinsed	1/2 cup diced tomatoes
1/2 cup kidney beans, rinsed	1 bay leaf
2 carrots, diced	1/2 red chili, sliced
1 celery stalk, diced	1/2 teaspoon cumin powder
2 garlic cloves, chopped	2 cups vegetable stock
2 tablespoons tomato paste	1 cup water
	Salt and pepper to taste

Directions:
Combine the beans, carrots, celery, onion and garlic in your Crock Pot.   Add the remaining ingredients and season with salt and pepper. Cook the chili on low settings for 8 hours.   The dish is best served warm.

---

201.   Chicken Stroganoff

Servings: 6   Cooking Time: 6 1/4 Hours

Ingredients:

3 chicken breasts, cubed	2 shallots, chopped
2 tablespoons butter	1 cup cream cheese
2 celery stalks, sliced	2 cups sliced mushrooms
2 garlic cloves, chopped	1 cup vegetable stock
1 teaspoon dried Italian herbs	Salt and pepper to taste
	Cooked pasta of your choice for serving

Directions:
Melt the butter in a skillet and add the chicken. Cook on all sides until golden then transfer in your crock pot.   Add the remaining ingredients and season with salt and pepper.   Cook on low settings for 6 hours.   The stroganoff tastes better warm over cooked pasta of your choice.

---

202.   Cream Cheese Button Mushroom Chicken Stew

Servings: 6   Cooking Time: 6 1/4 Hours

Ingredients:

2 chicken breasts, cubed	4 cups button mushrooms
2 tablespoons canola oil	1 cup cream cheese
2 garlic cloves, minced	1 cup vegetable stock
1 shallot, chopped	1 thyme sprig
	Salt and pepper to taste

Directions:
Heat the oil in a skillet and add the chicken. Cook on medium flame until golden brown, about 5 minutes.   Transfer in your Crock Pot and add the remaining ingredients.   Adjust the taste with salt and pepper and cook on low settings for 6 hours. Serve the chicken stew warm and fresh.

---

203.   Creamy Chicken

Servings: 6   Cooking Time: 8 Hours And 30 Minutes

Ingredients:

10 ounces canned cream of chicken soup	3 tablespoons flour
Salt and black pepper to the taste	1 celery rib, chopped
A pinch of cayenne pepper	½ cup green bell pepper, chopped
1 pound chicken breasts, skinless, boneless and cubed	¼ cup yellow onion, chopped
	10 ounces peas
	2 tablespoons pimientos, chopped

Directions:
In your Crock Pot, mix cream of chicken with salt, pepper, cayenne and flour and whisk well.   Add chicken, celery, bell pepper and onion, toss, cover and cook on Low for 8 hours.   Add peas and pimientos, stir, cover and cook on Low for minutes more.   Divide into bowls and serve for lunch.
Nutrition Info: calories 200, fat 3, fiber 4, carbs 16, protein 17

---

204.   Farro Pumpkin Stew

Servings: 6   Cooking Time: 6 1/4 Hours

Ingredients:

2 tablespoons butter	1 shallot, chopped
1 cup farro, rinsed	1/4 cup white wine
2 cups pumpkin cubes	2 1/2 cups vegetable stock
1 garlic clove, minced	Salt and pepper to taste
1/4 teaspoon cumin	

seeds
1/4 teaspoon fennel seeds

1/2 cup grated Parmesan cheese

Directions:
Combine the butter, faro, pumpkin, shallot, garlic, cumin seeds, fennel seeds, wine and stock in your crock pot.   Add salt and pepper to taste and cook on low settings for 6 hours.   Serve the stew warm or chilled.

205.	**Chicken Tikka Masala**

Servings: 4   Cooking Time: 2 1/2 Hours

Ingredients:

4 chicken thighs	1 cup diced tomatoes
2 tablespoons canola oil	1 lime, juiced
2 shallots, chopped	1 cup coconut milk
4 garlic cloves, minced	1/2 cup chicken stock
2 tablespoons tomato paste	Salt and pepper to taste
1 tablespoon garam masala	Cooked rice for serving
	Chopped cilantro for serving

Directions:
Heat the oil in a skillet and add the chicken. Cook on all sides until golden then transfer the chicken in your Crock Pot.   Add the rest of the ingredients and season with salt and pepper. Cook on high settings for 2 hours.   Serve the tikka masala warm, topped with chopped cilantro, over cooked rice.

206.	**Cream Cheese Chicken**

Servings: 4   Cooking Time: 4 1/4 Hours

Ingredients:

4 chicken breasts	2 tablespoons butter
1 teaspoon dried Italian herbs	1 can cream of chicken soup
1 sweet onion, chopped	1 cup cream cheese
4 garlic cloves, minced	1/2 cup chicken stock
	Salt and pepper

Directions:
Season the chicken with salt, pepper and Italian herbs. Melt the butter in a skillet and add the chicken. Cook on each side until golden then transfer the chicken in your crock pot.   Add the remaining ingredients and adjust the taste with salt and pepper.   Cook on low settings for 4 hours. Serve the chicken warm.

207.	**White Beans Stew**

Servings: 10   Cooking Time: 4 Hours

Ingredients:

2 pounds white beans	1 teaspoon oregano, dried
3 celery stalks,	

chopped
2 carrots, chopped
1 bay leaf
1 yellow onion, chopped
3 garlic cloves, minced
1 teaspoon rosemary, dried

1 teaspoon thyme, dried
10 cups water
Salt and black pepper to the taste
28 ounces canned tomatoes, chopped
6 cups chard, chopped

Directions:
In your Crock Pot, mix white beans with celery, carrots, bay leaf, onion, garlic, rosemary, oregano, thyme, water, salt, pepper, tomatoes and chard, cover and cook on High for 4 hours.   Stir, divide into bowls and serve for lunch,
Nutrition Info: calories 341, fat 8, fiber 12, carbs 20, protein 6

208.	**Balsamic Roasted Root Vegetables**

Servings: 4   Cooking Time: 3 1/4 Hours

Ingredients:

1/2 pound baby carrots	2 parsnips, sliced
2 sweet potatoes, peeled and cubed	1 tablespoon brown sugar
1 turnip, peeled and sliced	2 tablespoons balsamic vinegar
1 large red onion, sliced	1/4 cup vegetable stock
2 tablespoons olive oil	Salt and pepper to taste

Directions:
Combine all the ingredients in your crock pot. Add salt and pepper to taste and cook on high settings for 3 hours.   Serve the vegetables warm and fresh.

209.	**White Bean Casoulet**

Servings: 6   Cooking Time: 6 1/2 Hours

Ingredients:

2 tablespoons olive oil	1 parsnip, diced
1 large onion, chopped	1 cup vegetable stock
2 carrots, diced	1 thyme sprig
2 garlic cloves, chopped	1 1/2 cups diced tomatoes
2 cans white beans, drained	1 bay leaf
	Salt and pepper to taste

Directions:
Heat the oil in a skillet and add the onion, carrot and garlic. Sauté for 2 minutes until softened and translucent then transfer in your Crock Pot.   Add the remaining ingredients and cook on low settings for 6 hours.   Serve the cassoulet warm.

Beef, Pork & Lamb Recipes

210. Mexican Lamb Fillet

Servings: 4   Cooking Time: 8 Hrs.

Ingredients:

1 chili pepper, deseeded and chopped	1 tsp salt
	1 tsp ground black pepper
1 jalapeno pepper, deseeded and chopped	1 tbsp ground paprika
	1 tsp grated ginger
1 cup sweet corn	1 cup tomato juice
1 cup chicken stock	1 tbsp white sugar
14 oz lamb fillet	

Directions:

Add the peppers, ginger, and ground paprika to the blender jug.   Blend this peppers mixture for 30 seconds until smooth.   Place the lamb fillet to the insert of the Crock Pot.   Add pepper mixture, tomato juice, white sugar, black pepper, and salt to the lamb.   Lastly, add sweet corn and chicken stock.   Put the cooker's lid on and set the cooking time to 8 hours on Low settings.   Shred the cooked lamb and return the cooker.   Mix well and serve warm.

Nutrition Info: Per Serving: Calories: 348, Total Fat: 18.3g, Fiber: 3g, Total Carbs: 19.26g, Protein: 28g

211. Beef Mac&cheese

Servings: 4   Cooking Time: 4.5 Hours

Ingredients:

½ cup macaroni, cooked	1 cup Mozzarella, shredded
10 oz ground beef	½ cup of water
½ cup marinara sauce	

Directions:

Mix the ground beef with marinara sauce and water and transfer in the Crock Pot.   Cook it on High for 4 hours.   After this, add macaroni and Mozzarella.   Carefully mix the meal and cook it for 30 minutes more on high.

Nutrition Info: Per Serving: 218 calories, 25.4g protein, 12.4g carbohydrates, 1.2g fat, 68g fiber, 63mg cholesterol, 219mg sodium, 408mg potassium.

212. Crockpot Ground Beef Minestrone Soup

Servings: 4   Cooking Time: 8 Hours

Ingredients:

1-pound ground beef	1 stalk of celery, diced
2 zucchinis, diced	1 clove of garlic, minced
1 onion, diced	
½ cup homemade vegetable broth or water	½ teaspoon dried basil

Directions:

Place all ingredients in the CrockPot.   Give a good stir.   Close the lid and cook on high for 6 hours or on low for 8 hours.

Nutrition Info: Calories per serving: 312; Carbohydrates: 4.8g; Protein: 29.6g; Fat: 18.7g; Sugar: 0.9g; Sodium: 781mg; Fiber: 3.1g

213. Beef And Scallions Bowl

Servings: 4   Cooking Time: 5 Hours

Ingredients:

1 teaspoon chili powder	1 cup corn kernels, frozen
2 oz scallions, chopped	2 tablespoons tomato paste
1-pound beef stew meat, cubed	1 teaspoon minced garlic
1 cup of water	

Directions:

Mix water with tomato paste and pour the liquid in the Crock Pot.   Add chili powder, beef, corn kernels, and minced garlic.   Close the lid and cook the meal on high for 5 hours.   When the meal is cooked, transfer the mixture in the bowls and top with scallions.

Nutrition Info: Per Serving: 258 calories, 36.4g protein, 10.4g carbohydrates, 7.7g fat, 2g fiber, 101mg cholesterol, 99mg sodium, 697mg potassium.

214. Balsamic Beef

Servings: 4   Cooking Time: 9 Hours

Ingredients:

1 pound beef stew meat, cubed	4 tablespoons balsamic vinegar
1 teaspoon cayenne pepper	½ cup of water
	2 tablespoons butter

Directions:

Toss the butter in the skillet and melt it.   Then add meat and roast it for minutes per side on medium heat.   Transfer the meat with butter in the Crock Pot.   Add balsamic vinegar, cayenne pepper, and water.   Close the lid and cook the meal on Low for 9 hours.

Nutrition Info: Per Serving: 266 calories, 34.5g protein, 0.4g carbohydrates, 12.9g fat, 0.1g fiber, 117mg cholesterol, 117mg sodium, 479mg potassium.

215. Simple Pork Chop Casserole

Servings: 4   Cooking Time: 10 Hours

Ingredients:

4 pork chops, bones removed and cut into bite-sized pieces	½ cup water
3 tablespoons minced onion	Salt and pepper to taste
	1 cup heavy cream

Directions:

Place the pork chop slices, onions, and water in the crockpot.   Season with salt and pepper to taste. Close the lid and cook on low for 10 hours or on high for 8 hours.   Halfway through the cooking time, pour in the heavy cream.
Nutrition Info: Calories per serving: 515; Carbohydrates: 2.5g; Protein: 39.2g; Fat: 34.3g; Sugar: 0g; Sodium: 613mg; Fiber:0.9 g

216.	**Balsamic Lamb Chops**

Servings: 2   Cooking Time: 6 Hours
Ingredients:

2 tablespoons balsamic vinegar	1 pound lamb chops
1 tablespoon chives, chopped	4 garlic cloves, minced
1 tablespoon olive oil	½ cup beef stock
	A pinch of salt and black pepper

Directions:
In your Crock Pot, mix the lamb chops with the vinegar and the other ingredients, toss, put the lid on and cook on Low for 6 hours.   Divide everything between plates and serve.
Nutrition Info:calories 292, fat 12, fiber 3, carbs 7, protein 16

217.	**Lamb And Cabbage**

Servings: 2   Cooking Time: 5 Hours
Ingredients:

2 pounds lamb stew meat, cubed	1 cup beef stock
1 cup red cabbage, shredded	2 tablespoons tomato paste
1 teaspoon avocado oil	A pinch of salt and black pepper
1 teaspoon sweet paprika	1 tablespoon cilantro, chopped

Directions:
In your Crock Pot, mix the lamb with the cabbage, stock and the other ingredients, toss, put the lid on and cook on High for 5 hours.   Divide everything between plates and serve.
Nutrition Info:calories 254, fat 12, fiber 3, carbs 6, protein 16

218.	**Lavender And Orange Lamb**

Servings: 4   Cooking Time: 7 Hours
Ingredients:

2 tablespoons rosemary, chopped	1 tablespoon lavender, chopped
1 and ½ pounds lamb chops	2 garlic cloves, minced
Salt and black pepper to the taste	1 red orange, cut into halves
2 red oranges, peeled and cut into segments	2 small pieces of orange peel
	1 teaspoon butter

Directions:
In a bowl, mix lamb chops with salt, pepper, rosemary, lavender, garlic and orange peel, toss to

coat and leave aside for a couple of hours in the fridge.   Put the butter in your Crock Pot, add lamb chops, squeeze 1 orange over them, add the rest of the oranges over the lamb, cover Crock Pot and cook on Low for 7 hours.   Divide lamb and sauce all over and serve.
Nutrition Info:calories 250, fat 5, fiber 7, carbs 15, protein 20

219.	**Beer Sausages**

Servings: 4   Cooking Time: 7 Hours
Ingredients:

1-pound beef sausages	3 tablespoons butter
1 teaspoon ground black pepper	1 teaspoon salt
	1 cup beer

Directions:
Toss the butter in the skillet and melt it.   Add beef sausages and roast them on high heat for minutes per side.   Transfer the beef sausages in the Crock Pot.   Add ground black pepper, salt, and beer.   Close the lid and cook the meal on Low for 7 hours.
Nutrition Info: Per Serving: 552 calories, 16.1g protein, 5.5g carbohydrates, 49.8g fat, 0.1g fiber, 103mg cholesterol, 1558mg sodium, 240mg potassium.

220.	**Hamburger Style Stuffing**

Servings: 4   Cooking Time: 3 Hours
Ingredients:

1-pound ground pork	¼ cup onion, minced
½ cup Cheddar cheese, shredded	1 cup of water
½ cup fresh cilantro, chopped	¼ cup tomato juice
	1 bell pepper, diced
	1 teaspoon salt

Directions:
Mix ground pork with cilantro, onion, and diced pepper.   Then transfer the mixture in the Crock Pot.   Add all remaining ingredients and mix. Close the lid and cook the stuffing on High for 3 hours.
Nutrition Info: Per Serving: 235 calories, 33.7g protein, 3.8g carbohydrates, 8.8g fat, 0.7g fiber, 98mg cholesterol, 778mg sodium, 604mg potassium

221.	**Classic Pork Adobo**

Servings: 6   Cooking Time: 12 Hours
Ingredients:

2 pounds pork chops, sliced	¼ cup soy sauce
4 cloves of garlic, minced	½ cup lemon juice, freshly squeezed
1 onion, chopped	4 quail eggs, boiled and peeled
2 bay leaves	

Directions:
Place all ingredients except the quail eggs in the CrockPot.   Give a good stir.   Close the lid and cook on high for 10 hours or on low for 12 hours.

Add in quail eggs an hour before the cooking time ends.
Nutrition Info: Calories per serving: 371; Carbohydrates: 6.4g; Protein: 40.7g; Fat: 24.1g; Sugar: 0g; Sodium: 720mg; Fiber: 3.9g

222. Pork Ragu With Basil

Servings: 4   Cooking Time: 4 Hours
Ingredients:

8 oz pork loin, chopped	½ cup carrot, chopped
1 cup russet potatoes	1 teaspoon salt
3 oz fennel bulb, chopped	3 cups of water
1 tablespoon dried basil	½ cup plain yogurt
	1 teaspoon tomato paste

Directions:
In the mixing bowl mix tomato paste with plain yogurt, salt, dried basil, and pork loin.   Transfer the mixture in the Crock Pot and close the lid. Cook the meat on high for 2 hours.   Then add water and all remaining ingredients. Carefully mix the mixture.   Close the lid and cook the ragu on low for hours.
Nutrition Info: Per Serving: 198 calories, 18.3g protein, 11.2g carbohydrates, 8.4g fat, 2g fiber, 47mg cholesterol, 667mg sodium, 613mg potassium

223. Blanked Hot Dogs

Servings: 4   Cooking Time: 4 Hours
Ingredients:

4 mini (cocktail) pork sausages	1 tablespoon olive oil
1 teaspoon cumin seeds	1 egg, beaten
	4 oz puff pastry

Directions:
Roll up the puff pastry and cut into strips.   Put the pork sausages on every strip.   Roll the puff pastry and brush with egg.   Then top the blanked hot dogs with cumin seeds.   Brush the Crock Pot with olive oil from inside.   Add the blanked hot dogs and close the lid.   Cook them on high for 4 hours.
Nutrition Info: Per Serving: 225 calories, 4.4g protein, 14.1g carbohydrates, 16.9g fat, 0.6g fiber, 41mg cholesterol, 120mg sodium, 42mg potassium

224. Crockpot Lamb Chops

Servings: 6   Cooking Time: 10 Hours
Ingredients:

6 lamb shanks	1 tablespoon dried oregano
1 tablespoon olive oil	
2 teaspoons salt	1 ½ cups chicken stock
2 teaspoons pepper	
2 stalks of celery, chopped	1 cup tomatoes, crushed
1 onion, chopped	3 bay leaves

Directions:

Place all ingredients in the CrockPot.   Give a good stir.   Close the lid and cook on high for 8 hours or on low for 10 hours.
Nutrition Info: Calories per serving: 762; Carbohydrates: 3.2g; Protein: 98g; Fat: 31g; Sugar: 0g; Sodium: 1816mg; Fiber: 2.1g

225. Balsamic Lamb Mix

Servings: 2   Cooking Time: 7 Hours
Ingredients:

1 pound lamb stew meat, cubed	½ teaspoon coriander, ground
2 teaspoons avocado oil	A pinch of salt and black pepper
1 tablespoon balsamic vinegar	1 cup beef stock

Directions:
In your Crock Pot, mix the lamb with the oil, vinegar and the other ingredients, toss, put the lid on and cook on Low for 7 hours.   Divide the mix between plates and serve with a side salad.
Nutrition Info:calories 243, fat 11, fiber 4, carbs 6, protein 10

226. Crockpot Pork Shanks

Servings: 10   Cooking Time: 10 Hours
Ingredients:

1 ½ tablespoons avocado oil	1 tablespoon oregano leaves, minced
3 pounds pork shanks, bone-in	2 teaspoons thyme leaves
3 cups onion, chopped	2 tablespoons basil leaves, finely
4 cloves of garlic, minced	¾ cup chicken broth
3 cups mushrooms, chopped	Salt and pepper to taste

Directions:
Place all ingredients in the CrockPot.   Give a good stir.   Close the lid and cook on high for 8 hours or on low for 10 hours.
Nutrition Info: Calories per serving: 233; Carbohydrates: 5.2g; Protein: 34.8g; Fat: 7.5g; Sugar: 0g; Sodium: 811mg; Fiber: 2.5g

227. Indian Style Cardamom Pork

Servings: 4   Cooking Time: 6 Hours
Ingredients:

1-pound pork steak, tenderized	½ cup of coconut milk
1 teaspoon ground cardamom	1 teaspoon ground turmeric
1 teaspoon chili powder	1 teaspoon cashew butter
	¼ cup of water

Directions:
Cut the pork steak into 4 servings and rub with ground cardamom, chili powder. And ground turmeric.   Place the meat in the Crock Pot.

Add cashew butter, water, and coconut milk. Close the lid and cook the pork on high for 6 hours.
Nutrition Info: Per Serving: 295 calories, 21g protein, 7.2g carbohydrates, 21.1g fat, 1.9g fiber, 69mg cholesterol, 569mg sodium, 118mg potassium

228. Beef With Spinach

Servings: 2   Cooking Time: 7 Hours
Ingredients:

1 red onion, sliced	Salt and black pepper
1 pound beef stew meat, cubed	to the taste
1 cup tomato passata	½ cup bee stock
1 cup baby spinach	1 tablespoon basil,
1 teaspoon olive oil	chopped

Directions:
In your Crock Pot, mix the beef with the onion, passata and the other ingredients except the spinach, toss, put the lid on and cook on Low for 6 hours and 30 minutes.   Add the spinach, toss, put the lid on, cook on Low for 30 minutes more, divide into bowls and serve.
Nutrition Info:calories 400, fat 15, fiber 4, carbs 25, protein 14

229. Beef With Peas And Corn

Servings: 2   Cooking Time: 7 Hours
Ingredients:

1 pound beef stew meat, cubed	2 scallions, chopped
½ cup corn	1 cup beef stock
½ cup fresh peas	2 tablespoons tomato paste
1 tablespoon lime juice	½ cup chives, chopped

Directions:
In your Crock Pot, mix the beef with the corn, peas and the other ingredients, toss, put the lid on and cook on Low for 7 hours.   Divide the mix between plates and serve right away.
Nutrition Info:calories 236, fat 12, fiber 2, carbs 7, protein 15

230. Pork Loin And Cauliflower Rice

Servings: 6   Cooking Time: 8 Hours
Ingredients:

3 bacon slices, cooked and chopped	Salt and black pepper to the taste
3 carrots, chopped	¼ cup olive oil
2 pounds pork loin roast	1 tablespoon garlic powder
1 rhubarb stalk, chopped	1 tablespoon Italian seasoning
2 bay leaves	24 ounces cauliflower rice
¼ cup red wine vinegar	1 teaspoon turmeric powder
4 garlic cloves, minced	1 cup beef stock

Directions:

In your Crock Pot, mix bacon with carrots, pork, rhubarb, bay leaves, vinegar, salt, pepper, oil, garlic powder, Italian seasoning, stock and turmeric, toss, cover and cook on Low for 7 hours.   Add cauliflower rice, cover, cook on Low for 1 more hour, divide between plates and serve.
Nutrition Info:calories 310, fat 6, fiber 3, carbs 14, protein 10

231. Cinnamon Lamb

Servings: 2   Cooking Time: 6 Hours
Ingredients:

1 pound lamb chops	1 tablespoon oregano, chopped
1 teaspoon cinnamon powder	½ cup beef stock
1 red onion, chopped	1 tablespoon chives, chopped
1 tablespoon avocado oil	

Directions:
In your Crock Pot, mix the lamb chops with the cinnamon and the other ingredients, toss, put the lid on and cook on Low for 6 hours.   Divide the chops between plates and serve with a side salad.
Nutrition Info:calories 253, fat 14, fiber 2, carbs 6, protein 18

232. Lamb's Feet Soup

Servings: 8   Cooking Time: 10 Hours
Ingredients:

1 ½ pounds lamb's feet	1 teaspoon black peppercorns
1 onion, chopped	1-inch ginger, grated
1 cup tomatoes, crushed	3 cloves of garlic, minced
1 teaspoon coriander seeds	1 bay leaf
	4 cups water

Directions:
Place all ingredients in the CrockPot.   Give a good stir.   Close the lid and cook on high for 8 hours or on low for 10 hours.
Nutrition Info: Calories per serving: 229; Carbohydrates: 2.4g; Protein: 21.6g; Fat:14.9 g; Sugar: 0g; Sodium: 528mg; Fiber: 1.7g

233. Lamb Cheese Casserole

Servings: 6   Cooking Time: 9 Hrs.
Ingredients:

1 cup of rice	3 carrots, chopped
4 cups of water	1 tbsp olive oil
13 oz lamb fillet	1 tsp salt
1 tbsp ground paprika	1 tsp ground cinnamon
1 onion	1 tbsp turmeric
9 oz Cheddar cheese, shredded	5 sweet potatoes

Directions:
Toss rice with turmeric and olive oil in the insert of the Crock Pot.   Spread the chopped carrot over the rice, then add a layer of the onion.   Place lamb fillet over the veggies and add the remaining ingredients.   Put the cooker's lid on and set the

cooking time to 9 hours on Low settings.   Serve warm.
Nutrition Info: Per Serving: Calories: 436, Total Fat: 20.8g, Fiber: 10g, Total Carbs: 42.77g, Protein: 26g

234.   Beef French Dip

Servings: 4   Cooking Time: 8 Hours
Ingredients:

1-pound beef chuck roast	1 cup onion, sliced
½ cup French onion soup	½ cup of water
1 teaspoon garlic powder	1 tablespoon coconut oil
	2 oz provolone cheese, shredded

Directions:
Dice the meat and put it in the Crock Pot.   Add all remaining ingredients and carefully mix. Close the lid and cook the dip on Low for 8 hours.
Nutrition Info: Per Serving: 520 calories, 32.4g protein, 6g carbohydrates, 39g fat, 0.9g fiber, 127mg cholesterol, 386mg sodium, 371mg potassium.

235.   Salsa Bean Pie

Servings: 6   Cooking Time: 7 Hrs
Ingredients:

8 tortillas	5 oz. Cheddar cheese, shredded
7 oz. ground beef	
7 oz. salsa	3 tbsp tomato sauce
5 oz. red beans, canned	¼ tbsp salt

Directions:
Spread 2 tortillas at the base of your Crock Pot. Mix beef with cheese, salt, and tomato sauce in a bowl.   Spread this beef mixture over the tortillas. Now place tortillas over the beef mixture.   Top them with red beans and spread evenly.   Place the remaining tortilla on top and finally add salsa. Put the cooker's lid on and set the cooking time to hours on Low settings.   Slice and serve.
Nutrition Info: Per Serving: Calories 433, Total Fat 16g, Fiber 6g, Total Carbs 53g, Protein 19g

236.   Pork Chops Under Peach Blanket

Servings: 4   Cooking Time: 4.5 Hours
Ingredients:

4 pork chops	1 onion, sliced
2 tablespoons butter, softened	1 cup of water
	1 cup peaches, pitted, halved
1 teaspoon salt	

Directions:
Sprinkle the pork chops with salt.   Grease the Crock Pot bottom with butter.   Put the pork chops inside in one layer.   Then top them with sliced onion and peaches.   Add water and close the lid.   Cook the meal on High for 4.5 hours.
Nutrition Info: Per Serving: 333 calories, 18.7g protein, 6.1g carbohydrates, 25.8g fat, 1.2g fiber,

84mg cholesterol, 681mg sodium, 389mg potassium

237.   Pork Marbella

Servings: 4   Cooking Time: 8 Hours
Ingredients:

2 oz prunes, chopped	½ teaspoon sugar
12 oz pork loin	1 garlic clove, peeled
¼ cup red wine	1 tablespoon sunflower oil
1 teaspoon capers	
1 teaspoon dried oregano	¼ cup of water

Directions:
Slice the pork loin and put it in the Crock Pot. Add all remaining ingredients and gently mix. Cook the meal on Low for 8 hours.   Then carefully mix the meat and cool it to the room temperature.
Nutrition Info: Per Serving: 287 calories, 23.7g protein, 10.5g carbohydrates, 15.4g fat, 1.2g fiber, 68mg cholesterol, 76mg sodium, 488mg potassium

238.   Italian Pork Chops

Servings: 6   Cooking Time: 10 Hours
Ingredients:

6 pork loin chops	3 cups sugar-free pasta sauce
1 onion, chopped	
3 cloves of garlic, minced	1 cup mozzarella cheese

Directions:
Place pork loin, onion, and garlic in the crockpot. Pour in the sugar-free pasta sauce.   Add the mozzarella cheese on top.   Close the lid and cook for low in 10 hours or on high for 7 hours.
Nutrition Info: Calories per serving: 420; Carbohydrates: 6.2g; Protein: 38.1g; Fat: 29.4g; Sugar: 0.9g; Sodium: 672mg; Fiber: 3.4g

239.   Jamaican Pork Mix

Servings: 4   Cooking Time: 4 Hours
Ingredients:

1 cup corn kernels, frozen	1 cup of water
	1 tomato, chopped
1 teaspoon Jamaican spices	1 teaspoon salt
	1 teaspoon avocado oil
10 oz pork sirloin, chopped	

Directions:
Roast the chopped pork sirloin in the avocado oil for minute per side.   Then mix the meat with Jamaican spices and transfer in the Crock Pot. Add all remaining ingredients and close the lid. Cook the meal on High for hours.
Nutrition Info: Per Serving: 174 calories, 23.5g protein, 7.9g carbohydrates, 5.4g fat, 1.3g fiber, 65mg cholesterol, 629mg sodium, 412mg potassium

240.   Asian Style Beef And Broccoli

Servings: 4   Cooking Time: 5 Hours
Ingredients:

2 tablespoons soy sauce
1 tablespoon liquid honey
1 tablespoon sesame seeds

1 cup of water
1 cup broccoli florets
1 garlic clove, diced
10 oz beef sirloin, chopped

Directions:
Mix the beef sirloin with garlic and soy sauce. Transfer the meat in the Crock Pot and water. Close the lid and cook it on high for hours.   Then add all remaining ingredients and gently mix. Cook the meal on High for 2 hours more.

Nutrition Info: Per Serving: 174 calories, 23.1g protein, 7.2g carbohydrates, 5.6g fat, 1g fiber, 63mg cholesterol, 507mg sodium, 392mg potassium.

241.	French Lamb

Servings: 4   Cooking Time: 8 Hours
Ingredients:

4 lamb chops
1 cup onion, chopped
2 cups canned tomatoes, chopped
2 tablespoons garlic, minced

1 cup leek, chopped
1 teaspoon herbs de Provence
Salt and black pepper to the taste
3 cups water

Directions:
In your Crock Pot mix, lamb chops with onion, tomatoes, leek, garlic, herbs de Provence, salt, pepper and water, stir, cover and cook on Low for 8 hours.   Divide lamb and veggies between plates and serve.

Nutrition Info:calories 430, fat 12, fiber 8, carbs 20, protein 18

242.	Filet Mignon With Fresh Basil Rub

Servings: 4   Cooking Time: 7 Hours
Ingredients:

1 ½ teaspoon fresh basil, minced
1 ½ teaspoon thyme, minced
2 teaspoons garlic, minced

Salt and pepper to taste
4 beef tenderloin steaks, cut to 1-inch thick

Directions:
Line the bottom of the crockpot with foil.   In a mixing bowl, combine the basil, thyme, and garlic. Season with salt and pepper.   Rub the steaks with the spice rub. Allow to marinate for at least minutes.   Place inside the crockpot and cook on high for 7 hours or on low for 10 hours.

Nutrition Info: Calories per serving: 424; Carbohydrates: 2.4g; Protein: 30.6g; Fat: 26.3g; Sugar: 0g; Sodium: 537mg; Fiber: 0.8g

243.	Pork Chops And Pineapple Mix

Servings: 4   Cooking Time: 6 Hours
Ingredients:

2 pounds pork chops
1/3 cup sugar
15 ounces pineapple, cubed
3 tablespoons apple cider vinegar

¼ cup ketchup
5 tablespoons soy sauce
2 teaspoons garlic, minced
3 tablespoons flour

Directions:
In a bowl, mix ketchup with sugar, vinegar, soy sauce and tapioca, whisk well, add pork chops, toss well and transfer everything to your Crock Pot Add pineapple and garlic, toss again, cover, cook on Low for 6 hours, divide everything between plates and serve.

Nutrition Info:calories 345, fat 5, fiber 6, carbs 13, protein 14

244.	Beef Casserole

Servings: 5   Cooking Time: 7 Hours
Ingredients:

7 oz ground beef
1 cup Cheddar cheese, shredded
½ cup cream

1 teaspoon Italian seasonings
½ cup broccoli, chopped

Directions:
Mix ground beef with Italian seasonings and put in the Crock Pot.   Top the meat with broccoli and Cheddar cheese.   Then pour the cream over the casserole mixture and close the lid.   Cook the casserole on Low for 7 hours.

Nutrition Info: Per Serving: 186 calories, 18.1g protein, 1.7g carbohydrates, 11.6g fat, 0.2g fiber, 64mg cholesterol, 178mg sodium, 220mg potassium.

245.	Stuffed Jalapenos

Servings: 3   Cooking Time: 4.5 Hours
Ingredients:

6 jalapenos, deseed
1 teaspoon garlic powder

4 oz minced beef
½ cup of water

Directions:
Mix the minced beef with garlic powder.   Then fill the jalapenos with minced meat and arrange it in the Crock Pot.   Add water and cook the jalapenos on High for 4.5 hours.

Nutrition Info: Per Serving: 55 calories, 7.5g protein, 2.3g carbohydrates, 1.9g fat, 0.9g fiber, 0mg cholesterol, 2mg sodium, 71mg potassium.

246.	Hot Sloppy Joes

Servings: 4   Cooking Time: 6 Hours
Ingredients:

2 cups ground pork
2 tablespoons hot sauce
½ cup bell pepper, chopped
1 cup white onion, diced

1 tablespoon tomato paste
½ cup tomato juice
1 teaspoon ground cumin
¼ cup of water

Directions:

Put the ground pork in the Crock Pot.   Add hot sauce, bell pepper, white onion, tomato paste, tomato juice, and ground cumin.   Carefully mix the meat mixture and add water.   Close the lid and cook the meal on Low for 6 hours.   Stir the meal well before serving.
Nutrition Info: Per Serving: 376 calories, 31.2g protein, 6.2g carbohydrates, 24.6g fat, 1.2g fiber, 110mg cholesterol, 364mg sodium, 625mg potassium

247.   Beef And Artichokes Bowls

Servings: 2   Cooking Time: 7 Hours
Ingredients:

6 oz beef sirloin, chopped	½ teaspoon white pepper
½ teaspoon cayenne pepper	4 artichoke hearts, chopped
1 cup of water	1 teaspoon salt

Directions:
Mix meat with white pepper and cayenne pepper. Transfer it in the Crock Pot bowl.   Add salt, artichoke hearts, and water.   Close the lid and cook the meal on Low for 7 hours.
Nutrition Info: Per Serving: 313 calories, 36.5g protein, 34.6g carbohydrates, 5.9g fat, 17.8g fiber, 76mg cholesterol, 1527mg sodium, 1559mg potassium

248.   Lamb And Lime Zucchinis

Servings: 2   Cooking Time: 4 Hours
Ingredients:

1 pound lamb stew meat, roughly cubed	1 red onion, chopped
2 small zucchinis, cubed	½ cup beef stock
Juice of 1 lime	1 tablespoon garlic, minced
½ teaspoon rosemary, dried	A pinch of salt and black pepper
2 tablespoons avocado oil	1 tablespoon cilantro, chopped

Directions:
In your Crock Pot, mix the lamb with the zucchinis, lime juice and the other ingredients, toss, put the lid on and cook on High for 4 hours.   Divide the mix between plates and serve.
Nutrition Info:calories 274, fat 9, fiber 5, carbs 6, protein 12

249.   Sweet Lamb Ribs

Servings: 3   Cooking Time: 9 Hours
Ingredients:

8 oz lamb ribs, chopped	2 teaspoons liquid honey
1 teaspoon tomato paste	½ cup butter
	¼ cup of water

Directions:
Rub the lamb ribs with tomato paste and liquid honey.   Then place them in the Crock Pot.   Add butter and water.   Close the lid and cook the meat on low for 9 hours.
Nutrition Info: Per Serving: 414 calories, 15.8g protein, 4.2g carbohydrates, 37.4g fat, 0.1g fiber, 132mg cholesterol, 274mg sodium, 30mg potassium.

250.   Beef Chops With Sprouts

Servings: 5   Cooking Time: 7 Hours
Ingredients:

1-pound beef loin	1 cup of water
½ cup bean sprouts	1 teaspoon chili powder
1 tablespoon tomato paste	1 teaspoon salt

Directions:
Cut the beef loin into 5 beef chops and sprinkle the beef chops with chili powder and salt.   Then place them in the Crock Pot.   Add water and tomato paste. Cook the meat on low for 7 hours. Then transfer the cooked beef chops in the plates, sprinkle with tomato gravy from the Crock Pot, and top with bean sprouts.
Nutrition Info: Per Serving: 175 calories,25.2g protein, 1.6g carbohydrates, 7.8g fat, 0.3g fiber, 64mg cholesterol, 526mg sodium, 386mg potassium.

251.   Indian Harissa Pork

Servings: 8   Cooking Time: 5 Hrs.
Ingredients:

21 oz pork steak, tenderized	1 tsp ground black pepper
2 tbsp curry	1 tsp salt
1 tsp harissa	1 tsp sugar
1 tbsp garam masala	1 cup cashew, crushed
1 tsp chili flakes	
½ cup cream	1 tsp ground nutmeg

Directions:
Season the pork steaks with harissa, curry, chili flakes, and garam masala.   Place the pork steak in the insert of the Crock Pot.   Add cream, salt, sugar, nutmeg, and black pepper to the pork.   Put the cooker's lid on and set the cooking time to 5 hours on High settings.   Serve warm.
Nutrition Info: Per Serving: Calories: 434, Total Fat: 33.4g, Fiber: 2g, Total Carbs: 12.27g, Protein: 23g

252.   Lamb Leg Mushrooms Satay

Servings: 8   Cooking Time: 8 Hrs.
Ingredients:

1 and ½ lbs. lamb leg, bone-in	6 garlic cloves, minced
2 carrots, sliced	2 tbsp tomato paste
½ lbs. mushrooms, sliced	1 tsp olive oil
4 tomatoes, chopped	Salt and black pepper to the taste
1 small yellow onion, chopped	Handful parsley, chopped

Directions:

Add lamb, carrots, and all other ingredients to the Crock Pot.   Put the cooker's lid on and set the cooking time to 8 hours on Low settings.   Serve warm.
Nutrition Info: Per Serving: Calories: 372, Total Fat: 12g, Fiber: 7g, Total Carbs: 18g, Protein: 22g

253.   Crockpot Beef Rendang

Servings: 8   Cooking Time: 10 Hours
Ingredients:

½ cup desiccated coconut, toasted	1 teaspoon salt
6 dried birds eye chilies, chopped	½ cup water
1 teaspoon ground cumin	1 tablespoon coconut oil
2 teaspoon ground coriander	6 kafir lime leaves
1 teaspoon turmeric powder	2 stalks lemon grass
6 cloves of garlic, minced	1 cup coconut cream
	1 beef shoulder, cut into chunks
	½ cup cilantro leaves, chopped

Directions:
Place all ingredients except the cilantro leaves in the CrockPot.   Give a good stir.   Close the lid and cook on high for 8 hours or on low for 10 hours.   Garnish with cilantro once cooked.
Nutrition Info: Calories per serving:305; Carbohydrates: 6.5g; Protein: 32.3g; Fat: 18.7g; Sugar: 0g; Sodium: 830mg; Fiber: 3.7g

254.   Honey Beef Sausages

Servings: 4   Cooking Time: 4.5 Hours
Ingredients:

1-pound beef sausages	1 teaspoon dried dill
2 tablespoons of liquid honey	½ teaspoon salt
	¼ cup heavy cream

Directions:
In the mixing bowl mix liquid honey with dried dill and salt.   Then add cream and whisk until smooth.   Pour the liquid in the Crock Pot.   Add beef sausages and close the lid.   Cook the meal on High for 4.hours.
Nutrition Info: Per Serving: 507 calories, 15.9g protein, 12.1g carbohydrates, 43.9g fat, 0.1g fiber, 91mg cholesterol, 1207mg sodium, 234mg potassium.

255.   Beef Onions Mix

Servings: 6   Cooking Time: 6 Hrs. 5 Minutes
Ingredients:

3 lbs. beef roast, trimmed and boneless	1/3 cup sun-dried tomatoes, chopped
1 tbsp Italian seasoning	½ cup beef stock
Salt and black pepper to the taste	½ cup kalamata olives pitted and halved
1 garlic clove, minced	1 cup yellow onions

chopped
1 tbsp olive oil
Directions:
Add oil to a suitable pan and place it over medium-high heat.   Stir in beef and sauté for 5 minutes then transfer to the insert of the Crock Pot.   Stir in Italian seasoning, black pepper, onions, stock, and tomatoes.   Put the cooker's lid on and set the cooking time to 6 hours on Low settings.   Slice the cooked meat and return to the tomato sauce. Mix well and serve warm.
Nutrition Info: Per Serving: Calories: 300, Total Fat: 5g, Fiber: 5g, Total Carbs: 12g, Protein: 25g

256.   Oregano Pork Chops

Servings: 4   Cooking Time: 8 Hours
Ingredients:

4 pork chops	15 ounces canned tomatoes, chopped
1 tablespoon oregano, chopped	1 tablespoon tomato paste
2 garlic cloves, minced	Salt and black pepper to the taste
1 tablespoon olive oil	¼ cup tomato juice

Directions:
In your Crock Pot, mix pork with oregano, garlic, oil, tomatoes, tomato paste, salt, pepper and tomato juice, cover and cook on Low for 8 hours. Divide everything between plates and serve.
Nutrition Info:calories 210, fat 10, fiber 2, carbs 15, protein 25

257.   Lettuce And Pork Wraps

Servings: 2   Cooking Time: 3.5 Hours
Ingredients:

2 lettuce leaves	3 tablespoons water
4 oz ground pork	1 teaspoon white pepper
1 teaspoon ketchup	
1 tablespoon butter	

Directions:
Mix ground pork with water, butter, and white pepper.   Put the meat mixture in the Crock Pot. Close the lid and cook it on High for 5 hours. After this, mix ground pork with ketchup.   Fill the lettuce leaves with ground pork.
Nutrition Info: Per Serving: 138 calories, 15.1g protein, 1.5g carbohydrates, 7.8g fat, 0.3g fiber, 57mg cholesterol, 10mg sodium, 270mg potassium

258.   Pork And Olives Mix

Servings: 2   Cooking Time: 8 Hours
Ingredients:

1 pound pork roast, sliced	Juice of ½ lime
½ cup tomato passata	¼ cup beef stock
1 red onion, sliced	Salt and black pepper to the taste
1 cup kalamata olives, pitted and halved	1 tablespoon chives, hopped

Directions:

In your Crock Pot, mix the pork slices with the passata, onion, olives and the other ingredients, toss, put the lid on and cook on Low for 8 hours. Divide the mix between plates and serve.
Nutrition Info: calories 360, fat 4, fiber 3, carbs 17, protein 27

259. Pork Casserole

Servings: 4   Cooking Time: 8 Hours
Ingredients:

1 cup cauliflower, chopped	7 oz pork mince
1 teaspoon ground black pepper	1 cup Cheddar cheese, shredded
1 teaspoon cayenne pepper	½ cup cream
	1 teaspoon sesame oil

Directions:
Brush the Crock Pot bowl with sesame oil from inside.   Then mix minced pork with ground black pepper and cayenne pepper.   Place the meat in the Crock Pot and flatten gently.   After this, top it with cauliflower and Cheddar cheese.   Add cream and close the lid.   Cook the casserole on Low for 8 hours.
Nutrition Info: Per Serving: 288 calories, 7.9g protein, 34g carbohydrates, 14.3g fat, 1.4g fiber, 35mg cholesterol, 193mg sodium, 130mg potassium

260. Peppercorn Beef Steak

Servings: 4   Cooking Time: 8 Hours
Ingredients:

4 beef steaks	1 tablespoon butter
1 teaspoon salt	1 cup of water
1 teaspoon peppercorns	1 teaspoon dried rosemary

Directions:
Rub the beef steaks with salt and dried rosemary. Then rub the meat with butter and transfer in the Crock Pot.   Add water and peppercorns.   Close the lid and cook the beef steaks on Low for 8 hours.
Nutrition Info: Per Serving: 186 calories, 25.9g protein, 0.5g carbohydrates, 8.3g fat, 0.3g fiber, 84mg cholesterol, 660mg sodium, 354mg potassium.

261. Oregano Lamb(1)

Servings: 2   Cooking Time: 6 Hours
Ingredients:

1 pound lamb stew meat, roughly cubed	½ teaspoon turmeric powder
1 teaspoon hot paprika	4 scallions, chopped
1 tablespoon oregano, chopped	A pinch of salt and black pepper
	1 cup beef stock

Directions:
In your Crock Pot, mix the lamb with the paprika, oregano and the other ingredients, toss, put the lid on and cook on Low for 6 hours.   Divide the mix between plates and serve with a side salad.

Nutrition Info: calories 200, fat 9, fiber 2, carbs 6, protein 12

262. Beef And Corn Mix

Servings: 2   Cooking Time: 8 Hours
Ingredients:

2 teaspoons olive oil	½ cup beef stock
3 scallions, chopped	Salt and black pepper to the taste
1 pound beef stew meat, cubed	1 tablespoon soy sauce
1 cup corn	
½ cup heavy cream	1 tablespoon parsley, chopped
2 garlic cloves, minced	

Directions:
In your Crock Pot, combine the beef with the corn, oil, scallions and the other ingredients except the cream, toss, put the lid on and cook on Low for 7 hours.   Add the cream, toss, cook on Low for 1 more hour, divide into bowls and serve.
Nutrition Info: calories 400, fat 10, fiber 4, carbs 15, protein 20

263. Beef And Peppers

Servings: 2   Cooking Time: 4 Hours
Ingredients:

1 pound lamb stew meat, cubed	2 teaspoons olive oil
1 red bell pepper, cut into strips	A pinch of salt and black pepper
1 green bell pepper, cut into strips	1 cup beef stock
1 orange bell pepper, cut into strips	1 tablespoon chives, chopped
	½ teaspoon sweet paprika

Directions:
In your Crock Pot, mix the lamb with the peppers and the other ingredients, toss, put the lid on and cook on High for 4 hours.   Divide the mix between plate sand serve.
Nutrition Info: calories 263, fat 14, fiber 3, carbs 6, protein 20

264. Bacon-wrapped Pork Tenderloin

Servings: 4   Cooking Time: 4 Hours
Ingredients:

3 oz bacon, sliced	1 tablespoon avocado oil
1-pound pork tenderloin	1 teaspoon salt
1 tablespoon maple syrup	½ cup of water
1 teaspoon white pepper	1 tablespoon mayonnaise

Directions:
Cut the pork tenderloin into 4 servings.   Then sprinkle the meat with white pepper, salt, and mayonnaise.   Wrap the pork cuts in the bacon and sprinkle with maple syrup and avocado oil. Put the meat in the Crock Pot.   Add water and close the lid.   Cook the meal on High for 4 hours.

Nutrition Info:Per Serving: 311 calories, 37.7g protein, 5.1g carbohydrates, 14.6g fat, 0.3g fiber, 107mg cholesterol, 1165mg sodium, 626mg potassium

265.   Beef-stuffed Peppers

Servings: 8   Cooking Time: 5 Hours
Ingredients:

1-pound lean ground beef	8 medium sweet peppers, top and seeds removed
1 can tomatoes and chilies	2 cups Mexican cheese blend
1 teaspoon cumin	

Directions:
Heat skillet over medium flame and add the ground beef.   Stir for 3 minutes until lightly brown.   Add the tomatoes and cumin. Turn off the heat and allow to cool.   Spoon the beef mixture into the sweet peppers. Top with the Mexican cheese blend.   Place inside the crockpot and close the lid.   Cook on low for hours or on high for 3 hours.
Nutrition Info: Calories per serving: 301; Carbohydrates: 2.5g; Protein:29 g; Fat: 14g; Sugar:0.3 g; Sodium: 797mg; Fiber: 3g

266.   Shredded Meat Dip With Pickles

Servings: 4   Cooking Time: 4 Hours
Ingredients:

1 tablespoon ketchup	1 teaspoon ground cinnamon
2 oz dill pickles, shredded	1 teaspoon brown sugar
1 cup of water	
9 oz pork tenderloin	

Directions:
Pour water in the Crock Pot.   Add pork tenderloin and ground cinnamon.   Cook the meat on High for 4 hours.   Then remove the meat from the Crock Pot and put it in the big bowl.   Shred the meat with the help of the fork.   Add ketchup, brown sugar, and dill pickles.   Carefully mix the meal.
Nutrition Info: Per Serving: 101 calories, 16.8g protein, 2.5g carbohydrates, 2.3g fat, 0.5g fiber, 47mg cholesterol, 251mg sodium, 290mg potassium

267.   Fall Pork

Servings: 4   Cooking Time: 10 Hours
Ingredients:

9 oz pork tenderloin, chopped	1 cup tomatoes, chopped
½ cup carrot, chopped	1 teaspoon Italian seasonings
½ cup pumpkin, chopped	1 teaspoon salt
2 cups of water	

Directions:
Put all ingredients in the Crock Pot.   Close the lid and cook the meal on Low for 10 hours.   Carefully mix the cooked meal before serving.

Nutrition Info:Per Serving: 119 calories, 17.5g protein, 5.7g carbohydrates, 2.8g fat, 1.8g fiber, 47mg cholesterol, 635mg sodium, 484mg potassium

268.   Oregano Beef

Servings: 2   Cooking Time: 4 Hours
Ingredients:

1 pound beef stew meat, cubed	1 tablespoon oregano, chopped
1 tablespoon olive oil	½ cup tomato sauce
1 tablespoon balsamic vinegar	1 red onion, chopped
½ tablespoon lemon juice	A pinch of salt and black pepper
	½ teaspoon chili powder

Directions:
In your Crock Pot, mix the beef with the oil, vinegar, lemon juice and the other ingredients, toss, put the lid on and cook on High for 4 hours.   Divide the mix between plates and serve right away.
Nutrition Info:calories 263, fat 14, fiber 4, carbs 6, protein 18

269.   Beef Stifado

Servings: 4   Cooking Time: 7 Hours
Ingredients:

1-pound beef stew meat	1 teaspoon ground nutmeg
1 onion, chopped	1 cup red wine
1 tablespoon sunflower oil	½ cup ketchup
1 cup tomatoes, canned, diced	1 teaspoon dried rosemary

Directions:
Mix red wine with ketchup and dried rosemary and pour it in the Crock Pot.   Then add tomatoes and ground nutmeg.   Add onion.   Heat the sunflower oil in the skillet well.   Add beef stew meat and roast it on high heat for 3 minutes per side.   Then add the meat in the Crock Pot, close the lid, and cook on Low for 7 hours.
Nutrition Info: Per Serving: 343 calories, 35.7g protein, 13.9g carbohydrates, 11g fat, 1.5g fiber, 101mg cholesterol, 415mg sodium, 781mg potassium.

270.   Dijon Basil Pork Loin

Servings: 4   Cooking Time: 10 Hours
Ingredients:

1 pork loin roast, trimmed from excess fat	1 teaspoon marjoram
	Salt and pepper to taste
2 tablespoons Dijon mustard	¼ cup basil, chopped

Directions:
Rub the pork loin roast with mustard, marjoram, salt and pepper.   Use your hands to massage the pork.   Place in the crockpot and sprinkle with

chopped basil.   Close the lid and cook on low for 10 hours or on high for 8 hours.
Nutrition Info: Calories per serving: 449; Carbohydrates: 3g; Protein: 38.2g; Fat:33.1g; Sugar:0 g; Sodium: 764mg; Fiber: 1.3g

271.Swedish Style Meatballs

Servings: 4   Cooking Time: 5.5 Hours
Ingredients:

½ cup of water	1 teaspoon salt
½ cup cream	1 tablespoon
1 tablespoon flour	breadcrumbs
9 oz minced pork	1 tablespoon fresh
1 teaspoon ground	parsley, chopped
black pepper	

Directions:
Make the meatballs: mix minced pork with ground black pepper, salt, and breadcrumbs.   Make the small meatballs and place them in the Crock Pot in one layer.   After this, mix water with cream and flour.   Pour the liquid over the meatballs and cook them on High for 5.5 hours.
Nutrition Info: Per Serving: 126 calories, 17.5g protein, 4.1g carbohydrates, 4.1g fat, 0.3g fiber, 52mg cholesterol, 642mg sodium, 297mg potassium.

272.   Short Ribs With Tapioca Sauce

Servings: 6   Cooking Time: 10 Hrs.
Ingredients:

3 lbs. beef short ribs	1 cup dry red wine
1 fennel bulb, cut into wedges	2 tbsp tapioca, crushed
2 yellow onions, cut into wedges	2 tbsp tomato paste
1 cup carrot, sliced	1 tsp rosemary, dried
14 oz. canned tomatoes, chopped	Salt and black pepper to the taste
	4 garlic cloves, minced

Directions:
Add short ribs, onion, and all other ingredients to the insert of Crock Pot.   Put the cooker's lid on and set the cooking time to 10 hours on Low settings.   Serve warm.
Nutrition Info: Per Serving: Calories: 432, Total Fat: 14g, Fiber: 6g, Total Carbs: 25g, Protein: 42g

273.   Meatballs In Vodka Sauce

Servings: 4   Cooking Time: 6 Hours
Ingredients:

1-pound ground pork	1 tablespoon
1 onion, diced	semolina
1 teaspoon ground	1 cup vodka sauce
black pepper	2 tablespoons sesame oil

Directions:
In the mixing bowl mix ground pork with onion, ground black pepper, and semolina.   Make the small meatballs.   Brush the Crock Pot bottom with sesame oil and put the meatballs inside in one

layer.   Add vodka sauce and close the lid.   Cook the meatballs on low for 6 hours.
Nutrition Info: Per Serving: 299 calories, 32.9g protein, 10.3g carbohydrates, 13.4g fat, 0.8g fiber, 85mg cholesterol, 286mg sodium, 529mg potassium

274.   Simple Roast Beef

Servings: 4   Cooking Time: 12 Hours
Ingredients:

2 pounds rump roast	Salt and pepper to
1 cup onion, chopped	taste
3 tablespoons butter	¼ cup water

Directions:
Place all ingredients in the crockpot.   Give a good stir.   Close the lid and cook on low for 12 hours or on high for 10 hours.   Once cooked, shred the pot roast using two forks.   Return to the crockpot and continue cooking on high for 1 hour.
Nutrition Info: Calories per serving: 523; Carbohydrates:1.8g; Protein: 43.6g; Fat: 32.6g; Sugar: 0g; Sodium: 734mg; Fiber:1.2 g

275.   Roast And Pepperoncinis

Servings: 4   Cooking Time: 8 Hours
Ingredients:

5 pounds beef chuck roast	10 pepperoncinis
1 tablespoon soy sauce	1 cup beef stock
	2 tablespoons butter, melted

Directions:
In your Crock Pot, mix beef roast with soy sauce, pepperoncinis, stock and butter, toss well, cover and cook on Low for 8 hours.   Transfer roast to a cutting board, shred usingforks, return to Crock Pot, toss, divide between plates and serve.
Nutrition Info:calories 362, fat 4, fiber 8, carbs 17, protein 17

276.   Lamb And Potatoes

Servings: 2   Cooking Time: 4 Hours
Ingredients:

1 pound lamb stew meat, roughly cubed	½ cup tomato sauce
2 sweet potatoes, peeled and cubed	1 tablespoon avocado oil
½ cup beef stock	1 tablespoon balsamic vinegar
½ teaspoon sweet paprika	1 tablespoon cilantro, chopped
½ teaspoon coriander, ground	A pinch of salt and black pepper

Directions:
In your Crock Pot, mix the lamb with the potatoes, stock, sauce and the other ingredients, toss, put the lid on and cook on High for 4 hours   Divide everything between plates and serve.
Nutrition Info:calories 253, fat 14, fiber 3, carbs 7, protein 17

277. Herbed Lamb Fillet

Servings: 4   Cooking Time: 5 Hrs.

Ingredients:

1 lemon, chopped	3 tbsp olive oil
3 tbsp lemon juice	1/3 cup fresh dill, chopped
1 tbsp lemon zest	1 tsp salt
1 tbsp minced garlic	1 lb. lamb fillet, sliced
1 tsp paprika	
1 tsp dried rosemary	
1 cup chicken stock	

Directions:

Mic lemon, lemon zest, and minced garlic in a small bowl.   Rub the lamb slices with lemon mixture liberally.   Place the lamb meat in the insert of the Crock Pot.   Top the lamb with chicken stock, dill, and rest of the ingredients. Put the cooker's lid on and set the cooking time to hours on High settings.   Serve warm.

Nutrition Info: Per Serving: Calories: 413, Total Fat: 30.1g, Fiber: 0g, Total Carbs: 5.1g, Protein: 30g

278. Jalapeno Mississippi Roast

Servings: 4   Cooking Time: 8 Hours

Ingredients:

3 pepperoncini	2 tablespoons flour
1-pound beef chuck roast	½ teaspoon salt
1 teaspoon ground black pepper	2 tablespoons avocado oil
	2 cups of water

Directions:

Put all ingredients in the Crock Pot.   Close the lid and cook the meal on Low for 8 hours.   Then open the lid and shred the beef.

Nutrition Info: Per Serving: 440 calories, 30.4g protein, 4.3g carbohydrates, 32.6g fat, 1g fiber, 117mg cholesterol, 369mg sodium, 322mg potassium.

279. Sausage Mix

Servings: 4   Cooking Time: 4 Hours

Ingredients:

1 cup yellow onion, chopped	5 pounds kale, chopped
1 and ½ pound Italian pork sausage, sliced	1 teaspoon garlic, minced
½ cup red bell pepper, chopped	¼ cup red hot chili pepper, chopped
Salt and black pepper to the taste	1 cup water

Directions:

In your Crock Pot, mix onion with sausage, bell pepper, salt, pepper, garlic, chili pepper and water, cover and cook on High for 3 hours.   Add kale, toss a bit, cover and cook on High for 1 more hour. Divide between plates and serve.

Nutrition Info: calories 250, fat 4, fiber 1, carbs 12, protein 20

280. Cauliflower Beef Soup

Servings: 4   Cooking Time: 6 Hrs.

Ingredients:

1 lb. beef, ground	15 oz. tomato sauce
2 cups cauliflower, chopped	3 cups beef stock
1 cup yellow onion, chopped	½ tsp basil, dried
2 red bell peppers, chopped	½ tsp oregano, dried
15 oz. tomatoes, chopped	3 garlic cloves, minced
	Salt and black pepper to the taste

Directions:

Add cauliflower and beef along with all other ingredients to the insert of Crock Pot.   Put the cooker's lid on and set the cooking time to 6 hours on Low settings.   Serve warm.

Nutrition Info: Per Serving: Calories: 214, Total Fat: 6g, Fiber: 6g, Total Carbs: 18g, Protein: 7g

281. Fennel Seeds Pork Chops

Servings: 4   Cooking Time: 6 Hours

Ingredients:

1 tablespoon fennel seeds	4 pork chops
3 tablespoons avocado oil	1 teaspoon garlic, diced
	½ cup of water

Directions:

Mix fennel seeds with avocado oil and garlic. Mash the mixture.   Then rub the pork chops with fennel seeds mixture and transfer in the Crock Pot. Add water and close the lid.   Cook the meat on low for 6 hours.

Nutrition Info: Per Serving: 276 calories, 18.4g protein, 1.6g carbohydrates, 21.4g fat, 1.1g fiber, 69mg cholesterol, 59mg sodium, 336mg potassium

282. Tender Beef Goulash

Servings: 4   Cooking Time: 8 Hours

Ingredients:

1 teaspoon flour	1 carrot, chopped
2 cups of water	1 teaspoon ground black pepper
¼ cup cream	1 tablespoon sunflower oil
1-pound beef brisket, chopped	

Directions:

Mix the cream with flour until smooth and pour in the Crock Pot.   Add water, chopped beef, carrot, ground black pepper, and sunflower oil.   Close the lid and cook the goulash for 8 hours on Low.

Nutrition Info: Per Serving: 261 calories, 34.8g protein, 2.8g carbohydrates, 11.4g fat, 0.5g fiber, 104mg cholesterol, 94mg sodium, 520mg potassium.

283. Saucy Beef Cheeks

Servings: 4   Cooking Time: 4 Hrs.

Ingredients:

4 beef cheeks, halved	1 tbsp balsamic vinegar
2 tbsp olive oil	

Salt and black pepper to the taste
1 white onion, chopped
4 garlic cloves, minced
2 cup beef stock
5 cardamom pods

3 bay leaves
7 cloves
2 vanilla beans, split
1 and ½ tbsp tomato paste
1 carrot, sliced

Directions:
Add beef cheeks and all remaining ingredients to the insert of your Crock Pot.   Put the cooker's lid on and set the cooking time to 4 hours on High settings.   Mix gently and serve warm.
Nutrition Info: Per Serving: Calories: 321, Total Fat: 5g, Fiber: 7g, Total Carbs: 18g, Protein: 12g

284.   Ketchup Pork Ribs

Servings: 4   Cooking Time: 4 Hours
Ingredients:
1-pound pork ribs, roughly chopped
1 tablespoon fresh dill

4 tablespoons ketchup
1 tablespoon avocado oil
½ cup beef broth

Directions:
Mix pork ribs with ketchup and avocado oil.   Put them in the Crock Pot.   Add beef broth and dill. Close the pork ribs on High for hours.
Nutrition Info: Per Serving: 336 calories, 31.1g protein, 4.5g carbohydrates, 20.8g fat, 0.3g fiber, 117mg cholesterol, 330mg sodium, 447mg potassium

285.   Crockpot Polish Hunter's Stew

Servings: 8   Cooking Time: 12 Hours
Ingredients:
½ ounce porcini mushrooms, sliced
2 pounds pork stew meat, bones removed
½ pound smoked nitrate-free sausages, chopped
2 onions, diced

1 teaspoon caraway seeds
2 bay leaves
1 cup tomatoes, chopped
6 cups beef stock
Salt and pepper to taste

Directions:
Place all ingredients in the CrockPot.   Give a good stir.   Close the lid and cook on high for 10 hours or on low for 12 hours.
Nutrition Info: Calories per serving: 312; Carbohydrates: 5.4g; Protein: 42.8g; Fat: 15.5g; Sugar: 0g; Sodium: 711mg; Fiber: 3.2g

286.   Rosemary Pork

Servings: 4   Cooking Time: 7 Hours
Ingredients:
4 pork chops, bone in
1 cup chicken stock
Salt and black pepper to the taste

1 teaspoon rosemary, dried
3 garlic cloves, minced

Directions:
Season pork chops with salt and pepper and place in your Crock Pot.   Add rosemary, garlic and stock, cover and cook on Low for 7 hours.   Divide pork between plates and drizzle cooking juices all over.
Nutrition Info:calories 165, fat 2, fiber 1, carbs 12, protein 26

287.   Fajita Beef

Servings: 4   Cooking Time: 4.5 Hours
Ingredients:
1 sweet pepper, cut into strips
1 red onion, sliced
1-pound beef sirloin, cut into strips

1 teaspoon fajita seasonings
½ cup of water
1 tablespoon butter

Directions:
Put the beef strips in the Crock Pot.   Add fajita seasonings, butter, and water.   Close the lid and cook the beef on high for 5 hours.   Add onion and sweet pepper.   Carefully mix the beef mixture and cook for 1 hour on High.
Nutrition Info: Per Serving: 259 calories, 35g protein, 5.4g carbohydrates, 10.1g fat, 1g fiber, 109mg cholesterol, 142mg sodium, 554mg potassium.

288.   Lamb In Curry Sauce

Servings: 4   Cooking Time: 5 Hours
Ingredients:
1 teaspoon curry paste
1-pound lamb fillet, sliced
1 tablespoon pomegranate juice

½ cup of water
½ cup of coconut milk
1 onion, sliced
1 teaspoon lemongrass
1 tablespoon coconut oil

Directions:
Melt the coconut oil in the skillet.   Add lamb fillet and roast it for minutes per side on low heat. After this, transfer the lamb in the Crock Pot.   In the bowl mix curry paste, pomegranate juice, coconut milk, water, and lemongrass.   Pour the liquid over the lamb.   Add sliced onion and cook the meal on High for 5 hours.
Nutrition Info: Per Serving: 329 calories, 32.9g protein, 4.7g carbohydrates, 19.6g fat, 1.3g fiber, 102mg cholesterol, 93mg sodium, 503mg potassium.

289.   Caribbean Pork Chop

Servings: 4   Cooking Time: 10 Hours
Ingredients:
1 tablespoon curry powder
Salt and pepper to taste

1 teaspoon cumin
1-pound pork loin roast, bones removed
½ cup chicken broth

Directions:
Place all ingredients in the crockpot. Give a good stir.   Close the lid and cook on low for 8 to 10 hours or on high for 7 hours.
Nutrition Info: Calories per serving: 471; Carbohydrates: 0.9g; Protein: 43.8g; Fat: 35g; Sugar: 0g; Sodium:528mg; Fiber: 0g

---

290. Bbq Ribs

Servings: 4   Cooking Time: 4 Hours
Ingredients:

- 1-pound pork ribs, roughly chopped
- 1 teaspoon minced garlic
- ½ cup BBQ sauce
- 1 tablespoon olive oil
- ¼ cup plain yogurt

Directions:
Mix BBQ sauce with plain yogurt and minced garlic and pour it in the Crock Pot.   Then pour olive oil in the skillet and heat well.   Add pork ribs and roast them for minutes per side on high heat.   Transfer the pork ribs in the Crock Pot and carefully mix.   Close the lid and cook them on High for 4 hours.
Nutrition Info: Per Serving: 398 calories, 31g protein, 12.6g carbohydrates, 23.9g fat, 0.2g fiber, 118mg cholesterol, 426mg sodium, 430mg potassium

---

291. Simple Crockpot Meatballs

Servings: 4   Cooking Time: 10 Hours
Ingredients:

- 2 tablespoons olive oil
- 2 tablespoons almonds, slivered
- 1-pound ground pork
- 1 tablespoon organic tomato paste
- 2 cloves of garlic, minced
- 1 teaspoon salt
- 1 teaspoon ground cinnamon
- ½ teaspoon dried oregano leaves
- ¼ teaspoon ground black pepper
- 2 tablespoons warm water
- ¼ teaspoon baking soda

Directions:
Line the bottom of the CrockPot with aluminum foil. Grease the foil with olive oil.   Place all ingredients in a mixing bowl. Form small meatballs using your hands.   Place in the CrockPot.   Close the lid and cook on high for 8 hours or on low for 10 hours.   Halfway through the cooking time, flip the meatballs to brown the other side.   Close the lid and continue cooking until the meat is cooked through.
Nutrition Info: Calories per serving:407; Carbohydrates: 1.9g; Protein: 29.6g; Fat: 30.7g; Sugar: 0g; Sodium: 825mg; Fiber:0.6g

---

292. Sesame Short Ribs

Servings: 4   Cooking Time: 8 Hours
Ingredients:

- 4 tablespoons mirin
- 1 tablespoon sesame oil
- 1 teaspoon sesame seeds
- ¼ cup of soy sauce
- 1-pound pork ribs
- ½ teaspoon brown sugar
- ¼ cup of water

Directions:
In the mixing bowl mix sesame oil with mirin, sesame seeds, brown sugar, and soy sauce.   Add the pork ribs in the soy sauce mixture and leave for 30 minutes to marinate.   After this, transfer the ingredients in the Crock Pot.   Add water and close the lid.   Cook the short ribs on Low for 8 hours.
Nutrition Info: Per Serving: 379 calories, 31.2g protein, 8.8g carbohydrates, 23.9g fat, 0.2g fiber, 117mg cholesterol, 1095mg sodium, 365mg potassium

---

293. Beef In Wine Sauce

Servings: 4   Cooking Time: 6 Hours
Ingredients:

- 1 tablespoon flour
- 1 tablespoon butter
- 1 cup red wine
- 1 teaspoon brown sugar
- ½ cup of water
- 1 onion, peeled, chopped
- 12 oz beef tenderloin, chopped

Directions:
Sprinkle the beef with flour.   Then toss the butter in the skillet. Melt it.   Add the beef and roast it on high heat for minutes per side.   Then transfer the meat in the Crock Pot.   Add onion, water, brown sugar, and red wine.   Close the lid and cook the meal on Low for hours.
Nutrition Info: Per Serving: 271 calories, 25.2g protein, 6.4g carbohydrates, 10.7g fat, 0.6g fiber, 86mg cholesterol, 76mg sodium, 406mg potassium.

---

294. Pork Chops And Spinach

Servings: 2   Cooking Time: 4 Hours
Ingredients:

- 1 pound pork chops
- 1 cup baby spinach
- ½ cup beef stock
- ½ teaspoon sweet paprika
- ½ teaspoon coriander, ground
- ¼ cup tomato passata
- 4 scallions, chopped
- 2 teaspoons olive oil
- A pinch of salt and black pepper
- 1 tablespoon chives, chopped

Directions:
In your Crock Pot, mix the pork chops with the stock, passata and the other ingredients except the spinach, toss, put the lid on and cook on High for 3 hours and 30 minutes.   Add the spinach, cook on High for 30 minutes more, divide the mix between plates and serve.
Nutrition Info:calories 274, fat 14, fiber 2, carbs 6, protein 16

295. Taco Pork

Servings: 5   Cooking Time: 5 Hours

Ingredients:

1-pound pork shoulder, chopped	1 tablespoon lemon juice
1 tablespoon taco seasonings	1 cup of water

Directions:

Mix pork shoulder with taco seasonings and place in the Crock Pot.   Add water and cook it on High for 5 hours.   After this, transfer the cooked meat in the bowl and shred gently with the help of the fork.   Add lemon juice and shake gently.

Nutrition Info: Per Serving: 274 calories, 21.1g protein, 1.7g carbohydrates, 19.4g fat, 0g fiber, 82mg cholesterol, 232mg sodium, 303mg potassium

296. Mint Lamb Chops

Servings: 2   Cooking Time: 4 Hours

Ingredients:

2 tablespoons olive oil	½ cup coconut cream
1 pound lamb chops	1 red onion, chopped
1 tablespoon mint, chopped	2 tablespoons garlic, minced
½ teaspoon garam masala	½ cup beef stock
	A pinch of salt and black pepper

Directions:

In your Crock Pot, mix the lamb chops with the oil, mint and the other ingredients, toss, put the lid on and cook on High for 4 hours.   Divide the mix between plates and serve warm.

Nutrition Info:calories 263, fat 14, fiber 3, carbs 7, protein 20

297. Cilantro Meatballs

Servings: 6   Cooking Time: 4 Hours

Ingredients:

1-pound minced beef	2 teaspoons dried cilantro
1 teaspoon minced garlic	1 tablespoon semolina
1 egg, beaten	½ cup of water
1 teaspoon chili flakes	1 tablespoon sesame oil

Directions:

In the bowl mix minced beef, garlic, egg, chili flakes, cilantro, and semolina.   Then make the meatballs.   After this, heat the sesame oil in the skillet.   Cook the meatballs in the hot oil on high heat for 1 minute per side.   Transfer the roasted meatballs in the Crock Pot, add water, and close the lid.   Cook the meatballs on High for 4 hours.

Nutrition Info: Per Serving: 178 calories, 24.1g protein, 1.5g carbohydrates, 7.7g fat, 0.1g fiber, 95mg cholesterol, 61mg sodium, 321mg potassium.

298. Pork And Beans Mix

Servings: 2   Cooking Time: 8 Hours

Ingredients:

1 red bell pepper, chopped	½ cup tomato sauce
1 pound pork stew meat, cubed	1 yellow onion, chopped
1 tablespoon olive oil	1 teaspoon Italian seasoning
1 cup canned black beans, drained and rinsed	Salt and black pepper to the taste
	1 tablespoon oregano, chopped

Directions:

In your Crock Pot, mix the pork with the bell pepper, oil and the other ingredients, toss, put the lid on and cook on Low for 8 hours.   Divide the mix between plates and serve.

Nutrition Info:calories 385, fat 12, fiber 5, carbs 18, protein 40

299. Succulent Pork Ribs

Servings: 4   Cooking Time: 8 Hours

Ingredients:

12 oz pork ribs, roughly chopped	1 teaspoon ground nutmeg
¼ cup of orange juice	1 teaspoon salt
1 cup of water	

Directions:

Pour water and orange juice in the Crock Pot. Then sprinkle the pork ribs with ground nutmeg and salt.   Put the pork ribs in the Crock Pot and close the lid.   Cook the meat on low for 8 hours.

Nutrition Info: Per Serving: 242 calories, 22.7g protein, 1.9g carbohydrates, 15.3g fat, 0.1g fiber, 88mg cholesterol, 633mg sodium, 279mg potassium

300. Shredded Pork

Servings: 4   Cooking Time: 5 Hours

Ingredients:

10 oz pork loin	1 teaspoon coriander seeds
½ cup cream	1 teaspoon salt
1 cup of water	

Directions:

Put all ingredients in the Crock Pot.   Cook it on High for 5 hours.   Then open the lid and shredded pork with the help of 2 forks.

Nutrition Info: Per Serving: 191 calories, 19.6g protein, 0.9g carbohydrates, 11.5g fat, 0g fiber, 62mg cholesterol, 367mg sodium, 312mg potassium

301. Italian Pork Roast

Servings: 10   Cooking Time: 12 Hours

Ingredients:

5 pounds pork shoulder, bone in	1 teaspoon dried basil
7 cloves of garlic, slivered	1 teaspoon dried rosemary
1 tablespoon salt	

1 teaspoon dried oregano   ½ teaspoon black pepper

Directions:
Place all ingredients in the CrockPot.   Give a good stir.   Close the lid and cook on high for 10 hours or on low for 12 hours.
Nutrition Info: Calories per serving:610; Carbohydrates: 0.9g; Protein: 57.1g; Fat: 40.8g; Sugar: 0g; Sodium: 1240mg; Fiber: 0.2g

---

302.   Kebab Cubes

Servings: 4   Cooking Time: 5 Hours
Ingredients:

1 teaspoon curry powder	1 teaspoon dried mint
1 teaspoon cayenne pepper	½ cup plain yogurt
	1-pound beef tenderloin, cubed

Directions:
In the mixing bowl, mix beef cubes with plain yogurt, cayenne pepper, dried mint, and curry powder.   Then put the mixture in the Crock Pot. Add water if there is not enough liquid and close the lid.   Cook the meal on High for 5 hours.
Nutrition Info: Per Serving: 259 calories, 34.7g protein, 2.7g carbohydrates, 10.9g fat, 0.3g fiber, 106mg cholesterol, 89mg sodium, 495mg potassium.

---

303.   Chili Lamb

Servings: 2   Cooking Time: 4 Hours
Ingredients:

1 pound lamb chops	1 teaspoon chili powder
2 teaspoons avocado oil	½ cup veggie stock
2 scallions, chopped	2 garlic cloves, minced
1 green chili pepper, minced	A pinch of salt and black pepper
½ teaspoon turmeric powder	

Directions:
In your Crock Pot, mix the lamb chops with the oil, scallions and the other ingredients, toss, put the lid on and cook on High for 4 hours.   Divide everything between plates and serve.
Nutrition Info:calories 243, fat 15, fiber 3, carbs 6, protein 20

---

304.   Pork Chops And Peppers

Servings: 4   Cooking Time: 10 Hours
Ingredients:

4 pork chops	½ cup chicken broth
1 onion, chopped	½ teaspoon thyme leaves
2 cups red and green bell peppers	

Directions:
Place all ingredients in the crockpot.   Mix to combine all ingredients.   Close the lid and cook on low for 10 hours or on high for 7 hours.

Nutrition Info: Calories per serving: 592; Carbohydrates: 0.5g; Protein: 47.1g; Fat: 39.2g; Sugar: 0g; Sodium:601 mg; Fiber:0 g

---

305.   Pepsi Pork Tenderloin

Servings: 4   Cooking Time: 6 Hours
Ingredients:

1-pound pork tenderloin	1 cup Pepsi
1 teaspoon cumin seeds	1 teaspoon olive oil
	2 tablespoons soy sauce

Directions:
Chop the pork tenderloin roughly and put it in the mixing bowl.   Add cumin seeds, soy sauce, Pepsi, and olive oil. Leave the meat for 30 minutes to marinate.   After this, transfer the meat and all Pepsi liquid in the Crock Pot and close the lid. Cook the meat on low for 6 hours.
Nutrition Info: Per Serving: 179 calories, 30.3g protein, 0.8g carbohydrates, 5.3g fat, 0.1g fiber,83mg cholesterol, 523mg sodium, 514mg potassium

---

306.   Braised Beef Strips

Servings: 4   Cooking Time: 5 Hours
Ingredients:

½ cup mushroom, sliced	1 teaspoon salt
1 onion, sliced	1 teaspoon white pepper
1 cup of water	10 oz beef loin, cut into strips
1 tablespoon coconut oil	

Directions:
Melt the coconut oil in the skillet.   Add mushrooms and roast them for 5 minutes on medium heat.   Then transfer the mushrooms in the Crock Pot.   Add all remaining ingredients and close the lid.   Cook the meal on High for hours
Nutrition Info: Per Serving: 173 calories, 19.6g protein, 3.2g carbohydrates, 9.4g fat, 0.8g fiber, 50mg cholesterol, 624mg sodium, 316mg potassium.

---

307.   Oregano Lamb(2)

Servings: 4   Cooking Time: 7 Hours
Ingredients:

2 teaspoons paprika	¼ cup parsley, chopped
2 garlic cloves, minced	2 teaspoons harissa
2 teaspoons oregano, dried	1 tablespoon red wine vinegar
2 tablespoons sumac	Salt and black pepper to the taste
12 lamb cutlets	2 tablespoons black olives, pitted and sliced
¼ cup olive oil	
2 tablespoons water	
2 teaspoons cumin, ground	
4 carrots, sliced	6 radishes, thinly sliced

Directions:

In a bowl, mix cutlets with paprika, garlic, oregano, sumac, salt, pepper, half of the oil and the water and rub well.   Put carrots in your Crock Pot and add olives and radishes.   In another bowl, mix harissa with the rest of the oil, parsley, cumin, vinegar and a splash of water and stir well.   Add this over carrots mix, season with salt and pepper and toss to coat.   Add lamb cutlets, cover, cook on Low for 7 hours, divide everything between plates and serve.

Nutrition Info:calories 245, fat 32, fiber 6, carbs 12, protein 34

308.   Rosemary Beef

Servings: 2   Cooking Time: 7 Hours
Ingredients:

1 pound beef roast, sliced	1 tablespoon olive oil
1 tablespoon rosemary, chopped	½ cup tomato sauce
Juice of ½ lemon	A pinch of salt and black pepper

Directions:
In your Crock Pot, mix the roast with the rosemary, lemon juice and the other ingredients, toss, put the lid on and cook on Low for 7 hours.   Divide everything between plates and serve.

Nutrition Info:calories 210, fat 5, fiber 3, carbs 8, protein 12

309.   Pork Roast With Apples

Servings: 4   Cooking Time: 8 Hours
Ingredients:

1-pound pork shoulder, boneless	1 teaspoon thyme
1 teaspoon brown sugar	1 cup apples, chopped
1 teaspoon allspices	1 yellow onion, sliced
	2 cups of water

Directions:
Sprinkle the pork shoulder with allspices, thyme, and brown sugar. Transfer it in the Crock Pot. Add all remaining ingredients and close the lid. Cook the pork roast on Low for 8 hours.

Nutrition Info: Per Serving: 376 calories, 26.9g protein, 11.5g carbohydrates, 24.5g fat, 2.1g fiber, 102mg cholesterol, 83mg sodium, 482mg potassium

Dessert Recipes

310. Vanilla Buns

Servings: 4   Cooking Time: 3 Hours

Ingredients:

1 cup flour
½ teaspoon fresh yeast
3 tablespoons sugar
¼ cup milk
2 tablespoons olive oil
1 teaspoon vanilla extract

Directions:

Mix sugar with fresh yeast and leave for 5 minutes. Then mix the mixture with milk, flour, and vanilla extract.   Knead it and add olive oil.   Knead the dough until smooth and cut into buns.   Leave the buns for 30 minutes in a warm place to rise. Then line the Crock Pot bowl with baking paper. Put the buns inside and close the lid.   Cook them on High for 3 hours.

Nutrition Info: Per Serving: 220 calories, 3.9g protein, 33.9g carbohydrates, 7.6g fat, 1g fiber, 1mg cholesterol, 8mg sodium, 54mg potassium.

311. Cherry And Rhubarb Mix

Servings: 2   Cooking Time: 2 Hours

Ingredients:

2 cups rhubarb, sliced
½ cup cherries, pitted
1 tablespoon butter, melted
¼ cup coconut cream
½ cup sugar

Directions:

In your Crock Pot, mix the rhubarb with the cherries and the other ingredients, toss, put the lid on and cook on High for 2 hours.   Divide the mix into bowls and serve cold.

Nutrition Info: calories 200, fat 2, fiber 3, carbs 6, protein 1

312. Amaranth Bars

Servings: 7   Cooking Time: 1 Hour

Ingredients:

½ cup amaranth
4 oz peanuts, chopped
¼ cup of coconut oil
3 oz milk chocolate, chopped

Directions:

Put all ingredients in the Crock Pot and cook on High for hour.   Then transfer the melted amaranth mixture in the silicone mold, flatten it, and refrigerate until solid.   Cut the dessert into bars.

Nutrition Info: Per Serving: 276 calories, 7.1g protein, 19.1g carbohydrates, 20.3g fat, 3.1g fiber, 3mg cholesterol, 15mg sodium, 210mg potassium.

313. Mixed Nuts Brownies

Servings: 12   Cooking Time: 4 1/4 Hours

Ingredients:

8 oz. dark chocolate, chopped
1/2 cup butter
1 cup white sugar
3 eggs
1 teaspoon vanilla extract
1 cup all-purpose flour
1/2 cup cocoa powder
1/2 teaspoon salt
1 cup mixed nuts, chopped

Directions:

Mix the chocolate and butter in a bowl and place over a hot water bath. Melt them together until smooth.   Remove from heat and add the eggs, vanilla, flour, cocoa powder and salt and mix gently.   Fold in the nuts then pour the batter in your Crock Pot (greased or lined with baking paper).   Cover and bake for hours on low settings.   Allow to cool before cutting into small squares.

314. Lemon Bars

Servings: 10   Cooking Time: 6 1/2 Hours

Ingredients:

Crust:
1/2 cup butter, softened
1/4 cup white sugar
2 egg yolks
1 teaspoon vanilla extract
1 1/2 cups all-purpose flour
1 pinch salt
1/4 teaspoon baking powder
Filling:
6 egg yolks
1/2 cup lemon juice
1 tablespoon lemon zest
2/3 cup white sugar

Directions:

To make the crust, mix the butter and sugar in a bowl for 5 minutes. Add the egg yolks and vanilla and give it a quick mix.   Fold in the flour, salt and baking powder and knead the dough for a few times.   Place the dough on a floured working surface then roll it into a thin sheet. Transfer in your Crock Pot and trim the edges if needed.   For the filling, mix the ingredients in a bowl. Pour the filling into the crust.   Bake for 6 hours on low settings.   Allow to cool in the pot before serving.

315. Brownie Bars

Servings: 8   Cooking Time: 5 Hours

Ingredients:

1/2 cup of cocoa powder
1/2 cup flour
1 teaspoon baking powder
1/4 cup butter, melted
1 teaspoon vanilla extract
3 eggs, beaten
1/4 cup of sugar
2 oz chocolate chips

Directions:

Mix all ingredients in the bowl and stir until smooth.   Line the Crock Pot with baking paper and transfer the mixture inside.   Close the lid and cook the brownie on low for 5 hours.   When the

brownie is cooked, let it cool little.   Cut the dessert into bars.
Nutrition Info: Per Serving: 178 calories, 4.5g protein, 19.9g carbohydrates, 10.3g fat, 2.1g fiber, 78mg cholesterol, 71mg sodium, 258mg potassium.

316.   Cranberry Stuffed Apples

Servings: 4   Cooking Time: 4 1/4 Hours
Ingredients:

4 large Granny Smith apples	2 tablespoons honey
1/2 cup dried cranberries	1/4 cup pecans, chopped
1/4 cup ground almonds	1/4 teaspoon cinnamon powder
	1/2 cup apple cider

Directions:
Carefully remove the core of each apple and place them in your Crock Pot.   Mix the cranberries, honey, almonds, pecans and cinnamon in a bowl. Stuff the apples with this mixture then pour in the apple cider.   Cover the pot and cook on low settings for hours.   The apples are best served warm.

317.Panna Cotta

Servings: 2   Cooking Time: 1.5 Hours
Ingredients:

1 tablespoon gelatin	2 tablespoons strawberry jam
1 cup cream	
¼ cup of sugar	

Directions:
Pour cream in the Crock Pot.   Add sugar and close the lid.   Cook the liquid on High for 1.5 hours.   Then cool it to the room temperature, add gelatin, and mix until smooth.   Pour the liquid in the glasses and refrigerate until solid.   Top every cream jelly with jam.
Nutrition Info: Per Serving: 270 calories, 7g protein, 47.4g carbohydrates, 6.7g fat, 0g fiber, 23mg cholesterol, 53mg sodium, 45mg potassium.

318.   Maple Roasted Pears

Servings: 4   Cooking Time: 6 1/4 Hours
Ingredients:

4 ripe pears, carefully peeled and cored	1 teaspoon grated ginger
1/4 cup maple syrup	1 cinnamon stick
1/4 cup white wine	2 cardamom pods, crushed
1/2 cup water	

Directions:
Combine all the ingredients in your Crock Pot. Cover with a lid and cook on low settings for 6 hours.   Allow to cool before serving.

319.   Chia Pudding

Servings: 4   Cooking Time: 1 Hour
Ingredients:

1 cup milk	¼ cup chia seeds
½ cup pumpkin puree	
2 tablespoons maple	½ teaspoon cinnamon powder

syrup
½ cup coconut milk

¼ teaspoon ginger, grated

Directions:
In your Crock Pot, mix milk with coconut milk, pumpkin puree, maple syrup, chia, cinnamon and ginger, stir, cover and cook on High for hour. Divide pudding into bowls and serve.
Nutrition Info:calories 105, fat 2, fiber 7, carbs 11, protein 4

320.   Passion Fruit Mousse

Servings: 6   Cooking Time: 1.5 Hours
Ingredients:

3 tablespoons corn starch	1 cup milk
5 oz passion fruit, puree	3 tablespoons sugar
	1 teaspoon vanilla extract

Directions:
Mix milk with sugar, vanilla extract, and corn starch.   Then pour the liquid in the Crock Pot and cook it on High for 1.5 hours.   Cool the liquid well and transfer in the serving glasses.   Top every glass with passion fruit puree.
Nutrition Info: Per Serving: 85 calories, 1.9g protein, 18.1g carbohydrates, 1g fat, 2.5g fiber, 3mg cholesterol, 26mg sodium, 107mg potassium.

321.   Apricot Marmelade

Servings: 6   Cooking Time: 2 Hours
Ingredients:

1 cup apricots, pitted, chopped	1 teaspoon vanilla extract
1 cup of sugar	1 tablespoon agar

Directions:
Put all ingredients in the Crock Pot and close the lid.   Cook the mixture on High for hours.   Then blend the mixture until smooth with the help of the immersion blender and pour in the silicone molds. Cool the marmalade until solid.
Nutrition Info: Per Serving: 139 calories, 0.3g protein, 36.3g carbohydrates, 0.2g fat, 0.5g fiber, 0mg cholesterol, 0mg sodium, 68mg potassium.

322.   Coffee Cookies

Servings: 12   Cooking Time: 4 Hours
Ingredients:

1 tablespoon coffee beans, grinded	2 eggs, beaten
1 teaspoon baking powder	2 cups flour
½ cup butter, softened	¼ cup of sugar
	1 teaspoon sunflower oil

Directions:
Brush the Crock Pot bowl with sunflower oil. Then mix all remaining ingredients in the mixing bowl.   Knead the dough and cut it into small pieces.   Roll the dough pieces into small balls and make the small cut in the center of every ball (to get the shape of the cocoa bean).   Put the cocoa beans in the Crock Pot in one layer and close the

lid.   Cook them on High for 2 hours.   Repeat the same steps with remaining cookies.
Nutrition Info: Per Serving: 174 calories, 3.2g protein, 20.3g carbohydrates, 9g fat, 0.6g fiber, 48mg cholesterol, 66mg sodium, 77mg potassium.

323.	Black Forest Cake

Servings: 8   Cooking Time: 4 1/4 Hours
Ingredients:

1 pound pitted cherries	3 eggs
2 tablespoons kirsch	1 cup all-purpose flour
1 tablespoon cornstarch	1/2 cup cocoa powder
1/2 cup butter, softened	1/2 teaspoon salt
3/4 cup white sugar	1 teaspoon baking powder
1 teaspoon vanilla extract	Whipped cream for serving

Directions:
Mix the cherries, kirsch and cornstarch in your Crock Pot.   For the batter, mix the butter, sugar and vanilla in a bowl until creamy. Add the eggs, one by one, then fold in the rest of the ingredients, trying to not over-mix the batter.   Spoon the batter over the cherries and cook for 4 hours on low settings.   Serve the cake chilled, topped with whipped cream.

324.	Double Chocolate Cake

Servings: 8   Cooking Time: 4 1/4 Hours
Ingredients:

1 1/2 cups all-purpose flour	1 cup water
1 1/2 teaspoons baking powder	1 cup sour cream
1/4 teaspoon salt	4 eggs
1/4 cup cocoa powder	1 teaspoon vanilla extract
1/2 cup vegetable oil	1 cup dark chocolate chips

Directions:
Mix the flour, baking powder, salt, cocoa powder in a bowl.   Stir in the water, oil, sour cream, eggs, vanilla extract and give it a quick mix.   Pour the batter in your Crock Pot and top with chocolate chips.   Cover and cook on low settings for hours. Allow the cake to cool before serving.

325.	Pear Apple Jam

Servings: 12   Cooking Time: 3 Hrs.
Ingredients:

8 pears, cored and cut into quarters	½ cup apple juice
2 apples, peeled, cored and quartered	1 tsp cinnamon, ground

Directions:
Toss pears, apples, apple juice, and cinnamon in the insert of Crock Pot.   Put the cooker's lid on and set the cooking time to 3 hours on High settings.   Blend this cooked pears-apples mixture to make a jam.   Allow it to cool them divide in the jars.   Serve.

Nutrition Info: Per Serving: Calories: 100, Total Fat: 1g, Fiber: 2g, Total Carbs: 20g, Protein: 3g

326.	Raspberry Poached Pears

Servings: 6   Cooking Time: 6 1/2 Hours
Ingredients:

1 cup fresh or frozen raspberries	1 cup white sugar
2 cups red wine	6 ripe but firm pears, peeled and cored
1 vanilla bean, split in half lengthwise	

Directions:
Combine all the ingredients in your Crock Pot. Cover and cook for 6 hours on low settings. Allow the pears to cool down before serving. Drizzle them with the sauce formed in the pot before serving.

327.	Crème Brule

Servings: 4   Cooking Time: 8 Hours
Ingredients:

6 egg yolks	½ cup of sugar
1 ½ cup heavy cream	1 teaspoon flour

Directions:
Blend the egg yolks with sugar until you get a smooth lemon color mixture.   Add heavy cream and flour. Mix the liquid until smooth.   Pour the liquid in the ramekins and place in the Crock Pot. Cover the ramekins with foil and close the lid of the Crock Pot.   Cook the dessert on Low for 8 hours.
Nutrition Info: Per Serving: 332 calories, 5g protein, 27.7g carbohydrates, 23.4g fat, 0g fiber, 376mg cholesterol, 29mg sodium, 62mg potassium.

328.	Rice Vanilla Pudding

Servings: 6   Cooking Time: 2 Hrs.
Ingredients:

1 tbsp butter	3 oz. sugar
7 oz. long-grain rice	1 egg
4 oz. water	1 tbsp cream
16 oz. milk	1 tsp vanilla extract

Directions:
Add rice, water, egg, cream, sugar, butter, milk, and vanilla to the insert of Crock Pot.   Put the cooker's lid on and set the cooking time to hours on High settings.   Serve when chilled.
Nutrition Info: Per Serving: Calories: 152, Total Fat: 4g, Fiber: 4g, Total Carbs: 6g, Protein: 4g

329.	Chocolate Mocha Bread Pudding

Servings: 6   Cooking Time: 4 1/4 Hours
Ingredients:

6 cups bread cubed	2 egg yolks
1 cup heavy cream	2 whole eggs
1 cup whole milk	1/2 cup white sugar
1 cup brewed coffee	

Directions:
Mix the cream, milk, coffee, egg yolks, eggs and sugar in a bowl.   Place the bread cubes in a Crock

Pot and pour the coffee mixture over it.   Cover and cook on low settings for 4 hours.   Allow the pudding to cool slightly before serving.

330.   Tangerine Cream Pie

Servings: 6   Cooking Time: 4.5 Hrs.

Ingredients:

8 oz tangerines, peeled and separated into pieces	1 cup flour
	¼ tsp salt
1 tsp baking soda	5 tbsp white sugar
1 tbsp vinegar	1 tsp vanilla extract
1 cup sour cream	2 eggs
	1 tsp butter

Directions:

Grease the insert of Crock Pot with butter and place tangerine pieces in it.   Whisk flour, baking soda, salt, sour cream whisked eggs, and vinegar in a bowl until smooth.   Spread this sour cream batter over the tangerines.   Put the cooker's lid on and set the cooking time to 5 hours on High settings.   Serve when chilled.

Nutrition Info: Per Serving: Calories: 201, Total Fat: 8.7g, Fiber: 1g, Total Carbs: 23.21g, Protein: 7g

331.   Lemon Poppy Seed Cake

Servings: 8   Cooking Time: 4 1/2 Hours

Ingredients:

3/4 cup butter, softened	1 teaspoon baking soda
3/4 cup white sugar	1/2 teaspoon baking powder
1 large lemon, zested and juiced	1/2 teaspoon salt
2 eggs	2 tablespoons poppy seeds
1 cup all-purpose flour	1 cup buttermilk
1/2 cup fine cornmeal	

Directions:

Mix the flour, cornmeal, baking soda, baking powder, salt and poppy seeds in a bowl. Combine the butter, sugar and lemon zest in a bowl and mix well for 5 minutes.   Add the eggs and lemon zest and mix well.   Fold in the flour mixture, alternating it with the buttermilk. Spoon the batter in your crock pot and cook on low settings for 4 hours.   Allow the cake to cool in the pot before slicing and serving.

332.   Milk Fondue

Servings: 3   Cooking Time: 4 Hours

Ingredients:

5 oz milk chocolate, chopped	1 teaspoon vanilla extract
1 tablespoon butter	¼ cup milk

Directions:

Put the chocolate in the Crock Pot in one layer. Then top it with butter, vanilla extract, and milk. Close the lid and cook the dessert on Low for 4 hours.   Gently stir the cooked fondue and transfer in the ramekins.

Nutrition Info: Per Serving: 301 calories, 4.3g protein, 29.3g carbohydrates, 18.3g fat, 1.6g fiber, 23mg cholesterol, 74mg sodium, 191mg potassium.

333.   Cheesecake With Lime Filling

Servings: 10   Cooking Time: 1 Hr.

Ingredients:

2 tbsp butter, melted	For the filling:
2 tsp sugar	1 lb. cream cheese
4 oz. almond meal	Zest of 1 lime
¼ cup coconut, shredded	Juice from 1 lime
	2 sachets lime jelly
Cooking spray	2 cup hot water

Directions:

Whisk coconut with butter, sugar, and almond meal in a bowl.   Grease the insert of Crock Pot with cooking spray.   Spread the coconut mixture in the greased cooker.   Now beat cream cheese with lime zest, lime juice, and jelly in a separate bowl.   Spread this cream cheese mixture over the coconut crust.   Put the cooker's lid on and set the cooking time to 1 hour on High settings. Refrigerate the cooked cheesecake for 2 hours. Slice and serve.

Nutrition Info: Per Serving: Calories: 300, Total Fat: 23g, Fiber: 2g, Total Carbs: 5g, Protein: 7g

334.   Berry Pudding

Servings: 2   Cooking Time: 5 Hours

Ingredients:

¼ cup strawberries, chopped	1 tablespoon corn starch
2 tablespoons sugar	1 teaspoon vanilla extract
2 cups of milk	

Directions:

Mix milk with corn starch and pour liquid in the Crock Pot.   Add vanilla extract, sugar, and strawberries.   Close the lid and cook the pudding on low for 5 hours.   Carefully mix the dessert before serving.

Nutrition Info: Per Serving: 196 calories, 8.1g protein, 30.2g carbohydrates, 5.1g fat, 0.4g fiber, 20mg cholesterol, 115mg sodium, 171mg potassium.

335.   Nutty Pear Streusel Dessert

Servings: 4   Cooking Time: 4 1/2 Hours

Ingredients:

4 large apples, peeled and cubed	1 cup ground almonds
1/2 cup golden raisins	2 tablespoons all-purpose flour
1 teaspoon cinnamon powder	2 tablespoons melted butter
1/2 cup pecans, chopped	2 tablespoons brown sugar
	1 pinch salt

Directions:

Mix the apples, raisins and cinnamon in your Crock Pot.   For the topping, combine the pecans, almonds, flour, melted butter, sugar and salt and rub the mix well with your fingertips.   Spread this mixture over the pears and cook for 4 hours on low settings.   This dessert is best served chilled.

336.   Cinnamon Plums

Servings: 2   Cooking Time: 2 Hours
Ingredients:
- ½ pound plums, pitted and halved
- 2 tablespoons sugar
- 1 teaspoon cinnamon, ground
- ½ cup orange juice

Directions:
In your Crock Pot, mix the plums with the cinnamon and the other ingredients, toss, put the lid on and cook on Low for 2 hours.   Divide into bowls and serve as a dessert.
Nutrition Info:calories 180, fat 2, fiber 1, carbs 8, protein 8

337.   Mint Cookies

Servings: 6   Cooking Time: 3.5 Hours
Ingredients:
- 1 teaspoon dried mint
- ½ cup buttermilk
- 1 tablespoon olive oil
- 2 eggs, beaten
- 1 cup flour
- 4 tablespoons brown sugar
- 4 tablespoons flax meal
- 1 teaspoon baking powder

Directions:
Put all ingredients in the mixing bowl.   Knead the soft dough.   Then line the Crock Pot with baking paper.   Cut the dough into small pieces and roll them in the balls.   Put the balls in the Crock Pot one-by-one.   Close the lid and cook the cookies on High for 3.5 hours.
Nutrition Info: Per Serving: 169 calories, 5.7g protein, 24.6g carbohydrates, 5.8g fat, 1.9g fiber, 55mg cholesterol, 45mg sodium, 204mg potassium.

338.   Banana Chia Seeds Pudding

Servings: 2   Cooking Time: 5 Hours
Ingredients:
- 4 tablespoons chia seeds
- 1 cup milk
- 2 bananas, chopped

Directions:
Mix milk with chia seeds and pour in the Crock Pot. Cook the liquid on Low for 5 hours.   Meanwhile, put the chopped bananas in the bottom of glass jars.   When the pudding is cooked, pour it over the bananas.
Nutrition Info: Per Serving: 304 calories, 10g protein, 44.9g carbohydrates, 11.6g fat, 12.8g fiber, 10mg cholesterol, 63mg sodium, 608mg potassium.

339.   Rhubarb Muffins

Servings: 4   Cooking Time: 3 Hours
Ingredients:
- 1 egg, beaten
- ½ cup skim milk
- 1 teaspoon baking powder
- ½ cup flour
- ½ cup rhubarb, diced
- 1 tablespoon olive oil

Directions:
Put all ingredients except rhubarb in the mixing bowl.   Stir them carefully until you get a smooth mass.   After this, add rhubarb and mix.   Fill ½ part of every muffin mold with muffin batter and transfer in the Crock Pot.   Cook the muffin on High for 3 hours.
Nutrition Info: Per Serving: 118 calories, 4.1g protein, 14.8g carbohydrates, 4.8g fat, 0.7g fiber, 42mg cholesterol, 34mg sodium, 249mg potassium.

340.   Hazelnut Crumble Cheesecake

Servings: 8   Cooking Time: 6 1/2 Hours
Ingredients:
Crust and topping:
- 3/4 cup butter, chilled and cubed
- 1 1/4 cups all-purpose flour
- 1 cup ground hazelnuts
- 1/4 cup buttermilk
- 1 pinch salt
- 2 tablespoons light brown sugar

Filling:
- 20 oz. cream cheese
- 1/2 cup sour cream
- 1/2 cup white sugar
- 1 teaspoon vanilla extract
- 2 tablespoons Grand Marnier
- 1 tablespoon cornstarch
- 2 eggs

Directions:
For the crust and topping, combine all the ingredients in a food processor and pulse until a dough comes together. Cut the dough in half. Wrap one half in plastic wrap and place in the fridge. The remaining dough, roll it into a thin sheet and place it in your Crock Pot, trimming the edges if needed. For the filling, mix all the ingredients in a large bowl. Pour this mixture over the crust.   For the topping, remove the dough from the fridge then grate it on a large grater over the cheesecake filling. Cover the pot and bake for 6 hours on low settings. Allow to cool completely before slicing and serving.

341.   Dulce De Leche

Servings: 4   Cooking Time: 8 Hours
Ingredients:
- 1 can (14 oz.) sweetened condensed milk
- Water as needed

Directions:
Make 2-3 holes in the condensed milk can, preferably on the top side.   Place the can in your Crock Pot and add enough water to cover it 3/4. Cover the crock pot with its lid and cook on low settings for 8 hours.   Serve the dulce de leche chilled.

342.   Sweet Chai Latte

Servings: 4   Cooking Time: 4 Hours
Ingredients:

2 tablespoons black tea	2 cups of water
2 tablespoons chai latte spices	1 cup milk
	4 teaspoons sugar

Directions:
Put black tea in the Crock Pot.   Add water, milk, and sugar.   Close the lid and cook the mixture on High for 2 hours.   Then sieve the liquid and return in the Crock Pot.   Add spices and carefully mix them.   Cook the drink on Low for 2 hours.
Nutrition Info: Per Serving: 68 calories, 2.3g protein, 11g carbohydrates, 1.6g fat, 0g fiber, 5mg cholesterol, 38mg sodium, 39mg potassium.

343.   Apricot Marmalade

Servings: 2   Cooking Time: 3 Hours
Ingredients:

1 cup apricots, chopped	2 tablespoons lemon juice
½ cup water	1 teaspoon fruit pectin
1 teaspoon vanilla extract	2 cups sugar

Directions:
In your Crock Pot, mix the apricots with the water, vanilla and the other ingredients, whisk, put the lid on and cook on High for 3 hours.   Stir the marmalade, divide into bowls and serve cold.
Nutrition Info:calories 100, fat 1, fiber 2, carbs 20, protein 1

344.   Maple Plums And Mango

Servings: 2   Cooking Time: 1 Hour
Ingredients:

2 teaspoons orange zest	1 cup mango, peeled and cubed
1 tablespoon orange juice	1 tablespoon maple syrup
1 cup plums, pitted and halved	3 tablespoons sugar

Directions:
In your Crock Pot, mix the plums with the mango and the other ingredients, toss, put the lid on and cook on High for hour.   Divide into bowls and serve cold
Nutrition Info:calories 123, fat 1, fiber 2, carbs 20, protein 3

345.   Pear Walnut Cake

Servings: 8   Cooking Time: 4 1/2 Hours
Ingredients:

1 cup butter, softened	1/4 teaspoon salt
1 cup white sugar	1 teaspoon baking powder
3 eggs	
1 cup all-purpose flour	1/2 teaspoon cinnamon powder
1 cup ground walnuts	4 ripe pears, peeled, cored and sliced
1/4 cup cocoa powder	

Directions:
Mix the butter and sugar in a bowl until creamy and pale. Add the eggs one by one and mix well. Fold in the flour, walnuts, cocoa powder, salt, baking powder and cinnamon with a spatula. Spoon the batter in your Crock Pot and top with pear slices.   Bake in the crock pot for hours on low settings.   Allow the cake to cool in the pot before slicing.

346.   Vanilla And Cocoa Pudding

Servings: 2   Cooking Time: 7 Hours
Ingredients:

1 cup of coconut milk	1 tablespoon brown sugar
1 tablespoon cornflour	1 tablespoon butter
1 teaspoon vanilla extract	2 tablespoons cocoa powder

Directions:
Mix coconut milk with cocoa powder, brown sugar, vanilla extract, and cornflour.   Whisk the mixture until smooth and transfer in the Crock Pot.   Add butter and close the lid.   Cook the pudding on Low for 7 hours.   Then transfer it in the serving bowls and cool to the room temperature.
Nutrition Info: Per Serving: 375 calories, 4.1g protein, 17.1g carbohydrates, 35.2g fat, 4.5g fiber, 15mg cholesterol, 62mg sodium, 473mg potassium.

347.   Glazed Bacon

Servings: 4   Cooking Time: 2 Hours
Ingredients:

4 bacon slices	5 tablespoons maple syrup
1 tablespoon butter	
3 tablespoons water	

Directions:
Put all ingredients in the Crock Pot.   Close the lid and cook the dessert on High for hours.   Then transfer the bacon in the serving plates and top with maple syrup mixture from the Crock Pot.
Nutrition Info: Per Serving: 193 calories, 7.1g protein, 17g carbohydrates, 10.9g fat, 0g fiber, 29mg cholesterol, 462mg sodium, 159mg potassium.

348.   Strawberry Marmalade

Servings: 8   Cooking Time: 4 Hours
Ingredients:

| 2 cups strawberries, chopped | ¼ cup lemon juice |
| 1 cup of sugar | 2 oz water |

Directions:
Put all ingredients in the Crock Pot and gently mix. Then close the lid and cook the mixture on low for 4 hours.   Transfer the cooked mixture in the silicone molds and leave to cool for up to 8 hours.
Nutrition Info: Per Serving: 107 calories, 0.3g protein, 27.9g carbohydrates, 0.2g fat, 0.8g fiber, 0mg cholesterol, 2mg sodium, 65mg potassium.

349.   Coconut Pudding

Servings: 4   Cooking Time: 1 Hour
Ingredients:

1 and 2/3 cups coconut milk
1 tablespoon gelatin
6 tablespoons sugar

3 egg yolks
½ teaspoon vanilla extract

Directions:
In a bowl, mix gelatin with tablespoon coconut milk and stir.   Put the rest of the milk in your Crock Pot, add whisked egg yolks, gelatin, vanilla and sugar, stir everything, cover, cook on High for 1 hour, divide into bowls and serve cold.
Nutrition Info:calories 170, fat 2, fiber 0, carbs 6, protein 2

350.   Raisin Bake

Servings: 4   Cooking Time: 6 Hours
Ingredients:
1 cup cottage cheese
2 oz raisins, chopped
1 egg, beaten
3 tablespoons sugar, powdered

1 teaspoon vanilla extract
1 teaspoon peanuts, chopped

Directions:
The Crock Pot with baking paper.   Then mix all ingredients in the bowl and mix until smooth. Transfer the mixture in the Crock Pot and flatten the surface of it well.   Close the lid and cook the bake on Low for 6 hours.
Nutrition Info: Per Serving: 150 calories, 9.8g protein, 22.6g carbohydrates, 2.6g fat, 0.6g fiber, 45mg cholesterol, 247mg sodium, 182mg potassium.

351.   Plum Pie

Servings: 6   Cooking Time: 2 Hours
Ingredients:
1 cup flour
¼ cup butter, melted
2 eggs, beaten
¼ cup of sugar

1 teaspoon ground nutmeg
½ cup plums, pitted, chopped

Directions:
Put flour, eggs, butter, and sugar in the food processor.   Blend the mixture until smooth. Add ground nutmeg and stir it.   Then transfer the mixture in the Crock Pot and top with plums. Close the lid and cook the pie on High for 2 hours.
Nutrition Info: Per Serving: 200 calories, 4.1g protein, 25.2g carbohydrates, 9.5g fat, 0.7g fiber, 75mg cholesterol, 76mg sodium, 54mg potassium.

352.   Rich Chocolate Peanut Butter Cake

Servings: 8   Cooking Time: 2 3/4 Hours
Ingredients:
1 1/2 cups all-purpose flour
1/4 cup cocoa powder
1 teaspoon baking powder
1/2 teaspoon baking

1 cup smooth peanut butter
1/4 cup butter, softened
3/4 cup white sugar
3 eggs
3/4 cup sour cream

soda
1/4 teaspoon salt
Directions:
Mix the peanut butter, butter and sugar in a bowl until creamy.   Add the eggs, one by one, then fold in the flour, cocoa powder, baking powder, baking soda and salt.   Finally, add the sour cream and mix on high speed for   seconds.   Spoon the batter in your Crock Pot and cook on high settings for 2 1/hours.   The cake is best served chilled.

353.   Cinnamon Apples

Servings: 2   Cooking Time: 2 Hours
Ingredients:
2 tablespoons brown sugar
1 pound apples, cored and cut into wedges
1 tablespoon cinnamon powder
2 tablespoons walnuts, chopped

A pinch of nutmeg, ground
½ tablespoon lemon juice
¼ cup water
2 apples, cored and tops cut off

Directions:
In your Crock Pot, mix the apples with the sugar, cinnamon and the other ingredients, toss, put the lid on and cook on High for 2 hours.   Divide the mix between plates and serve.
Nutrition Info:calories 189, fat 4, fiber 7, carbs 19, protein 2

354.   Braised Pears

Servings: 6   Cooking Time: 2.5 Hours
Ingredients:
6 pears
2 cups wine

1 tablespoon sugar
1 cinnamon stick

Directions:
Cut the pears into halves and put them in the Crock Pot.   Add all remaining ingredients and close the lid.   Cook the pears on High for 2.5 hours. Serve the pears with hot wine mixture.
Nutrition Info: Per Serving: 210 calories, 1.1g protein, 38g carbohydrates, 1.1g fat, 6.5g fiber, 0mg cholesterol, 29mg sodium, 320mg potassium.

355.   Chocolate Pear Crumble

Servings: 6   Cooking Time: 4 1/2 Hours
Ingredients:
6 ripe pears, peeled, cored and sliced
1/4 cup light brown sugar
1 tablespoon cornstarch
1/2 cup cocoa powder

3/4 cup all-purpose flour
1/4 teaspoon salt
1/2 teaspoon baking powder
1/2 cup butter, chilled and cubed

Directions:
Mix the pears, sugar and cornstarch in your Crock Pot.   For the crumble topping, mix the flour, cocoa powder, salt and baking powder in a bowl. Add the butter and mix well until the mixture looks grainy.   Spread this mixture over the pears then

cover the pot and cook for hours on low settings. The dessert is best served slightly warm or chilled.

356. Spiced Peach Crisp

Servings: 6   Cooking Time: 3.5 Hrs.

Ingredients:

1 lb. peaches, pitted and sliced	1 tsp vinegar
¼ cup of sugar	1/3 cup flour
4 tbsp lemon juice	3 tbsp butter
1 tsp vanilla extract	1 tsp ground ginger
5 oz oats	½ tsp pumpkin pie seasoning
1 tsp baking soda	

Directions:

Grease the insert of Crock Pot with butter.   Place the peach slices in the insert and top them with sugar and lemon juice.   Toss oats with vanilla extract, vinegar, baking soda, flour, ground ginger, pumpkin pie seasoning in a bowl.   Spread this oats spice mixture on top of the peaches.   Put the cooker's lid on and set the cooking time to 1.hours on High settings.   Remove the lid and stir the cooked mixture well.   Cover again and continue cooking for another 2 hours on High settings. Serve.

Nutrition Info: Per Serving: Calories: 212, Total Fat: 7.6g, Fiber: 5g, Total Carbs: 41.26g, Protein: 5g

357. Stuffed Apples

Servings: 5   Cooking Time: 1 Hour And 30 Minutes

Ingredients:

5 apples, tops cut off and cored	¼ teaspoon nutmeg, ground
5 figs	½ teaspoon cinnamon powder
1/3 cup sugar	1 tablespoon lemon juice
1 teaspoon dried ginger	1tablespoon vegetable oil
¼ cup pecans, chopped	½ cup water
2 teaspoons lemon zest, grated	

Directions:

In a bowl, mix figs with sugar, ginger, pecans, lemon zest, nutmeg, cinnamon, oil and lemon juice, whisk really well, stuff your apples with this mix and put them in your Crock Pot.   Add the water, cover, cook on High for 1 hour and 30 minutes, divide between dessert plates and serve.

Nutrition Info: calories 200, fat 1, fiber 2, carbs 4, protein 7

358. Creamy Caramel Dessert

Servings: 2   Cooking Time: 2 Hrs.

Ingredients:

1 and ½ tsp caramel extract	For the caramel sauce:
1 cup of water	2 tbsp sugar
2 oz. cream cheese	2 tbsp butter, melted
2 eggs	¼ tsp caramel extract
1 and ½ tbsp sugar	

Directions:

Blend cream cheese with ½ tbsp sugar, 1 ½ tsp caramel extract, water, and eggs in a blender. Transfer this mixture to the insert of Crock Pot. Put the cooker's lid on and set the cooking time to 2 hours on High settings.   Divide this cream cheese mixture into the serving cups.   Now mix melted butter with caramel extract and sugar in a bowl. Pour this caramel sauce over the cream cheese mixture.   Refrigerate the caramel cream for 1 hour.   Serve.

Nutrition Info: Per Serving: Calories: 254, Total Fat: 24g, Fiber: 1g, Total Carbs: 6g, Protein: 8g

359. Avocado Peppermint Pudding

Servings: 3   Cooking Time: 1 Hr.

Ingredients:

½ cup vegetable oil	14 oz. coconut milk
½ tbsp sugar	1 avocado, pitted, peeled and chopped
1 tbsp cocoa powder	1 tbsp sugar
For the pudding:	
1 tsp peppermint oil	

Directions:

Start by mixing vegetable oil, ½ tbsp sugar, and cocoa powder in a bowl.   Spread this mixture in a container and refrigerate for 1 hour.   Blend this mixture with coconut milk, avocado, 1 tbsp sugar, peppermint oil in a blender.   Transfer this mixture to the insert of the Crock Pot.   Put the cooker's lid on and set the cooking time to 1 hour on Low settings.   Stir in chocolate chips then divide the pudding the serving bowls. Refrigerate for 1 hour then enjoy.

Nutrition Info: Per Serving: Calories: 140, Total Fat: 3g, Fiber: 2g, Total Carbs: 3g, Protein: 4g

360. Carrot Cake

Servings: 12   Cooking Time: 2 3/4 Hours

Ingredients:

3/4 cup white sugar	1/2 teaspoon ground ginger
1/4 cup dark brown sugar	1 teaspoon cinnamon powder
2 eggs	1/4 teaspoon cardamom powder
1/2 cup canola oil	1/2 teaspoon salt
1 teaspoon vanilla extract	1 cup grated carrots
1 1/2 cups all-purpose flour	1 cup crushed pineapple, drained
1 teaspoon baking powder	1/2 cup pecans, chopped
1/2 teaspoon baking soda	

Directions:

Mix the two types of sugar, eggs, canola oil and vanilla in a bowl until creamy.   Fold in the flour, baking powder, baking soda, ginger, cinnamon, cardamom powder and salt then add the carrots, crushed pineapple and pecans.   Pour the batter in your Crock Pot and cook for 2 1/4 hours on high settings.   Allow the cake to cool in the pot before slicing and serving.

361.   Rhubarb Stew

Servings: 2   Cooking Time: 2 Hours
Ingredients:

½ pound rhubarb, roughly sliced	½ teaspoon lemon extract
2 tablespoons sugar	1 tablespoon lemon juice
½ teaspoon vanilla extract	¼ cup water

Directions:
In your Crock Pot, mix the rhubarb with the sugar, vanilla and the other ingredients, toss, put the lid on and cook on Low for 2 hours.   Divide the mix into bowls and serve cold.
Nutrition Info:calories 60, fat 1, fiber 0, carbs 10, protein 1

362.   Pear Blueberry Cake

Servings: 8   Cooking Time: 4 1/2 Hours
Ingredients:

3/4 cup butter, softened	1/4 cup cornstarch
1 cup white sugar	1 teaspoon baking powder
1 teaspoon vanilla extract	1/2 teaspoon salt
3 eggs	2 ripe pears, peeled, cored and diced
1 cup all-purpose flour	1 cup fresh or frozen blueberries

Directions:
Mix the butter, sugar and vanilla in a bowl for 5 minutes until creamy.   Stir in the eggs, one by one, then add the dry ingredients.   Fold in the pears and blueberries then spoon the batter in a greased Crock Pot.   Cover the pot and cook on low settings for hours.   Allow the cake to cool in the pot before serving.

363.   Cherry Bowls

Servings: 2   Cooking Time: 1 Hour
Ingredients:

1 cup cherries, pitted	1 tablespoon sugar
½ cup red cherry juice	2 tablespoons maple syrup

Directions:
In your Crock Pot, mix the cherries with the sugar and the other ingredients, toss gently, put the lid on, cook on High for hour, divide into bowls and serve.
Nutrition Info:calories 200, fat 1, fiber 4, carbs 5, protein 2

364.   Vegan Mousse

Servings: 3   Cooking Time: 2 Hours
Ingredients:

2 tablespoons corn starch	1 cup of coconut milk
1 teaspoon vanilla extract	1 avocado, pitted, pilled

Directions:
Mix coconut milk and corn starch until smooth and pour in the Crock Pot.   Add vanilla extract and cook it on High for hours.   Then cool the mixture till room temperature and mix with avocado. Blend the mousse until fluffy and smooth.
Nutrition Info: Per Serving: 348 calories, 3.1g protein, 16.4g carbohydrates, 32.1g fat, 6.3g fiber, 0mg cholesterol, 16mg sodium, 537mg potassium.

365.   Marshmallow Hot Drink

Servings: 3   Cooking Time: 5 Hours
Ingredients:

½ cup of chocolate chips	1 teaspoon butter
4 oz marshmallows	2 cups of milk

Directions:
Put all ingredients in the Crock Pot and close the lid.   Cook the drink on Low for 5 hours. Stir it every hours.
Nutrition Info: Per Serving: 364 calories, 7.8g protein, 54.g carbohydrates, 13g fat, 1g fiber, 23mg cholesterol, 138mg sodium, 200mg potassium.

366.   Dump Cake

Servings: 8   Cooking Time: 5 Hours
Ingredients:

1 teaspoon vanilla extract	1 cupcake mix
½ teaspoon ground nutmeg	2 eggs, beaten
1 tablespoon butter, melted	1 teaspoon lemon zest, grated
	½ cup heavy cream
	4 pecans, chopped

Directions:
In the bowl mix all ingredients except pecans. The line the Crock Pot with baking paper and pour the dough inside.   Flatten the batter and top with pecans.   Close the lid and cook the dump cake for 5 hours on Low.   Cook the cooked cake well before serving.
Nutrition Info: Per Serving: 245 calories, 3.8g protein, 27g carbohydrates, 13.9g fat, 1.1g fiber, 55mg cholesterol, 246mg sodium, 90mg potassium

367.   Cashew Cake

Servings: 6   Cooking Time: 2 Hours
Ingredients:

For the crust:	
½ cup dates, pitted	2 and ½ cups cashews, soaked for 8 hours
1 tablespoon water	
½ teaspoon vanilla	1 cup blueberries
½ cup almonds	¾ cup maple syrup
For the cake:	1 tablespoon vegetable oil

Directions:
In your blender, mix dates with water, vanilla and almonds, pulse well, transfer dough to a working surface, flatten and arrange on the bottom of your Crock Pot.   In your blender, mix maple syrup

with the oil, cashews and blueberries, blend well, spread over crust, cover and cook on High for hours. Leave the cake to cool down, slice and serve.
Nutrition Info:calories 200, fat 3, fiber 5, carbs 12, protein 3

368. Cinnamon Giant Cookie

Servings: 6   Cooking Time: 4 Hours
Ingredients:

5 tablespoons coconut oil	5 tablespoons sugar
1 tablespoon ground ginger	1 cup flour
½ teaspoon ground cinnamon	1 egg, beaten
	1 teaspoon baking powder
	½ cup half and half

Directions:
Put all ingredients in the food processor. Blend the mixture until you get a smooth dough. Then line the bottom of the Crock Pot with baking paper and put the dough inside. Flatten it in the shape of a cookie. Cook the cookie on Low for 4 hours. Then cool the cookie and cut it into servings.
Nutrition Info: Per Serving: 252 calories, 3.8g protein, 28g carbohydrates, 14.6g fat, 0.8g fiber, 35mg cholesterol, 20mg sodium, 155mg potassium.

369. Vanilla Cookies

Servings: 12   Cooking Time: 2 Hours And 30 Minutes
Ingredients:

2 eggs	1 cup sugar
¼ cup vegetable oil	1 and ½ cups almond meal
½ teaspoon vanilla extract	½ cup almonds, chopped
1 teaspoon baking powder	

Directions:
In a bowl, mix oil with sugar, vanilla extract and eggs and whisk. Add baking powder, almond meal and almonds and stir well. Line your Crock Pot with parchment paper, spread cookie mix on the bottom of the Crock Pot, cover and cook on Low for 2 hours and minutes. Leave cookie sheet to cool down, cut into medium pieces and serve.
Nutrition Info:calories 220, fat 2, fiber 1, carbs 3, protein 6

370. Honey Pasta Casserole

Servings: 6   Cooking Time: 3 Hours
Ingredients:

8 oz pasta, cooked, chopped	½ cup plain yogurt
3 tablespoons of liquid honey	2 eggs, beaten
2 tablespoons ricotta cheese	1 teaspoon vanilla extract
	1 tablespoon butter, melted

Directions:
Mix pasta with eggs, yogurt, and vanilla extract. Add ricotta cheese and stir it little. Then pour butter in the Crock Pot. Add pasta mixture and flatten it. Close the lid and cook the casserole on High for 3 hours. Then cut the casserole into servings and top with honey.
Nutrition Info: Per Serving: 202 calories, 7.9g protein, 31.3g carbohydrates, 4.9g fat, 0g fiber, 31.3mg cholesterol, 65mg sodium, 149mg potassium.

371.Mango Cream Dessert

Servings: 4   Cooking Time: 1 Hr.
Ingredients:

1 mango, sliced	14 oz. coconut cream

Directions:
Add mango and cream to the insert of Crock Pot. Put the cooker's lid on and set the cooking time to 1 hour on High settings. Serve.
Nutrition Info: Per Serving: Calories: 150, Total Fat: 12g, Fiber: 2g, Total Carbs: 6g, Protein: 1g

372. White Chocolate Apricot Bread Pudding

Servings: 8   Cooking Time: 5 1/2 Hours
Ingredients:

8 cups one day old bread cubes	1 cup heavy cream
1 cup dried apricots, diced	4 eggs
	1 teaspoon vanilla extract
1 cup white chocolate chips	1 teaspoon orange zest
2 cups milk	1/2 cup white sugar

Directions:
Mix the bread, apricots and chocolate chips in your Crock Pot. Combine the milk, cream, eggs, vanilla, orange zest and sugar in a bowl. Pour this mixture over the bread pudding then cover the pot with a lid and cook on low settings for 5 hours. The pudding is best served slightly warm.

373. Apple Dump Cake

Servings: 8   Cooking Time: 4 1/2 Hours
Ingredients:

6 Granny Smith apples, peeled, cored and sliced	1 teaspoon cinnamon
	1 box yellow cake mix
1/4 cup light brown sugar	1/2 cup butter, melted

Directions:
Mix the apples, brown sugar and cinnamon in a Crock Pot. Top with the cake mix and drizzle with butter. Cover the pot and cook on low settings for 4 hours. Allow the cake to cool in the pot before serving.

374. Mexican Chocolate Cake

Servings: 8   Cooking Time: 6 1/4 Hours
Ingredients:

1 cup all-purpose flour	1 cup buttermilk
1/2 cup cocoa powder	2 eggs
1 teaspoon baking	1/2 cup corn oil
	1 teaspoon vanilla

soda
1/4 teaspoon salt
1/4 teaspoon chili powder

extract
1 cup dulce de leche
to frost the cake

Directions:
Mix the dry ingredients in your Crock Pot.   Add the wet ingredients and give it a quick mix just until combined.   Pour the batter in a grease Crock Pot and bake for 6 hours on low settings. Allow the cake to cool completely then frost it with dulce de leche.   Slice and serve fresh.

375.   Coconut And Mango Mousse

Servings: 3   Cooking Time: 7 Hours
Ingredients:
1 cup coconut cream
3 egg yolks
1 teaspoon vanilla extract

3 tablespoons sugar
1 mango, peeled, chopped, pureed

Directions:
Mix egg yolks with sugar and blend until smooth. Pour the liquid in the Crock Pot, add coconut cream, and stir carefully.   Close the lid and cook it on Low for 7 hours.   After this, stir the mixture well and pour in the glasses.   Add mango puree.
Nutrition Info: Per Serving: 354 calories, 5.5g protein, 34g carbohydrates, 24g fat, 3.6g fiber, 210mg cholesterol, 21mg sodium, 419mg potassium.

376.   Nuts Brownies

Servings: 6   Cooking Time: 2.5 Hours
Ingredients:
3 tablespoons cocoa powder
1 tablespoon apple cider vinegar
1 teaspoon baking powder

3 oz nuts, chopped
1 cup flour
4 eggs, beaten
½ cup skim milk
½ cup of sugar

Directions:
Mix cocoa powder with flour and sugar.   Add apple cider vinegar, baking powder, and skim milk. Mix the mixture until you get the smooth batter. Then add nuts and carefully mix the batter.   Put the baking paper at the bottom of the Crock Pot. Add chocolate batter and close the lid.   Cook the brownies on High for 2.5 hours.   Then cool the dessert well and cut into bars.
Nutrition Info: Per Serving: 279 calories, 9.5g protein, 39.3g carbohydrates, 10.8g fat, 2.7g fiber, 110mg cholesterol, 149mg sodium, 331mg potassium.

377.   Coconut Shaped Cake

Servings: 6   Cooking Time: 1.5 Hours
Ingredients:
1 cup cream
4 tablespoons coconut shred

¼ cup condensed milk
2 tablespoons gelatin
2 tablespoons agar

Directions:
Pour cream in the Crock Pot. Add agar and mix it until smooth.   Close the lid and cook it on high for 1.5 hours.   When the time is finished, pour ½ part of all cream in the silicone mold and freeze it until solid.   Then mix condensed milk with gelatin and microwave for 2 minutes.   Carefully mix and cool the mixture.   Pour it over the frozen cream and return in the freezer for 25 minutes. Pour the remaining cream over the condensed milk.   Add coconut shred.   Refrigerate the cake until solid.
Nutrition Info: Per Serving: 108 calories, 3.3g protein, 9.6g carbohydrates, 6.7g fat, 0.7g fiber, 12mg cholesterol, 36mg sodium, 66mg potassium.

378.   Autumnal Bread Pudding

Servings: 8   Cooking Time: 5 1/2 Hours
Ingredients:
2 red apples, peeled and diced
2 pears, peeled and diced
1/2 cup golden raisins
1/4 cup butter, melted

16 oz. bread cubes
2 cups whole milk
4 eggs, beaten
1/2 cup white sugar
1 teaspoon vanilla extract
1/2 teaspoon cinnamon powder

Directions:
Mix the bread cubes, apples, pears and raisins in your Crock Pot.   Combine the butter, milk, eggs, sugar, vanilla and cinnamon in a bowl. Pour this mixture over the bread.   Cover the pot and cook on low settings for 5 hours.   Serve the bread pudding slightly warm.

379.   Avocado Pudding

Servings: 3   Cooking Time: 1 Hour
Ingredients:
½ cup vegetable oil
½ tablespoon sugar
1 tablespoon cocoa powder
1 teaspoon peppermint oil

For the pudding:
14 ounces coconut milk
1 avocado, pitted, peeled and chopped
1 tablespoon sugar

Directions:
In a bowl, mix vegetable oil with cocoa powder and ½ tablespoon sugar, stir well, transfer to a lined container, keep in the fridge for hour and chop into small pieces.   In your blender, mix coconut milk with avocado, 1 tablespoon sugar and peppermint oil, pulse well, transfer to your Crock Pot, cook on Low for 1 hour and mix with the chocolate chips you made at the beginning.   Divide pudding into bowls and keep in the fridge for 1 more hour before serving.
Nutrition Info:calories 140, fat 3, fiber 2, carbs 3, protein 4

380.   Cranberry Cookies

Servings: 6   Cooking Time: 2.5 Hours
Ingredients:

2 oz dried cranberries, chopped
3 tablespoons peanut butter
1 cup flour
1 teaspoon baking powder
3 tablespoons sugar
1 tablespoon cream cheese

Directions:
Mix peanut butter with flour, baking powder, and sugar.   Add cream cheese and cranberries and knead the dough.   Make the small balls and press them gently to get the shape of the cookies.   After this, line the Crock Pot bowl with baking paper. Put the cookies inside and close the lid.   Cook the cookies on high for 2.5 hours.

Nutrition Info: Per Serving: 157 calories, 4.3g protein, 24.8g carbohydrates, 4.8g fat, 1.4g fiber, 2mg cholesterol, 43mg sodium, 176mg potassium.

381.	Hazelnut Liqueur Cheesecake

Servings: 8   Cooking Time: 6 1/2 Hours
Ingredients:

Crust:
1 cup graham crackers, crushed
1 cup ground hazelnuts
1/4 cup butter, melted
Filling:
20 oz. cream cheese
1/2 cup hazelnut butter
1/4 cup hazelnut liqueur
1/4 cup light brown sugar
1/2 cup white sugar
4 eggs
1/2 cup heavy cream
1 pinch salt
1 teaspoon vanilla extract

Directions:
For the crust, mix the crackers, hazelnuts and butter in a bowl. Transfer the mix in your Crock Pot and press it well on the bottom of the pot.   For the filling, mix the cream cheese, hazelnut butter, liqueur, sugars, eggs, cream, salt and vanilla and mix well.   Pour the mixture over the crust and cook in the covered pot for 6 hours on low settings. Serve the cheesecake chilled.

382.	Chocolate Mango Mix

Servings: 2   Cooking Time: 1 Hour
Ingredients:

1/4 cup dark chocolate, cut into chunks
1 cup mango, peeled and chopped
1 cup crème fraiche
2 tablespoons sugar
1/2 teaspoon almond extract

Directions:
In your Crock Pot, mix the crème fraiche with the chocolate and the other ingredients, toss, put the lid on and cook on Low for hour.   Blend using an immersion blender, divide into bowls and serve.
Nutrition Info:calories 200, fat 12, fiber 4, carbs 7, protein 3

383.	Rice Pudding

Servings: 6   Cooking Time: 2 Hours
Ingredients:

1 tablespoon butter
7 ounces long grain rice
4 ounces water
16 ounces milk
3 ounces sugar
1 egg
1 tablespoon cream
1 teaspoon vanilla extract

Directions:
In your Crock Pot, mix butter with rice, water, milk, sugar, egg, cream and vanilla, stir, cover and cook on High for 2 hours.   Stir pudding one more time, divide into bowls and serve.
Nutrition Info:calories 152, fat 4, fiber 4, carbs 6, protein 4

384.	Browned Butter Pumpkin Cheesecake

Servings: 8   Cooking Time: 6 1/2 Hours
Ingredients:

Crust:
1 1/4 cups crushed graham crackers
1/2 cup butter
Filling:
1 cup pumpkin puree
24 oz. cream cheese
1/2 cup light brown sugar
4 eggs
1 pinch salt
1 teaspoon cinnamon powder
1 teaspoon ground ginger
1/2 teaspoon cardamom powder
1/4 cup butter

Directions:
To make the curst, start by browning the butter. Place the butter in a saucepan and cook for a few minutes until it starts to look golden. Allow to cool slightly.   Mix the browned butter with crushed crackers then transfer the mixture in your crock pot and press it well on the bottom of the pot.   For the filling, brown 1/4 cup butter as described above then stir in the pumpkin puree, cream cheese, eggs, sugar, salt, cinnamon, ginger and cardamom. Pour the mixture over the curst and cook on low settings for 6 hours.   Allow the cheesecake to cool down before slicing and serving.

385.	Strawberry Cake

Servings: 2   Cooking Time: 1 Hour
Ingredients:

1/4 cup coconut flour
1/4 teaspoon baking soda
1 tablespoon sugar
1/4 cup strawberries, chopped
1/2 cup coconut milk
1 teaspoon butter, melted
1/2 teaspoon lemon zest, grated
1/4 teaspoon vanilla extract
Cooking spray

Directions:
In a bowl, mix the coconut flour with the baking soda, sugar and the other ingredients except the cooking spray and stir well.   Grease your Crock Pot with the cooking spray, line it with parchment paper, pour the cake batter inside, put the lid on and cook on High for 1 hour.   Leave the cake to cool down, slice and serve.
Nutrition Info:calories 200, fat 4, fiber 4, carbs 10, protein 4

386.   Espresso Ricotta Cream

Servings: 10   Cooking Time: 1 Hr.
Ingredients:
- ½ cup hot coffee
- 2 cups ricotta cheese
- 2 and ½ tsp gelatin
- 1 tsp vanilla extract
- 1 tsp espresso powder
- 1 tsp sugar
- 1 cup whipping cream

Directions:
Whisk coffee with gelatin in a bowl and leave it for minutes.   Add espresso, ricotta, vanilla extract, sugar, cream, and coffee mixture to the insert of Crock Pot.   Put the cooker's lid on and set the cooking time to 1 hour on Low settings. Refrigerate this cream mixture for 2 hours. Serve.
Nutrition Info: Per Serving: Calories: 200, Total Fat: 13g, Fiber: 0g, Total Carbs: 5g, Protein: 7g

387.   Apple Cobbler

Servings: 2   Cooking Time: 2 Hours
Ingredients:
- 1 cup apples, diced
- 1 teaspoon ground cinnamon
- ½ cup flour
- 2 tablespoons coconut oil
- ½ cup cream

Directions:
Mix flour with sugar and coconut oil and knead the dough.   Then mix apples with ground cinnamon and place it in the Crock Pot in one layer.   Grate the dough over the apples and add cream.   Close the lid and cook the cobbler on High for 2 hours.
Nutrition Info: Per Serving: 330 calories, 4.1g protein, 42.1g carbohydrates, 17.5g fat, 4.2g fiber, 11mg cholesterol, 21mg sodium, 180mg potassium.

388.   Sweet Lemon Mix

Servings: 4   Cooking Time: 1 Hour
Ingredients:
- 2 cups heavy cream
- Sugar to the taste
- 2 lemons, peeled and roughly chopped

Directions:
In your Crock Pot, mix cream with sugar and lemons, stir, cover and cook on Low for hour. Divide into glasses and serve very cold.
Nutrition Info: calories 177, fat 0, fiber 0, carbs 6, protein 1

389.   Vanilla Blueberry Cream

Servings: 4   Cooking Time: 1 Hr.
Ingredients:
- 14 oz. canned coconut milk
- 1 tsp vanilla extract
- 2 tbsp sugar
- 4 oz. blueberries
- 2 tbsp walnuts, chopped

Directions:
Whisk coconut milk, vanilla extract, and sugar in a mixer.   Transfer this mixture to the insert of the Crock Pot.   Stir in berries and walnuts, then mix them gently.   Put the cooker's lid on and set the cooking time to 1 hour on Low settings.   Allow it to cool then serve.
Nutrition Info: Per Serving: Calories: 160, Total Fat: 23g, Fiber: 4g, Total Carbs: 6g, Protein: 7g

390.   Upside Down Banana Cake

Servings: 8   Cooking Time: 4 1/2 Hours
Ingredients:
- 2 ripe bananas, sliced
- 1/2 cup light brown sugar
- 2 tablespoons brandy
- 1/2 cup butter
- 3/4 cup sugar
- 2 eggs
- 3/4 cup sour cream
- 1 teaspoon vanilla extract
- 1 cup all-purpose flour
- 1/4 cup cornstarch
- 1 teaspoon baking soda
- 1 pinch salt

Directions:
Spread the brown sugar in your Crock Pot. Arrange the banana slices over the sugar and drizzle with brandy.   For the cake, mix the butter and 4 cup sugar in a bowl until creamy, at least 3 minutes.   Add the eggs, one by one, followed by the sour cream and vanilla.   Fold in the flour, cornstarch, baking soda and salt then spoon the batter over the banana slices.   Cover the pot and cook on low settings for 4 hours.   Allow the cake to cool for 10 minutes then carefully turn it upside down on a platter. You can also slice it and serve it straight from the pot.

391.   Caramelized Bananas

Servings: 6   Cooking Time: 2 Hours 15 Minutes
Ingredients:
- 6 bananas, peeled
- 2 tablespoons butter
- 3 tablespoons caramel

Directions:
Put butter in the Crock Pot.   Add bananas and cook them on High for 15 minutes.   Then add caramel and cook the dessert on Low for 2 hours. Carefully mix the cooked dessert and transfer it into the plates.
Nutrition Info: Per Serving: 159 calories, 1.6g protein, 29.3g carbohydrates, 5.3g fat, 3.1g fiber, 10mg cholesterol, 28mg sodium, 424mg potassium.

392.   Fluffy Vegan Cream

Servings: 6   Cooking Time: 1.5 Hours
Ingredients:
- 1 cup coconut cream
- 1 avocado, pitted, peeled, chopped
- ½ cup of soy milk
- 1 tablespoon corn starch

Directions:
Pour soy milk in the Crock Pot.   Add corn starch and stir until smooth.   Then close the lid and cook the liquid on high for 1.5 hours.   Meanwhile, whip the coconut cream and blend the avocado. Mix the blended avocado with thick soy milk mixture and then carefully mix it with whipped coconut cream.

Nutrition Info:Per Serving: 363 calories, 4.2g protein, 14.5g carbohydrates, 33.7g fat, 2.8g fiber, 0mg cholesterol, 13mg sodium, 206mg potassium.

393. Silky Chocolate Fondue

Servings: 6   Cooking Time: 2 1/4 Hours

Ingredients:

1 cup heavy cream	1/4 cup whole milk
1/4 cup sweetened condensed milk	Fresh fruits of your choice for serving
1 1/2 cups dark chocolate chips	(strawberries, grapes, bananas, kiwi fruits)
2 tablespoons dark rum	

Directions:

Combine the cream, two types of milk, chocolate chips and rum in your Crock Pot.   Cover and cook on low settings for hours.   Serve the fondue by dipping fresh fruits into it.

394. Lemon Buttermilk Cake

Servings: 8   Cooking Time: 4 1/4 Hours

Ingredients:

4 eggs	3/4 cup white sugar
1 cup buttermilk	1/2 cup all-purpose flour
1 tablespoon lemon zest	1/4 teaspoon salt
2 tablespoons lemon juice	1 teaspoon baking powder

Directions:

Mix the eggs, buttermilk, sugar, lemon zest and lemon juice in a bowl.   Add the flour, salt and baking powder and give it a quick mix just until combined.   Pour the batter in your crock pot and bake for 4 hours on low settings.   Allow the cake to cool in the pot before slicing and serving.

395. Spiced Poached Pears

Servings: 6   Cooking Time: 6 1/2 Hours

Ingredients:

6 ripe but firm pears	1 star anise
2 cups white wine	4 whole cloves
1 1/2 cups water	2 cinnamon stick
3/4 cup white sugar	2 cardamom pods, crushed
1-inch piece of ginger, sliced	

Directions:

Carefully peel and core the pears and place them in your crock pot.   Add the remaining ingredients and cook on low settings for 6 hours.   The pears are best served chilled.

396. Triple Chocolate Brownies

Servings: 12   Cooking Time: 4 1/2 Hours

Ingredients:

1 1/4 cups all-purpose flour	1 cup sugar
1/4 cup cocoa powder	2 eggs
1/2 teaspoon salt	1 egg yolk
1/2 cup butter, melted	1 teaspoon vanilla extract

8 oz. dark chocolate, chopped	1/2 cup dark chocolate chips

Directions:

Mix the dry ingredients in a bowl and place aside. Combine the butter and 8 oz. chocolate in a heatproof bowl and place over a hot water bath. Melt them together until smooth.   Remove from heat and add the sugar, eggs, yolk and vanilla. Fold in the flour mixture and the chocolate chips. Pour the batter in your crock pot and bake for 4 hours on low settings.   Allow to cool in the pot before cutting into small squares and serving.

397. Boozy Bread Pudding

Servings: 10   Cooking Time: 6 1/2 Hours

Ingredients:

1/4 cup dark chocolate chips	8 cups bread cubes
1/2 cup golden raisins	1/2 cup brandy
	4 eggs
1/2 cup dried apricots, chopped	2 cups whole milk
	1/2 cup fresh orange juice
1/2 cup dried cranberries	1/2 cup light brown sugar

Directions:

Combine the bread cubes and chocolate chips in your Crock Pot.   Mix the raisins, apricots, cranberries and brandy in a bowl and allow to soak up for 30 minutes at least, preferably overnight. In a bowl, mix the eggs, milk, orange juice and brown sugar.   Spoon the dried fruits and brandy over the bread cubes and top with the egg and milk mixture.   Cover the pot and bake for 6 hours on low settings.   The pudding is best served slightly warm.

398. Vanilla Peach Cream

Servings: 2   Cooking Time: 3 Hours

Ingredients:

¼ teaspoon cinnamon powder	1 tablespoon maple syrup
1 cup peaches, pitted and chopped	½ teaspoons vanilla extract
¼ cup heavy cream	2 tablespoons sugar
Cooking spray	

Directions:

In a blender, mix the peaches with the cinnamon and the other ingredients except the cooking spray and pulse well.   Grease the Crock Pot with the cooking spray, pour the cream mix inside, put the lid on and cook on Low for 3 hours.   Divide the cream into bowls and serve cold.

Nutrition Info:calories 200, fat 3, fiber 4, carbs 10, protein 9

399. Sweet Zucchini Pie

Servings: 6   Cooking Time: 4 Hours

Ingredients:

2 cups zucchini, chopped	4 eggs, beaten
½ cup of sugar	1 tablespoon butter, melted

| 2 cups all-purpose flour | 1 cup milk |
| 1 teaspoon baking powder | 1 teaspoon vanilla extract |

Directions:
Mix sugar with flour, baking powder, eggs, butter, milk, and vanilla extract. Stir the mixture until smooth. Then line the Crock Pot with baking paper and pour the smooth dough inside. Top the dough with zucchini and close the lid. Cook the pie on High for 4 hours.
Nutrition Info: Per Serving: 302 calories, 9.8g protein, 52.4g carbohydrates, 6.2g fat, 1.6g fiber, 118mg cholesterol, 79mg sodium, 291mg potassium.

400.   Berry Marmalade

Servings: 12   Cooking Time: 3 Hours
Ingredients:

1 pound cranberries	½ pound blueberries
1 pound strawberries	2 pounds sugar
3.5 ounces black currant	Zest of 1 lemon
	2 tablespoon water

Directions:
In your Crock Pot, mix strawberries with cranberries, blueberries, currants, lemon zest, sugar and water, cover, cook on High for 3 hours, divide into jars and serve cold.
Nutrition Info:calories 100, fat 4, fiber 3, carbs 12, protein 3

401.   Pumpkin Spices Hot Chocolate

Servings: 4   Cooking Time: 2 Hours
Ingredients:

| 3 cups of milk | 1 teaspoon pumpkin spices |
| ½ cup of chocolate chips | |

Directions:
Put all ingredients in the Crock Pot. Close the lid and cook the hot chocolate on high for hours. Then stir the cooked dessert well and pour it into glasses.
Nutrition Info: Per Serving: 205 calories, 7.6g protein, 21.8g carbohydrates, 10g fat, 0.8g fiber, 20mg cholesterol, 103mg sodium, 186mg potassium.

402.   Caramel

Servings: 10   Cooking Time: 7 Hours
Ingredients:

| 1 cup of sugar | 2 tablespoons butter |
| 1 cup heavy cream | |

Directions:
Put sugar in the Crock Pot. Add heavy cream and butter. Close the lid and cook the caramel on Low for 7 hours. Carefully mix the cooked caramel and transfer it in the glass cans.
Nutrition Info: Per Serving: 137 calories, 0.3g protein, 20.3g carbohydrates, 6.7g fat, 0g

fiber,23mg cholesterol, 21mg sodium, 10mg potassium.

403.   Caramel Cookies

Servings: 6   Cooking Time: 3 Hours
Ingredients:

2 tablespoons salted caramel	1 teaspoon baking powder
½ cup butter	3 tablespoon sugar
1 egg yolk	1 ½ cup flour

Directions:
Mix butter with egg yolk and baking powder. Then add sugar and flour. Knead the soft non-sticky dough. After this, line the Crock Pot bottom with baking paper. Make the small balls from the dough and press them gently. Put the dough balls in the Crock Pot in one layer and sprinkle with salted caramel. Close the lid and cook the cookies on High for 3 hours.
Nutrition Info: Per Serving: 282 calories, 3.9g protein, 30.4g carbohydrates, 16.4g fat, 0.9g fiber, 76mg cholesterol, 112mg sodium, 125mg potassium.

404.   No Crust Lemon Cheesecake

Servings: 8   Cooking Time: 6 1/4 Hours
Ingredients:

24 oz. cream cheese	4 eggs
1 lemon, zested and juiced	1 teaspoon vanilla extract
2 tablespoons cornstarch	1/4 cup butter, melted
1/2 cup white sugar	

Directions:
Mix all the ingredients in a bowl. Pour the cheesecake mix in a greased Crock Pot and cook on low settings for 6 hours. Allow the cheesecake to cool in the pot before slicing and serving.

405.   Spongy Banana Bread

Servings: 6   Cooking Time: 3 Hrs.
Ingredients:

¾ cup of sugar	1 and ½ cups flour
1/3 cup butter, soft	½ tsp baking soda
1 tsp vanilla extract	1/3 cupmilk
1 egg	1 and ½ tsp cream of tartar
2 bananas, mashed	Cooking spray
1 tsp baking powder	

Directions:
Whisk milk with cream of tartar, sugar, egg, butter, bananas, and vanilla in a bowl. Beat well, then add flour, baking soda, baking powder, and salt. Again, mix well until it forms a smooth tartar-banana batter, Grease the insert of Crock Pot with cooking spray and spread the bread batter in it. Put the cooker's lid on and set the cooking time to 3 hours on High settings. Slice and serve.
Nutrition Info: Per Serving: Calories: 300, Total Fat: 3g, Fiber: 4g, Total Carbs: 28g, Protein: 5g

406. Classic Banana Foster

Servings: 3   Cooking Time: 3 Hours

Ingredients:

3 bananas, peeled chopped

2 tablespoons sugar

2 tablespoons butter, melted

1 teaspoon vanilla extract

1 tablespoon rum

3 ice cream balls

Directions:

Put the bananas in the Crock Pot in one layer. Then sprinkle them with sugar, butter, vanilla extract, and rum.   Close the lid and cook on Low for hours.   Transfer the cooked bananas in the ramekins and top with ice cream balls.

Nutrition Info: Per Serving: 378 calories, 3.4g protein, 57.1g carbohydrates, 16.1g fat, 3.1g fiber, 40mg cholesterol, 106mg sodium, 532mg potassium.

407. Blueberry Dumpling Pie

Servings: 8   Cooking Time: 5 1/2 Hours

Ingredients:

1 1/2 pounds fresh blueberries

2 tablespoons cornstarch

1/4 cup light brown sugar

1 tablespoon lemon zest

1/2 cup butter, chilled and cubed

1 1/2 cups all-purpose flour

1/2 teaspoon salt

1 teaspoon baking powder

2 tablespoons white sugar

2/3 cup buttermilk, chilled

Directions:

Mix the blueberries, cornstarch, brown sugar and lemon zest in your Crock Pot.   For the dumpling topping, mix the flour, salt, baking powder, sugar and butter in a bowl and mix until sandy.   Stir in the buttermilk and give it a quick mix.   Drop spoonfuls of batter over the blueberries and cook on low settings for 5 hours.   Allow the dessert to cool completely before serving.

408. Almonds, Walnuts And Mango Bowls

Servings: 2   Cooking Time: 2 Hours

Ingredients:

1 cup walnuts, chopped

2 tablespoons almonds, chopped

1 cup mango, peeled and roughly cubed

1 cup heavy cream

½ teaspoon vanilla extract

1 teaspoon almond extract

1 tablespoon brown sugar

Directions:

In your Crock Pot, mix the nuts with the mango, cream and the other ingredients, toss, put the lid on and cook on High for 2 hours.   Divide the mix into bowls and serve.

Nutrition Info:calories 220, fat 4, fiber 2, carbs 4, protein 6

409. Cornmeal Apricot Pudding

Servings: 6   Cooking Time: 7 Hrs.

Ingredients:

4 oz. cornmeal

10 oz. milk

¼ tsp salt

2 oz. butter

1 egg

2 oz. molasses

1 tsp vanilla extract

1/3 tsp ground ginger

3 tbsp dried apricots, chopped

Directions:

Grease the insert of your Crock Pot with butter. Put the cooker's lid on and set the cooking time to 10 minutes on High settings.   Mix milk with cornmeal in a separate bowl.   Stir in vanilla extract, salt, ground ginger, molasses, and whisked egg then mix until smooth.   Spread this cornmeal batter in the greased insert of Crock Pot.   Add dried apricots on top of this batter.   Put the cooker's lid on and set the cooking time to hours on Low settings.   Serve when chilled.

Nutrition Info: Per Serving: Calories: 234, Total Fat: 11.2g, Fiber: 1g, Total Carbs: 28.97g, Protein: 5g

Fish & Seafood Recipes

410.   Mushrooms Snapper

Servings: 6   Cooking Time: 6 Hrs.

Ingredients:

1 cup sour cream	1 tsp ground
1 onion, diced	coriander
¼ cup almond milk	1 tsp kosher salt
1 tsp salt	1 tbsp lemon juice
7 oz cremini	1 tsp butter
mushrooms	1 lb. snapper,
1 tsp ground thyme	chopped
1 tbsp ground paprika	1 tsp lemon zest

Directions:

Season the snapper with thyme, paprika, coriander, salt, lemon zest, and lemon juice in a bowl. Cover the snapper and marinate it for 10 minutes. Grease the insert of Crock Pot with butter and add snapper mixture.   Add cremini mushrooms, onion, almond milk, and sour cream.   Put the cooker's lid on and set the cooking time to 6 hours on Low settings.   Serve warm.

Nutrition Info: Per Serving: Calories: 248, Total Fat: 6.3g, Fiber: 5g, Total Carbs: 31.19g, Protein: 20g

411. Orange Cod

Servings: 4   Cooking Time: 3 Hours

Ingredients:

1-pound cod fillet,	1 cup of water
chopped	1 garlic clove, diced
2 oranges, chopped	1 teaspoon ground
1 tablespoon maple	black pepper
syrup	

Directions:

Mix cod with ground black pepper and transfer in the Crock Pot.   Add garlic, water, maple syrup, and oranges.   Close the lid and cook the meal on High for hours.

Nutrition Info: Per Serving: 150 calories, 21.2g protein, 14.8g carbohydrates, 1.2g fat, 2.4g fiber, 56mg cholesterol, 73mg sodium, 187mg potassium.

412.   Shrimp Salad

Servings: 4   Cooking Time: 1 Hour

Ingredients:

2 tablespoons olive	3 tablespoons
oil	parsley, chopped
1 pound shrimp,	2 teaspoons mint,
peeled and deveined	chopped
Salt and black pepper	1 tablespoon
to the taste	tarragon, chopped
2 tablespoons lime	1 tablespoon lemon
juice	juice
3 endives, leaves	2 tablespoons
separated	mayonnaise
1 teaspoon lime zest	½ cup sour cream

Directions:

In a bowl, mix shrimp with salt, pepper and the olive oil, toss to coat and spread into the Crock Pot, Add lime juice, endives, parsley, mint, tarragon, lemon juice, lemon zest, mayo and sour cream, toss, cover and cook on High for 1 hour.   Divide into bowls and serve.

Nutrition Info: calories 200, fat 11, fiber 2, carbs 11, protein 13

413.   Cod With Shrimp Sauce

Servings: 4   Cooking Time: 2 Hrs.

Ingredients:

1 lb. cod fillets, cut	2 eggs, whisked
into medium pieces	2 oz. butter, melted
2 tbsp parsley,	½ pint milk
chopped	
4 oz. breadcrumbs	½ pint shrimp sauce
2 tsp lemon juice	Salt and black pepper
	to the taste

Directions:

Toss fish with crumbs, parsley, salt, black pepper, and lemon juice in a suitable bowl.   Add butter, milk, egg, and fish mixture to the insert of the Crock Pot.   Put the cooker's lid on and set the cooking time to 2 hours on High settings.   Serve warm.

Nutrition Info: Per Serving: Calories: 231, Total Fat: 3g, Fiber: 5g, Total Carbs: 10g, Protein: 5g

414.   Scallops With Sour Cream And Dill

Servings: 4   Cooking Time: 2 Hours

Ingredients:

1 ¼ pounds scallops	¼ cup sour cream
Salt and pepper to	1 tablespoon fresh dill
taste	
3 teaspoons butter	

Directions:

Add all ingredients into the crockpot.   Give a good stir to combine everything.   Close the lid and cook on high for   minutes or on low for 2 hours.

Nutrition Info: Calories per serving: 152; Carbohydrates: 4.3g; Protein: 18.2g; Fat: 5.7g; Sugar: 0.5g; Sodium: 231mg; Fiber: 2.3g

415.   Baked Cod

Servings: 2   Cooking Time: 5 Hours

Ingredients:

2 cod fillets	1 teaspoon salt
2 teaspoons cream	½ teaspoon cayenne
cheese	pepper
2 tablespoons bread	2 oz Mozzarella,
crumbs	shredded

Directions:

Sprinkle the cod fillets with cayenne pepper and salt.   Put the fish in the Crock Pot.   Then top it

with cream cheese, bread crumbs, and Mozzarella. Close the lid and cook the meal for 5 hours on Low.
Nutrition Info: Per Serving: 210 calories, 29.2g protein, 6.2g carbohydrates, 7.6g fat, 0.4g fiber, 74mg cholesterol, 1462mg sodium, 26mg potassium

416.   Pesto Salmon

Servings: 4   Cooking Time: 2.5 Hours
Ingredients:

1-pound salmon fillet	1 tablespoon butter
3 tablespoons pesto sauce	¼ cup of water

Directions:
Pour water in the Crock Pot.   Add butter and 1 tablespoon of pesto.   Add salmon and cook the fish on High for 2.5 hours.   Chop the cooked salmon and top with remaining pesto sauce.
Nutrition Info: Per Serving: 226 calories, 23.2g protein, 0.8g carbohydrates, 14.8g fat, 0.2g fiber, 60mg cholesterol, 142mg sodium, 436mg potassium

417.Cod Sticks

Servings: 2   Cooking Time: 1.5 Hour
Ingredients:

2 cod fillets	1/3 cup breadcrumbs
1 teaspoon ground black pepper	1 tablespoon coconut oil
1 egg, beaten	¼ cup of water

Directions:
Cut the cod fillets into medium sticks and sprinkle with ground black pepper.   Then dip the fish in the beaten egg and coat in the breadcrumbs.   Pour water in the Crock Pot.   Add coconut oil and fish sticks.   Cook the meal on High for 1.hours.
Nutrition Info: Per Serving: 254 calories, 25.3g protein, 13.8g carbohydrates, 11g fat, 1.1g fiber, 137mg cholesterol, 234mg sodium, 78mg potassium.

418.   Almond-crusted Tilapia

Servings: 4   Cooking Time: 4 Hours
Ingredients:

2 tablespoons olive oil	4 tilapia fillets
1 cup chopped almonds	Salt and pepper to taste
¼ cup ground flaxseed	

Directions:
Line the bottom of the crockpot with a foil.   Grease the foil with the olive oil.   In a mixing bowl, combine the almonds and flaxseed.   Season the tilapia with salt and pepper to taste.   Dredge the tilapia fillets with the almond and flaxseed mixture.   Place neatly in the foil-lined crockpot.   Close the lid and cook on high for 2 hours and on low for 4 hours.

Nutrition Info: Calories per serving: 233; Carbohydrates: 4.6g; Protein: 25.5g; Fat: 13.3g; Sugar: 0.4g; Sodium: 342mg; Fiber: 1.9g

419.   Seafood Bean Chili

Servings: 8   Cooking Time: 3.5 Hrs.
Ingredients:

1 lb. salmon, diced	1 cup fish stock
7 oz shrimps, peeled	1 tsp cayenne pepper
1 tbsp salt	1 cup bell pepper, chopped
1 cup tomatoes, canned	1 tbsp olive oil
1 tsp ground white pepper	1 tsp coriander
1 tbsp tomato sauce	1 cup of water
2 onions, chopped	6 oz Parmesan, shredded
1 cup carrot, chopped	1 garlic clove, sliced
1 can red beans	
½ cup tomato juice	

Directions:
Add tomatoes, white pepper, tomato sauce, red beans, carrots, tomato juice, bell pepper, fish stock, cayenne pepper, garlic, water and coriander to the insert of Crock Pot.   Put the cooker's lid on and set the cooking time to 3 hours on High settings.   Add olive oil and seafood to a suitable pan, then sauté for minutes.   Transfer the sautéed seafood to the Crock Pot.   Put the cooker's lid on and set the cooking time to 30 minutes on High settings.   Serve warm.
Nutrition Info: Per Serving: Calories: 281, Total Fat: 7.9g, Fiber: 4g, Total Carbs: 22.52g, Protein: 30g

420.   Hot Salmon And Carrots

Servings: 2   Cooking Time: 3 Hours
Ingredients:

1 pound salmon fillets, boneless	¼ cup chicken stock
1 cup baby carrots, peeled	2 scallions, chopped
½ teaspoon hot paprika	1 tablespoon smoked paprika
½ teaspoon chili powder	A pinch of salt and black pepper
	2 tablespoons chives, chopped

Directions:
In your Crock Pot, mix the salmon with the carrots, paprika and the other ingredients, toss, put the lid on and cook on Low for 3 hours.   Divide the mix between plates and serve.
Nutrition Info:calories 193, fat 7, fiber 3, carbs 6, protein 6

421.   Chili-rubbed Tilapia

Servings: 4   Cooking Time: 4 Hours
Ingredients:

2 tablespoons chili powder	2 tablespoons lemon juice
½ teaspoon garlic	2 tablespoons olive oil

powder
1-pound tilapia

Directions:
Place all ingredients in a mixing bowl. Stir to combine everything.   Allow to marinate in the fridge for at least 30 minutes.   Get a foil and place the fish including the marinade in the middle of the foil.   Fold the foil and crimp the edges to seal.   Place inside the crockpot.   Cook on high for 2 hours or on low for 4 hours.
Nutrition Info: Calories per serving: 183; Carbohydrates: 2.9g; Protein: 23.4g; Fat: 11.3g; Sugar: 0.3g; Sodium: 215mg; Fiber:1.4 g

422.	Fish Mix

Servings: 4   Cooking Time: 2 Hours And 30 Minutes
Ingredients:

½ teaspoon mustard seeds	4 white fish fillets, skinless and boneless
Salt and black pepper to the taste	1 small red onion, chopped
2 green chilies, chopped	1-inch turmeric root, grated
1 teaspoon ginger, grated	¼ cup cilantro, chopped
1 teaspoon curry powder	1 and ½ cups coconut cream
¼ teaspoon cumin, ground	3 garlic cloves, minced
2 tablespoons olive oil	

Directions:
Heat up a Crock Pot with half of the oil over medium heat, add mustard seeds, ginger, onion, garlic, turmeric, chilies, curry powder and cumin, stir and cook for 3-4 minutes.   Add the rest of the oil to your Crock Pot, add spice mix, fish, coconut milk, salt and pepper, cover and cook on High for hours and 30 minutes.   Divide into bowls and serve with the cilantro sprinkled on top.
Nutrition Info:calories 500, fat 34, fiber 7, carbs 13, protein 44

423.	Curry Shrimps

Servings: 4   Cooking Time: 45 Minutes
Ingredients:

1 teaspoon curry paste	16 oz shrimps, peeled
	½ cup fish stock

Directions:
Mix the curry paste with fish stock and pour it in the Crock Pot.   Add shrimps and cook them on High for 45 minutes.
Nutrition Info: Per Serving: 148 calories, 26.6g protein, 2.1g carbohydrates, 2.9g fat, 0g fiber, 239mg cholesterol, 322mg sodium, 234mg potassium

424.	Shrimp Scampi

Servings: 4   Cooking Time: 4 Hours

Ingredients:

1-pound shrimps, peeled	1 cup of water
2 tablespoons lemon juice	1 teaspoon dried parsley
2 tablespoons coconut oil	½ teaspoon white pepper

Directions:
Put all ingredients in the Crock Pot and gently mix. Close the lid and cook the scampi on Low for 4 hours.
Nutrition Info: Per Serving: 196 calories, 25.9g protein, 2.1g carbohydrates, 8.8g fat, 0.1g fiber, 239mg cholesterol, 280mg sodium, 207mg potassium

425.	Hot Calamari

Servings: 4   Cooking Time: 1 Hour
Ingredients:

12 oz calamari, sliced	1 garlic clove, crushed
¼ cup of soy sauce	1 teaspoon mustard
1 teaspoon cayenne pepper	½ cup of water
	1 teaspoon sesame oil

Directions:
In the bowl mix slices calamari, soy sauce, cayenne pepper, garlic, mustard, and sesame oil. Leave the ingredients for   minutes to marinate.   Then transfer the mixture in the Crock Pot, add water, and close the lid.   Cook the meal on high for 1 hour.
Nutrition Info: Per Serving: 103 calories, 14.6g protein, 4.6g carbohydrates, 2.6g fat, 0.4g fiber, 198mg cholesterol, 937mg sodium, 262mg potassium.

426.	Chili Bigeye Jack (tuna)

Servings: 4   Cooking Time: 3.5 Hours
Ingredients:

9 oz tuna fillet (bigeye jack), roughly chopped	1 teaspoon curry paste
1 teaspoon chili powder	½ cup of coconut milk
	1 tablespoon sesame oil

Directions:
Mix curry paste and coconut milk and pour the liquid in the Crock Pot.   Add tuna fillet and sesame oil.   Then add chili powder.   Cook the meal on High for 3.5 hours.
Nutrition Info: Per Serving: 341 calories, 14.2g protein, 2.4g carbohydrates, 31.2g fat, 0.9g fiber, 0mg cholesterol, 11mg sodium, 91mg potassium

427.	Cod And Broccoli

Servings: 2   Cooking Time: 3 Hours
Ingredients:

1 pound cod fillets, boneless	½ cup veggie stock
1 cup broccoli florets	1 red onion, minced
2 tablespoons tomato	½ teaspoon

paste

2 garlic cloves, minced

rosemary, dried

A pinch of salt and black pepper

1 tablespoon chives, chopped

Directions:

In your Crock Pot, mix the cod with the broccoli, stock, tomato paste and the other ingredients, toss, put the lid on and cook on Low for 3 hours. Divide the mix between plates and serve.

Nutrition Info:calories 200, fat 13, fiber 3, carbs 6, protein 11

---

428.   Thyme Mussels

Servings: 4   Cooking Time: 2.5 Hours

Ingredients:

1 teaspoon dried thyme

1 teaspoon ground black pepper

1-pound mussels

½ teaspoon salt

1 cup of water

½ cup sour cream

Directions:

In the mixing bowl mix mussels, dried thyme, ground black pepper, and salt.   Then pour water in the Crock Pot.   Add sour cream and cook the liquid on High for 1.5 hours.   After this, add mussels and cook them for 1 hour on High or until the mussels are opened.

Nutrition Info: Per Serving: 161 calories, 14.5g protein, 5.9g carbohydrates, 8.6g fat, 0.2g fiber, 44mg cholesterol, 632mg sodium, 414mg potassium.

---

429.   Seabass Balls

Servings: 4   Cooking Time: 2 Hours

Ingredients:

1 teaspoon ground coriander

½ teaspoon salt

2 tablespoons flour

½ cup chicken stock

1 teaspoon dried dill

10 oz seabass fillet

1 tablespoon sesame oil

Directions:

Dice the seabass fillet into tiny pieces and mix with salt, ground coriander, flour, and dill.   Make the medium size balls.   Preheat the skillet well. Add sesame oil and heat it until hot.   Add the fish balls and roast them on high heat for 1 minute per side.   Then transfer the fish balls in the Crock Pot. Arrange them in one layer.   Add water and close the lid.   Cook the meal on High for 2 hours.

Nutrition Info: Per Serving: 191 calories, 16.6g protein, 3.2g carbohydrates, 12.2g fat, 0.7g fiber, 0mg cholesterol, 387mg sodium, 15mg potassium.

---

430.   Crockpot Asian Shrimps

Servings: 2   Cooking Time: 3 Hours

Ingredients:

2 tablespoons soy sauce

½ teaspoon sliced ginger

½ cup chicken stock

2 tablespoons sesame oil

½ pound shrimps, cleaned and deveined

2 tablespoons rice vinegar

2 tablespoons toasted sesame seeds

2 tablespoons green onions, chopped

Directions:

Place the chicken stock, soy sauce, ginger, shrimps, and rice vinegar in the CrockPot.   Give a good stir.   Close the lid and cook on high for 2 hours or on low for hours.   Sprinkle with sesame oil, sesame seeds, and chopped green onions before serving.

Nutrition Info: Calories per serving: 352; Carbohydrates: 4.7g; Protein: 30.2g; Fat: 24.3g; Sugar: 0.4g; Sodium: 755mg; Fiber: 2.9g

---

431.   Mashed Potato Fish Casserole

Servings: 4   Cooking Time: 5 Hours

Ingredients:

1 cup potatoes, cooked, mashed

1 egg, beaten

½ cup Monterey Jack cheese, shredded

1 cup of coconut milk

1 tablespoon avocado oil

½ teaspoon ground black pepper

7 oz cod fillet, chopped

Directions:

Brush the Crock Pot bottom with avocado oil. Then mix chopped fish with ground black pepper and put in the Crock Pot in one layer.   Top it with mashed potato and cheese.   Add egg and coconut milk.   Close the lid and cook the casserole on Low for hours.

Nutrition Info: Per Serving: 283 calories, 16.9g protein, 9.8g carbohydrates, 20.7g fat, 2.4g fiber, 81mg cholesterol, 138mg sodium, 351mg potassium

---

432.   Chili Catfish

Servings: 4   Cooking Time: 6 Hours

Ingredients:

1 catfish, boneless and cut into 4 pieces

3 red chili peppers, chopped

½ cup sugar

1 tablespoon soy sauce

¼ cup water

1 shallot, minced

A small ginger piece, grated

1 tablespoon coriander, chopped

Directions:

Put catfish pieces in your Crock Pot.   Heat up a pan with the coconut sugar over medium-high heat and stir until it caramelizes.   Add soy sauce, shallot, ginger, water and chili pepper, stir, pour over the fish, add coriander, cover and cook on Low for 6 hours.   Divide fish between plates and serve with the sauce from the Crock Pot drizzled on top.

Nutrition Info:calories 200, fat 4, fiber 4, carbs 8, protein 10

---

433.   Mediterranean Octopus

Servings: 6   Cooking Time: 3 Hours

Ingredients:

1 octopus, cleaned and prepared
2 rosemary springs
2 teaspoons oregano, dried
½ yellow onion, roughly chopped
4 thyme springs
1 teaspoon black peppercorns
3 tablespoons extra virgin olive oil

½ lemon
For the marinade:
¼ cup extra virgin olive oil
Juice of ½ lemon
4 garlic cloves, minced
2 thyme springs
1 rosemary spring
Salt and black pepper to the taste

Directions:
Put the octopus in your Crock Pot, add oregano, 2 rosemary springs, 4 thyme springs, onion, lemon, 3 tablespoons olive oil, peppercorns and salt, stir, cover and cook on High for 2 hours.   Transfer octopus on a cutting board, cut tentacles, put them in a bowl, mix with ¼ cup olive oil, lemon juice, garlic, 1 rosemary springs, thyme springs, salt and pepper, toss to coat and leave aside for 1 hour. Transfer octopus and the marinade to your Crock Pot again, cover and cook on High for 1 more hour. Divide octopus on plates, drizzle the marinade all over and serve.
Nutrition Info:calories 200, fat 4, fiber 3, carbs 10, protein 11

434.   Mustard Cod
Servings: 4   Cooking Time: 3 Hours
Ingredients:
4 cod fillets
2 tablespoons sesame oil

4 teaspoons mustard
¼ cup of water

Directions:
Mix mustard with sesame oil.   Then brush the cod fillets with mustard mixture and transfer in the Crock Pot.   Add water and cook the fish on low for hours.
Nutrition Info: Per Serving: 166 calories, 20.8g protein, 1.2g carbohydrates, 8.8g fat, 0.5g fiber, 55mg cholesterol, 71mg sodium, 23mg potassium

435.   Apple Cider Vinegar Sardines
Servings: 4   Cooking Time: 4.5 Hours
Ingredients:
14 oz sardines
1 tablespoon butter
¼ cup apple cider vinegar

½ teaspoon cayenne pepper
4 tablespoons coconut cream

Directions:
Put sardines in the Crock Pot.   Add butter, apple cider vinegar, cayenne pepper, and coconut cream. Close the lid and cook the meal on Low for 4.5 hours.
Nutrition Info: Per Serving: 270 calories, 24.8g protein, 1.1g carbohydrates, 17.9g fat, 0.4g fiber, 149mg cholesterol,525mg sodium, 450mg potassium

436.   Basil Cod And Olives
Servings: 2   Cooking Time: 3 Hours
Ingredients:
1 pound cod fillets, boneless
1 cup black olives, pitted and halved
½ tablespoon tomato paste
1 tablespoon basil, chopped

¼ cup chicken stock
1 red onion, sliced
1 tablespoon lime juice
1 tablespoon chives, chopped
Salt and black pepper to the taste

Directions:
In your Crock Pot, mix the cod with the olives, basil and the other ingredients, toss, put the lid on and cook on Low for 3 hours.   Divide everything between plates and serve.
Nutrition Info:calories 132, fat 9, fiber 2, carbs 5, protein 11

437.   Sriracha Cod
Servings: 4   Cooking Time: 6 Hours
Ingredients:
2 tablespoons sriracha
1 tablespoon olive oil

4 cod fillets
1 teaspoon tomato paste
½ cup of water

Directions:
Sprinkle the cod fillets with sriracha, olive oil, and tomato paste.   Put the fish in the Crock Pot and add water.   Cook it on Low for 6 hours.
Nutrition Info: Per Serving: 129 calories, 20.1g protein, 1.8g carbohydrates, 4.5g fat, 0.1g fiber, 55mg cholesterol, 125mg sodium, 14mg potassium.

438.   Cream White Fish
Servings: 6   Cooking Time: 2 Hrs.
Ingredients:
17 oz. white fish, skinless, boneless and cut into chunks
1 yellow onion, chopped
13 oz. potatoes, peeled and cut into chunks

13 oz. milk
Salt and black pepper to the taste
14 oz. chicken stock
14 oz. water
14 oz. half and half cream

Directions:
Add onion, fish, potatoes, water, stock, and milk to the insert of Crock Pot.   Put the cooker's lid on and set the cooking time to hours on High settings. Add half and half cream, black pepper, and salt to the fish.   Mix gently, then serve warm.
Nutrition Info: Per Serving: Calories: 203, Total Fat: 4g, Fiber: 5g, Total Carbs: 20g, Protein: 15g

439.   Mozzarella Fish Casserole
Servings: 4   Cooking Time: 2.5 Hours
Ingredients:
1 cup Mozzarella, shredded

1 teaspoon salt
½ cup of water

1-pound salmon fillet, chopped
1 cup onion, sliced

1 teaspoon avocado oil

Directions:
Mix salmon with salt and put it in the Crock Pot. Add avocado oil and water.   After this, top the fish with sliced onion and Mozzarella.   Close the lid and cook the casserole on High for 2.5 hours.
Nutrition Info: Per Serving: 183 calories, 24.3g protein, 3g carbohydrates, 8.4g fat, 0.7g fiber, 54mg cholesterol, 676mg sodium, 482mg potassium

440.   Walnut Tuna Mix

Servings: 2   Cooking Time: 3 Hours
Ingredients:

1 pound tuna fillets, boneless
½ tablespoon walnuts, chopped
½ cup chicken stock
½ teaspoon chili powder

½ teaspoon sweet paprika
1 red onion, sliced
2 tablespoons parsley, chopped
A pinch of salt and black pepper

Directions:
In your Crock Pot, mix the tuna with the walnuts, stock and the other ingredients, toss, put the lid on and cook on High for 3 hours.   Divide everything between plates and serve.
Nutrition Info:calories 200, fat 10, fiber 2, carbs 5, protein 9

441.   Crockpot Seafood Cioppino

Servings: 8   Cooking Time: 4 Hours
Ingredients:

1-pound haddock fillets, cut into strips
1-pound shrimps, shelled and deveined
1 cup raw clam meat
1 cup crab meat
1 cup tomatoes, diced
2 onions, chopped
3 stalks of celery, chopped

2 cups clam juice
3 tablespoons tomato paste
5 cloves of garlic, minced
1 tablespoons olive oil
2 teaspoons Italian seasoning
1 bay leaf

Directions:
Place all ingredients in the CrockPot.   Give a good stir.   Close the lid and cook on high for hours or on low for 4 hours.   Garnish with parsley.
Nutrition Info: Calories per serving: 217; Carbohydrates: 5.2g; Protein: 26.8g; Fat: 8.1g; Sugar: 0g; Sodium: 620mg; Fiber: 3.5g

442.   Flavored Squid

Servings: 4   Cooking Time: 3 Hours
Ingredients:

17 ounces squids
1 and ½ tablespoons red chili powder
Salt and black pepper

4 garlic cloves, minced
½ teaspoons cumin seeds

to the taste
¼ teaspoon turmeric powder
2 cups water
5 pieces coconut, shredded

3 tablespoons olive oil
¼ teaspoon mustard seeds
1-inch ginger pieces, chopped

Directions:
Put squids in your Crock Pot, add chili powder, turmeric, salt, pepper and water, stir, cover and cook on High for 2 hours.   In your blender, mix coconut with ginger, oil, garlic and cumin and blend well.   Add this over the squids, cover and cook on High for 1 more hour.   Divide everything into bowls and serve.
Nutrition Info:calories 261, fat 3, fiber 8, carbs 19, protein 11

443.   Mussels And Vegetable Ragout

Servings: 4   Cooking Time: 5 Hours
Ingredients:

1 cup potato, chopped
½ onion, chopped
1 bell pepper, chopped
1 teaspoon peppercorns

2 cups of water
1 cup tomatoes, chopped
1 cup mussels
1 teaspoon salt

Directions:
Put all ingredients except mussels in the Crock Pot. Close the lid and cook the meal on High for 3 hours.   Then add mussels and mix the meal. Close the lid and cook the ragout on Low for 2 hours.
Nutrition Info: Per Serving: 71 calories, 5.8g protein, 10.3g carbohydrates, 1.1g fat, 1.8g fiber, 11mg cholesterol, 697mg sodium, 390mg potassium

444.   Coated Salmon Fillets

Servings: 3   Cooking Time: 2.5 Hours
Ingredients:

2 tablespoons coconut flakes
8 oz salmon fillet
1 egg white, whisked
1 teaspoon flour

½ teaspoon chili powder
1 teaspoon butter
1/3 cup water

Directions:
Sprinkle the salmon fillet with chili powder. Then dip it with egg and coat in the flour. Sprinkle with remaining egg mixture and top with coconut flakes.   Put the fish in the Crock Pot. Add butter and water.   Close the lid and cook the salmon on High for 2.5 hours.
Nutrition Info: Per Serving: 133 calories, 16.1g protein, 1.5g carbohydrates, 7.2g fat, 0.5g fiber, 37mg cholesterol, 59mg sodium, 330mg potassium

445.   Chipotle Salmon Fillets

Servings: 2   Cooking Time: 2 Hrs
Ingredients:

2 medium salmon fillets, boneless
A pinch of nutmeg, ground
A pinch of cloves, ground
A pinch of ginger powder
2 tsp sugar
Salt and black pepper to the taste
1 tsp onion powder
¼ tsp chipotle chili powder
½ tsp cayenne pepper
½ tsp cinnamon, ground
1/8 tsp thyme, dried

Directions:
Place the salmon fillets in foil wraps.   Drizzle ginger, cloves, salt, thyme, cinnamon, black pepper, cayenne, chili powder, onion powder, nutmeg, and coconut sugar on top.   Wrap the fish fillet with the aluminum foil.   Put the cooker's lid on and set the cooking time to 2 hours on Low settings. Unwrap the fish and serve warm.
Nutrition Info: Per Serving: Calories 220, Total Fat 4g, Fiber 2g, Total Carbs 7g, Protein 4g

446.	Crispy Mackerel

Servings: 4   Cooking Time: 2 Hrs.
Ingredients:
4 mackerels
3 oz. breadcrumbs
Juice and rind of 1 lemon
1 tbsp chives, finely chopped
Salt and black pepper to the taste
1 egg, whisked
1 tbsp butter
1 tbsp vegetable oil
3 lemon wedges

Directions:
Whisk breadcrumbs with lemon rinds, lemon juice, chives, egg, black pepper, and salt in a small bowl. Coat the mackerel with this breadcrumb's mixture liberally.   Brush the insert of your Crock Pot with butter and oil.   Place the mackerel along with breadcrumbs mixture to the cooker.   Put the cooker's lid on and set the cooking time to 2 hours on High settings.   Garnish with lemon wedges. Enjoy.
Nutrition Info: Per Serving: Calories: 200, Total Fat: 3g, Fiber: 1g, Total Carbs: 3g, Protein: 12g

447.	Mackerel Chops

Servings: 6   Cooking Time: 5 Hours
Ingredients:
24 oz mackerel fillet
1 teaspoon dried lemongrass
½ teaspoon ground nutmeg
1 teaspoon smoked paprika
1 teaspoon salt
1 tablespoon apple cider vinegar
1 tablespoon fish sauce
½ cup of water

Directions:
Cut the mackerel fillet into 6 servings.   Then sprinkle every mackerel fillet with dried lemongrass, ground nutmeg, smoked paprika, salt, apple cider vinegar, and fish sauce.   Put the fish fillets in the Crock Pot. Add water.   Cook the meal on Low for 5 hours.

Nutrition Info: Per Serving: 301 calories, 27.3g protein, 0.5g carbohydrates, 20.3g fat, 0.2g fiber, 85mg cholesterol, 714mg sodium, 476mg potassium.

448.	Miso Cod

Servings: 4   Cooking Time: 4 Hours
Ingredients:
1-pound cod fillet, sliced
½ teaspoon ground ginger
1 teaspoon miso paste
2 cups chicken stock
½ teaspoon ground nutmeg

Directions:
In the mixing bowl mix chicken stock, ground nutmeg, ground ginger, and miso paste.   Then pour the liquid in the Crock Pot.   Add cod fillet and close the lid.   Cook the fish on Low for hours.
Nutrition Info: Per Serving: 101 calories, 20.8g protein, 1.1g carbohydrates, 1.5g fat, 0.2g fiber, 56mg cholesterol, 506mg sodium, 14mg potassium.

449.	Chili Perch

Servings: 4   Cooking Time: 3 Hours
Ingredients:
1 chili pepper, chopped
1 carrot, grated
1 tablespoon coconut oil
1 onion, diced
1 teaspoon salt
½ cup chicken stock
1-pound perch fillet, chopped

Directions:
Put the chili pepper in the Crock Pot.   Add carrot, onion, and coconut oil.   Sprinkle the perch fillet with salt and transfer in the Crock Pot.   Add chicken stock and close the lid.   Cook the perch on High for 3 hours.
Nutrition Info: Per Serving: 159 calories, 21.6g protein, 4.3g carbohydrates, 5.6g fat, 1g fiber, 45mg cholesterol, 779mg sodium, 93mg potassium

450.	Hot Salmon

Servings: 4   Cooking Time: 3 Hours
Ingredients:
1-pound salmon fillet, sliced
2 chili peppers, chopped
1 onion, diced
1 tablespoon olive oil
½ cup cream
½ teaspoon salt

Directions:
Mix salmon with salt, onion, and olive oil.   Transfer the ingredients in the Crock Pot.   Add cream and onion.   Cook the salmon on high for 3 hours.
Nutrition Info: Per Serving: 211 calories, 22.6g protein, 3.7g carbohydrates, 12.2g fat, 0.7g fiber, 56mg cholesterol, 352mg sodium, 491mg potassium.

451.	Lemon Scallops

Servings: 4   Cooking Time: 1 Hour
Ingredients:

1-pound scallops
1 teaspoon salt
1 teaspoon ground white pepper
3 tablespoons lemon juice
½ teaspoon olive oil
1 teaspoon lemon zest, grated
1 tablespoon dried oregano
½ cup of water

Directions:
Sprinkle the scallops with salt, ground white pepper, lemon juice, and lemon zest and leave for - 15 minutes to marinate.   After this, sprinkle the scallops with olive oil and dried oregano.   Put the scallops in the Crock Pot and add water.   Cook the seafood on High for 1 hour.
Nutrition Info: Per Serving: 113 calories, 19.3g protein, 4.1g carbohydrates, 1.7g fat, 0.7g fiber, 37mg cholesterol, 768mg sodium, 407mg potassium

452.   Lobster Colorado

Servings: 4   Cooking Time: 6 Hours 30 Minutes
Ingredients:
½ teaspoon garlic powder
Salt and black pepper, to taste
4 (8 ounce) beef tenderloin
½ cup butter, divided
4 slices bacon
8 ounces lobster tail, cleaned and chopped
1 teaspoon Old Bay Seasoning

Directions:
Season the beef tenderloins with garlic powder, salt and black pepper.   Transfer the beef tenderloins in the crock pot and add butter.   Cover and cook on LOW for about hours.   Add lobster and bacon and cover the lid.   Cook on LOW for another 3 hours and dish out to serve hot.
Nutrition Info: Calories:825 Fat:52.2g Carbohydrates:0.6g

453.   Shrimp Mix

Servings: 4   Cooking Time: 1 Hour And 30 Minutes
Ingredients:
2 tablespoons olive oil
1 pound shrimp, peeled and deveined
1 tablespoon garlic, minced
¼ cup chicken stock
2 tablespoons parsley, chopped
Juice of ½ lemon
Salt and black pepper to the taste

Directions:
Put the oil in your Crock Pot, add stock, garlic, parsley, lemon juice, salt and pepper and whisk really well.   Add shrimp, stir, cover, cook on High for 1 hour and 30 minutes, divide into bowls and serve.
Nutrition Info:calories 240, fat 4, fiber 3, carbs 9, protein 3

454.   Salmon And Rice

Servings: 2   Cooking Time: 2 Hours

Ingredients:
2 wild salmon fillets, boneless
Salt and black pepper to the taste
½ cup jasmine rice
1 cup chicken stock
¼ cup veggie stock
1 tablespoon butter
A pinch of saffron

Directions:
In your Crock Pot mix stock with rice, stock, butter and saffron and stir.   Add salmon, salt and pepper, cover and cook on High for hours.   Divide salmon on plates, add rice mix on the side and serve.
Nutrition Info:calories 312, fat 4, fiber 6, carbs 20, protein 22

455.   Shrimp And Eggplant

Servings: 2   Cooking Time: 1 Hour
Ingredients:
1 pound shrimp, peeled and deveined
2 teaspoons avocado oil
1 eggplant, cubed
2 tomatoes, cubed
Juice of 1 lime
½ cup chicken stock
4 garlic cloves, minced
1 tablespoon coriander, chopped
1 tablespoon chives, chopped
A pinch of salt and black pepper

Directions:
In your Crock Pot, mix the shrimp with the oil, eggplant, tomatoes and the other ingredients, toss, put the lid on and cook on High for hour.   Divide the mix into bowls and serve.
Nutrition Info:calories 200, fat 11, fiber 4, carbs 5, protein 12

456.   Seabass Mushrooms Ragout

Servings: 8   Cooking Time: 8 Hrs.
Ingredients:
6 oz shiitake mushrooms, chopped
8 oz wild mushrooms, chopped
9 oz cremini mushrooms, chopped
2 white onions, chopped
1 tbsp balsamic vinegar
1 lb. seabass, boneless, cubed
1 tbsp ground celery
1 tsp salt
1 tsp ground nutmeg
2 tbsp sliced garlic
3 carrots, chopped
1 tbsp butter
½ tsp sage, chopped
2 cups of water
3 tbsp fresh dill, chopped
1 tbsp fresh celery, chopped

Directions:
Mix the mushrooms with ground celery, balsamic vinegar, and salt in a bowl.   Transfer the mushrooms along with butter to the insert of the Crock Pot.   Put the cooker's lid on and set the cooking time to 1 hour on Low settings.   Add seabass, nutmeg, garlic, carrots, sage, celery, dill, and water to the cooker.   Put the cooker's lid on and set the cooking time to 7 hours on Low settings.   Serve warm.
Nutrition Info: Per Serving: Calories: 313, Total Fat: 5g, Fiber: 9g, Total Carbs: 55.86g, Protein: 20g

457.   Turmeric Coconut Squid

Servings: 4   Cooking Time: 3 Hrs.

Ingredients:

17 oz. squids	2 cups of water
1 and ½ tbsp red chili powder	4 garlic cloves, minced
Salt and black pepper to the taste	½ tsp cumin seeds
¼ tsp turmeric powder	3 tbsp olive oil
	¼ tsp mustard seeds
5 pieces coconut, shredded	1-inch ginger pieces, chopped

Directions:

Add squids, turmeric, chili powder, water, black pepper, and salt to the insert of the Crock Pot. Put the cooker's lid on and set the cooking time to hours on High settings.   Add ginger, garlic, cumin, and oil to a blender jug and blend well. Transfer this ginger-garlic mixture to the squids in the cooker.   Cook again for 1 hour on High settings.   Serve warm.

Nutrition Info: Per Serving: Calories: 261, Total Fat: 3g, Fiber: 8g, Total Carbs: 19g, Protein: 11g

458.   Cod And Clams Saute

Servings: 2   Cooking Time: 4 Hours

Ingredients:

1 cod fillet	1 garlic clove, diced
1 cup clams	1 jalapeno pepper, diced
1 tablespoon fresh parsley, chopped	1 tablespoon olive oil
2 cups tomatoes, chopped	1 cup of water

Directions:

Slice the cod fillet and put it in the Crock Pot. Add all remaining ingredients and close the lid. Cook the saute on Low for 4 hours.

Nutrition Info: Per Serving: 200 calories, 12.6g protein, 21.3g carbohydrates, 8.2g fat, 2.9g fiber, 28mg cholesterol, 487mg sodium, 567mg potassium

459.   Fish Potato Cakes

Servings: 12   Cooking Time: 5 Hrs.

Ingredients:

1 lb. trout, minced	1 egg, beaten
6 oz mashed potato	1 tsp minced garlic
1 carrot, grated	1 onion, grated
½ cup fresh parsley	1 tsp olive oil
1 tsp salt	1 tsp ground black pepper
½ cup panko bread crumbs	¼ tsp cilantro

Directions:

Mix minced trout with mashed potatoes, carrot, salt, garlic, cilantro, onion, black pepper, and egg in a bowl.   Stir in breadcrumbs and olive oil, then mix well.   Make 12 balls out of this mixture then flatten the balls.   Place these fish cakes in the insert of Crock Pot.   Put the cooker's lid on and set the cooking time to hours on Low settings. Flip all the fish cakes when cooked halfway through.   Serve warm.

Nutrition Info: Per Serving: Calories: 93, Total Fat: 3.8g, Fiber: 1g, Total Carbs: 5.22g, Protein: 9g

460.   Shrimp And Mango Mix

Servings: 2   Cooking Time: 1 Hour

Ingredients:

1 pound shrimp, peeled and deveined	½ teaspoon rosemary, dried
½ cup mango, peeled and cubed	1 tablespoon olive oil
½ cup cherry tomatoes, halved	½ teaspoon chili powder
½ cup shallots, chopped	A pinch of salt and black pepper
1 tablespoon lime juice	1 tablespoon chives, chopped
½ cup chicken stock	

Directions:

In your Crock Pot, mix the shrimp with the mango, tomatoes and the other ingredients, toss, put the lid on and cook on High for hour.   Divide the mix into bowls and serve.

Nutrition Info: calories 210, fat 9, fiber 2, carbs 6, protein 7

461.   Ginger Tuna

Servings: 2   Cooking Time: 2 Hours

Ingredients:

1 pound tuna fillets, boneless and roughly cubed	Juice of 1 lime
	¼ cup chicken stock
1 tablespoon ginger, grated	1 tablespoon chives, chopped
1 red onion, chopped	A pinch of salt and black pepper
2 teaspoons olive oil	

Directions:

In your Crock Pot, mix the tuna with the ginger, onion and the other ingredients, toss, put the lid on and cook on High for 2 hours.   Divide the mix into bowls and serve.

Nutrition Info: calories 200, fat 11, fiber 4, carbs 5, protein 12

462.   Soy Sauce Scallops

Servings: 4   Cooking Time: 30 Minutes

Ingredients:

¼ cup of soy sauce	1 tablespoon butter
½ teaspoon white pepper	1-pound scallops

Directions:

Pour soy sauce in the Crock Pot.   Add butter and white pepper.   After this, add scallops and close the lid.   Cook them on High for 30 minutes.

Nutrition Info: Per Serving: 134 calories, 20.1g protein, 4.1g carbohydrates, 3.8g fat, 0.2g fiber, 45mg cholesterol, 1102mg sodium, 404mg potassium

463. Italian Clams

Servings: 6   Cooking Time: 2 Hours

Ingredients:

½ cup butter, melted
36 clams, scrubbed
1 teaspoon red pepper flakes, crushed
1 teaspoon parsley, chopped
5 garlic cloves, minced
1 tablespoon oregano, dried
2 cups white wine

Directions:

In your Crock Pot, mix butter with clams, pepper flakes, parsley, garlic, oregano and wine, stir, cover and cook on High for 2 hours.   Divide into bowls and serve.

Nutrition Info:calories 224, fat 15, fiber 2, carbs 7, protein 4

464. Cod And Peas

Servings: 4   Cooking Time: 2 Hours

Ingredients:

16 ounces cod fillets
1 tablespoon parsley, chopped
10 ounces peas
½ teaspoon oregano, dried
9 ounces wine
½ teaspoon paprika
2 garlic cloves, chopped
Salt and pepper to the taste

Directions:

In your food processor mix garlic with parsley, oregano, paprika and wine, blend well and add to your Crock Pot.   Add fish, peas, salt and pepper, cover and cook on High for hours.   Divide into bowls and serve.

Nutrition Info:calories 251, far 2, fiber 6, carbs 7, protein 22

465. Bbq Shrimps

Servings: 6   Cooking Time: 40 Minutes

Ingredients:

1/3 cup BBQ sauce
1-pound shrimps, peeled
¼ cup plain yogurt
1 tablespoon butter

Directions:

Melt butter and mix it with shrimps.   Put the mixture in the Crock Pot.   Add plain yogurt and BBQ sauce.   Close the lid and cook the meal on High for   minutes.

Nutrition Info: Per Serving: 135 calories, 17.8g protein, 6.9g carbohydrates, 3.4g fat, 0.1g fiber, 165mg cholesterol, 361mg sodium, 181mg potassium

466. Honey Mahi Mahi

Servings: 4   Cooking Time: 2 Hours

Ingredients:

2 tablespoons of liquid honey
2 tablespoons butter, softened
15 oz Mahi Mahi fillet
1 tablespoon olive oil
½ cup of water

½ teaspoon white pepper

Directions:

Slice the fish fillet and put it in the hot skillet.   Add olive oil and roast the fish for 3 minutes per side on high heat.   After this, transfer the fish in the Crock Pot.   Add all remaining ingredients and close the lid.   Cook the fish on high for 2 hours.

Nutrition Info: Per Serving: 208 calories, 20.2g protein, 8.8g carbohydrates, 10.3g fat, 0.1g fiber, 107mg cholesterol, 178mg sodium, 404mg potassium

467. Chili Shrimp And Zucchinis

Servings: 4   Cooking Time: 1 Hour

Ingredients:

1 pound shrimp, peeled and deveined
1 zucchini, cubed
2 scallions, minced
2 green chilies, chopped
1 cup tomato passata
A pinch of salt and black pepper
1 tablespoon chives, chopped

Directions:

In your Crock Pot, mix the shrimp with the zucchini and the other ingredients, toss, put the lid on and cook on High for hour.   Divide the shrimp mix into bowls and serve.

Nutrition Info:calories 210, fat 8, fiber 3, carbs 6, protein 14

468. Cider Dipped Clams

Servings: 4   Cooking Time: 2 Hrs.

Ingredients:

2 lbs. clams, scrubbed
3 oz. pancetta
1 tbsp olive oil
2 garlic cloves, minced
1 bottle infused cider
3 tbsp butter, melted
Salt and black pepper to the taste
Juice of ½ lemon
1 small green apple, chopped
2 thyme springs, chopped

Directions:

Place a suitable pan over medium-high heat and add oil.   Toss in pancetta and sauté for 3 minutes until brown.   Transfer the seared pancetta to the insert of the Crock Pot.   Stir in butter, garlic and rest of the ingredients to the cooker.   Put the cooker's lid on and set the cooking time to 2 hours on High settings.   Serve warm.

Nutrition Info: Per Serving: Calories: 270, Total Fat: 2g, Fiber: 1g, Total Carbs: 11g, Protein: 20g

469. Bigeye Jack Saute

Servings: 4   Cooking Time: 6 Hours

Ingredients:

7 oz (bigeye jack) tuna fillet, chopped
1 teaspoon ground black pepper
1 cup tomato, chopped
1 jalapeno pepper,

chopped

½ cup chicken stock

Directions:
Put all ingredients in the Crock Pot and close the lid.   Cook the saute on Low for 6 hours.
Nutrition Info: Per Serving: 192 calories, 11g protein, 2.4g carbohydrates, 15.6g fat, 0.8g fiber, 0mg cholesterol, 98mg sodium, 123mg potassium

470.   Stuffed Squid

Servings: 4   Cooking Time: 3 Hours
Ingredients:

4 squid	4 tablespoons soy
1 cup sticky rice	sauce
14 ounces dashi stock	1 tablespoon mirin
2 tablespoons sake	2 tablespoons sugar

Directions:
Chop tentacles from squid, mix with the rice, stuff each squid with this mix and seal ends with toothpicks.   Place squid in your Crock Pot, add stock, soy sauce, sake, sugar and mirin, stir, cover and cook on High for 3 hours.   Divide between plates and serve.
Nutrition Info:calories 230, fat 4, fiber 4, carbs 7, protein 11

471.Thai Coconut Shrimps

Servings: 2   Cooking Time: 3 Hours
Ingredients:

1 ½ cups coconut milk	1 tablespoon coconut oil
3 kaffir lime leaves	1 cup mushrooms, sliced
1 lemon grass stalk	
1 cup fresh cilantro	1 onion, sliced
1-inch ginger or galangal root	1 tablespoon fish sauce
1-pound shrimps, shelled and deveined	Juice from 1 lime

Directions:
Place all ingredients in the CrockPot.   Give a good stir.   Close the lid and cook on high for 2 hours or on low for hours.   Garnish with cilantro.
Nutrition Info: Calories per serving: 493; Carbohydrates: 4g; Protein: 11.5g; Fat: 45.3g; Sugar:0 g; Sodium: 940mg; Fiber: 1.7g

472.   Semolina Fish Balls

Servings: 11   Cooking Time: 8 Hrs.
Ingredients:

1 cup sweet corn	1 tsp ground black pepper
5 tbsp fresh dill, chopped	
1 tbsp minced garlic	1 tsp cumin
7 tbsp bread crumbs	1 tsp lemon zest
2 eggs, beaten	¼ tsp cinnamon
10 oz salmon, salmon	3 tbsp almond flour
2 tbsp semolina	3 tbsp scallion, chopped
2 tbsp canola oil	
1 tsp salt	3 tbsp water

Directions:

Mix sweet corn, dill, garlic, semolina, eggs, salt, cumin, almond flour, scallion, cinnamon, lemon zest, and black pepper in a large bowl.   Stir in chopped salmon and mix well.   Make small meatballs out of this fish mixture then roll them in the breadcrumbs.   Place the coated fish ball in the insert of the Crock Pot.   Add canola oil and water to the fish balls.   Put the cooker's lid on and set the cooking time to 8 hours on Low settings.   Serve warm.
Nutrition Info: Per Serving: Calories: 201, Total Fat: 7.9g, Fiber: 2g, Total Carbs: 22.6g, Protein: 11g

473.   Lamb Vegetable Curry

Servings: 4   Cooking Time: 4 Hrs
Ingredients:

1 and ½ tbsp sweet paprika	4 celery stalks, chopped
3 tbsp curry powder	1 onion, chopped
Salt and black pepper to the taste	4 celery stalks, chopped
2 lbs. lamb meat, cubed	1 cup chicken stock
2 tbsp olive oil	4 garlic cloves minced
3 carrots, chopped	1 cup of coconut milk

Directions:
Take oil in a non-stick skillet and heat it over medium-high heat.   Stir in lamb meat to sauté until brown.   Transfer this meat to the Crock Pot along with other ingredients.   Put the cooker's lid on and set the cooking time to hours on High settings.   Serve warm.
Nutrition Info: Per Serving: Calories 300, Total Fat 4g, Fiber 4g, Total Carbs 16g, Protein 13g

474.   Braised Tilapia With Capers

Servings: 4   Cooking Time: 5 Hours
Ingredients:

4 tilapia fillets	½ teaspoon salt
½ cup of water	
2 tablespoons sour cream	¼ teaspoon chili flakes
	1 tablespoon capers

Directions:
Put all ingredients in the Crock Pot and close the lid.   Cook the tilapia on Low for 5 hours.
Nutrition Info: Per Serving: 106 calories, 21.3g protein, 0.4g carbohydrates, 2.3g fat, 0.1g fiber, 58mg cholesterol, 399mg sodium, 10mg potassium

475.   Braised Lobster

Servings: 4   Cooking Time: 3 Hours
Ingredients:

2-pound lobster, cleaned	1 teaspoon Italian seasonings
1 cup of water	

Directions:
Put all ingredients in the Crock Pot.   Close the lid and cook the lobster in High for 3 hours.
Remove the lobster from the Crock Pot and cool it till room temperature

Nutrition Info:Per Serving: 206 calories, 43.1g protein, 0.1g carbohydrates, 2.2g fat, 0g fiber, 332mg cholesterol, 1104mg sodium, 524mg potassium.

476.   Mackerel And Lemon

Servings: 4   Cooking Time: 2 Hours
Ingredients:

4 mackerels	3 ounces breadcrumbs
Juice and rind of 1 lemon	1 egg, whisked
1 tablespoon chives, finely chopped	1 tablespoon butter
Salt and black pepper to the taste	1 tablespoon vegetable oil
	3 lemon wedges

Directions:
In a bowl, mix breadcrumbs with lemon juice, lemon rind, salt, pepper, egg and chives, stir very well and coat mackerel with this mix.   Add the oil and the butter to your Crock Pot and arrange mackerel inside.   Cover, cook on High for 2 hours, divide fish between plates and serve with lemon wedges on the side.
Nutrition Info:calories 200, fat 3, fiber 1, carbs 3, protein 12

477.   Salmon With Almond Crust

Servings: 2   Cooking Time: 2.5 Hours
Ingredients:

8 oz salmon fillet	1 teaspoon butter
2 tablespoons almond flakes	1 teaspoon salt
1 teaspoon ground black pepper	1 egg, beaten
	¼ cup of coconut milk

Directions:
Sprinkle the salmon fillet with ground black pepper and salt.   Then dip the fish in egg and coat in the almond flakes.   Put butter and coconut milk in the Crock Pot.   Then add salmon and close the lid.   Cook the salmon on High for 2.hours.
Nutrition Info:Per Serving: 301 calories, 26.6g protein, 3g carbohydrates, 20.9g fat, 1.5g fiber, 137mg cholesterol, 1262mg sodium, 558mg potassium

478.   Parsley Cod

Servings: 2   Cooking Time: 2 Hours
Ingredients:

1 pound cod fillets, boneless	Juice of 1 lime
3 scallions, chopped	Salt and black pepper to the taste
2 teaspoons olive oil	1 tablespoon parsley, chopped
1 teaspoon coriander, ground	

Directions:
In your Crock Pot, mix the cod with the scallions, the oil and the other ingredients, rub gently, put the lid on and cook on High for hour.   Divide everything between plates and serve.

Nutrition Info:calories 200, fat 12, fiber 2, carbs 6, protein 9

479.   Cinnamon Catfish

Servings: 2   Cooking Time: 2.5 Hours
Ingredients:

1 teaspoon ground cinnamon	2 catfish fillets
1 tablespoon lemon juice	½ teaspoon sesame oil
	1/3 cup water

Directions:
Sprinkle the fish fillets with ground cinnamon, lemon juice, and sesame oil.   Put the fillets in the Crock Pot in one layer.   Add water and close the lid.   Cook the meal on High for 2.5 hours.
Nutrition Info:Per Serving: 231 calories, 25g protein, 1.1g carbohydrates, 13.3g fat, 0.6g fiber, 75mg cholesterol, 88mg sodium, 528mg potassium.

480.   Nutmeg Trout

Servings: 4   Cooking Time: 3 Hours
Ingredients:

1 tablespoon ground nutmeg	1 teaspoon dried oregano
1 tablespoon butter, softened	1 teaspoon fish sauce
1 teaspoon dried cilantro	4 trout fillets
	½ cup of water

Directions:
In the shallow bowl mix butter with cilantro, dried oregano, and fish sauce. Add ground nutmeg and whisk the mixture.   Then grease the fish fillets with nutmeg mixture and put in the Crock Pot. Add remaining butter mixture and water.   Cook the fish on high for 3 hours.
Nutrition Info:Per Serving: 154 calories, 16.8g protein, 1.2g carbohydrates, 8.8g fat, 0.5g fiber, 54mg cholesterol, 178mg sodium, 305mg potassium.

481.   Tarragon Mahi Mahi

Servings: 4   Cooking Time: 2.5 Hours
Ingredients:

1-pound mahi-mahi fillet	1 tablespoon coconut oil
1 tablespoon dried tarragon	½ cup of water

Directions:
Melt the coconut oil in the skillet.   Add mahi-mahi fillet and roast it on high heat for minutes per side.   Put the fish fillet in the Crock Pot.   Add dried tarragon and water.   Close the lid and cook the fish on High for 2.hours.
Nutrition Info:Per Serving: 121 calories, 21.2g protein, 0.2g carbohydrates, 3.4g fat, 0g fiber, 40mg cholesterol, 97mg sodium, 14mg potassium

482.   Salmon And Relish

Servings: 2   Cooking Time: 2 Hours
Ingredients:

2 medium salmon fillets, boneless
Salt and black pepper to the taste
1 shallot, chopped
1 tablespoon lemon juice
1 big lemon, peeled and cut into wedges
¼ cup olive oil+ 1 teaspoon
2 tablespoons parsley, finely chopped

Directions:
Brush salmon fillets with the olive oil, sprinkle with salt and pepper, put in your Crock Pot, add shallot and lemon juice, cover and cook on High for 2 hours.   Shed salmon and divide into bowls. Add lemon segments to your Crock Pot, also add ¼ cup oil and parsley and whisk well.   Divide this mix over salmon, toss and serve.
Nutrition Info:calories 200, fat 10, fiber 1, carbs 5, protein 20

483.	Tuna With Potatoes

Servings: 8   Cooking Time: 4 Hrs
Ingredients:
4 large potatoes, cut in half
8 oz. tuna, canned
4 oz. Cheddar cheese, shredded
1 garlic clove, minced
½ cup cream cheese
1 tsp onion powder
½ tsp salt
1 tsp ground black pepper
1 tsp dried dill

Directions:
Wrap the potatoes with an aluminum foil and put them in the Crock Pot.   Put the cooker's lid on and set the cooking time to hours on High settings. Mix cream cheese with tuna, cheese, black pepper, salt, garlic, dill, and onion powder in a separate bowl.   Remove the potatoes from the foil and scoop out the flesh from each half.   Divide the tuna mixture in the potato shells then return then to the Crock Pot.   Put the cooker's lid on and set the cooking time to 2 hours on High settings. Serve warm.
Nutrition Info: Per Serving: Calories 247, Total Fat 5.9g, Fiber 4g, Total Carbs 35.31g, Protein 14g

484.	Flounder Cheese Casserole

Servings: 11   Cooking Time: 6 Hrs.
Ingredients:
8 oz rice noodles
2 cups chicken stock
12 oz flounder fillet, chopped
½ tsp ground black pepper
2 sweet peppers, chopped
3 sweet potatoes, chopped
1 cup carrot, cooked
2 tbsp butter, melted
3 tbsp chives
4 oz shallot, chopped
7 oz cream cheese
5 oz Parmesan, shredded
½ cup fresh cilantro, chopped
1 cup of water

Directions:
Brush the insert of your Crock Pot with melted butter.   Place the chopped flounder, carrots, sweet peppers, sweet potatoes, shallots, and chives

to the cooker.   Add cilantro, stock, black pepper, cream cheese, and water to the flounder.   Top the flounder casserole with shredded cheese.   Put the cooker's lid on and set the cooking time to 6 hours on Low settings.   Serve warm.
Nutrition Info: Per Serving: Calories: 202, Total Fat: 9.1g, Fiber: 2g, Total Carbs: 19.86g, Protein: 11g

485.	Clam Chowder

Servings: 4   Cooking Time: 2 Hours
Ingredients:
1 cup celery stalks, chopped
Salt and black pepper to the taste
1 teaspoon thyme, ground
2 cups chicken stock
14 ounces canned baby clams
2 cups whipping cream
1 cup onion, chopped
13 bacon slices, chopped

Directions:
Heat up a pan over medium heat, add bacon slices, brown them and transfer to a bowl.   Heat up the same pan over medium heat, add celery and onion, stir and cook for 5 minutes.   Transfer everything to your Crock Pot, also add bacon, baby clams, salt, pepper, stock, thyme and whipping cream, stir and cook on High for 2 hours.   Divide into bowls and serve.
Nutrition Info:calories 420, fat 22, fiber 0, carbs 5, protein 25

486.	Crockpot Garlic Shrimps

Servings: 5   Cooking Time: 3 Hours
Ingredients:
4 tablespoons butter
¼ cup olive oil
5 cloves of garlic, minced
½ teaspoon salt
¼ teaspoon black pepper
1 ½ pounds jumbo shrimps, shelled and deveined.

Directions:
Place all ingredients in the CrockPot.   Give a good stir.   Close the lid and cook on high for 2 hours or on low for hours.   Garnish with chopped parsley if desired.
Nutrition Info: Calories per serving: 292; Carbohydrates: 1.1g; Protein:27.6 g; Fat: 20.7g; Sugar: 0g; Sodium: 401mg; Fiber: 0.6g

487.	Salmon And Berries

Servings: 2   Cooking Time: 3 Hours
Ingredients:
1 pound salmon fillets, boneless and roughly cubed
½ cup blackberries
Juice of 1 lime
1 tablespoon avocado oil
2 scallions, chopped
½ teaspoon Italian seasoning
½ cup fish stock
A pinch of salt and black pepper

Directions:

In your Crock Pot, mix the salmon with the berries, lime juice and the other ingredients, toss, put the lid on and cook on Low for 3 hours.   Divide the mix between plates and serve.
Nutrition Info:calories 211, fat 13, fiber 2, carbs 7, protein 11

488.   Parsley Salmon

Servings: 6   Cooking Time: 5 Hours 30 Minutes
Ingredients:

¼ teaspoon ginger powder	Salt and black pepper, to taste
2 tablespoons olive oil	3 tablespoons fresh parsley, minced
24-ounce salmon fillets	

Directions:
Mix together all the ingredients except salmon fillets in a bowl.   Marinate salmon fillets in this mixture for about 1 hour.   Transfer the marinated salmon fillets into the crock pot and cover the lid. Cook on LOW for about 5 hours and dish out to serve hot.
Nutrition Info: Calories: 191 Fat: 11.7 g Carbohydrates: 0.2 g

489.   Cod With Asparagus

Servings: 4   Cooking Time: 2 Hrs
Ingredients:

4 cod fillets, boneless	Salt and black pepper to the taste
1 bunch asparagus	2 tbsp olive oil
12 tbsp lemon juice	

Directions:
Place the cod fillets in separate foil sheets.   Top the fish with asparagus spears, lemon pepper, oil, and lemon juice.   Wrap the fish with its foil sheet then place them in Crock Pot.   Put the cooker's lid on and set the cooking time to 2 hours on High settings.   Unwrap the fish and serve warm.
Nutrition Info: Per Serving: Calories 202, Total Fat 3g, Fiber 6g, Total Carbs 7g, Protein 3g

490.   Seafood Gravy

Servings: 4   Cooking Time: 5 Hours
Ingredients:

8 oz shrimps, peeled, chopped	1 cup cream
1 bell pepper, diced	1 teaspoon butter
1 onion, diced	¼ cup Cheddar cheese, shredded

Directions:
Put all ingredients in the Crock Pot and gently mix with the help of the spoon.   Close the lid and cook the meal on low for 5 hours.   Carefully mix the meal before serving.
Nutrition Info: Per Serving: 163 calories, 15.8g protein, 7.6g carbohydrates, 7.7g fat, 1g fiber, 141mg cholesterol, 210mg sodium, 221mg potassium

491.   Asian Salmon Mix

Servings: 2   Cooking Time: 3 Hours
Ingredients:

2 medium salmon fillets, boneless	16 ounces mixed broccoli and cauliflower florets
Salt and black pepper to the taste	2 tablespoons lemon juice
2 tablespoons soy sauce	1 teaspoon sesame seeds
2 tablespoons maple syrup	

Directions:
Put the cauliflower and broccoli florets in your Crock Pot and top with salmon fillets.   In a bowl, mix maple syrup with soy sauce and lemon juice, whisk well, pour this over salmon fillets, season with salt, pepper, sprinkle sesame seeds on top and cook on Low for 3 hours.   Divide everything between plates and serve.
Nutrition Info:calories 230, fat 4, fiber 2, carbs 12, protein 6

492.   Coriander Cod Balls

Servings: 3   Cooking Time: 2 Hours
Ingredients:

½ teaspoon minced garlic	2 tablespoons cornflour
8 oz cod fillet, grinded	1 teaspoon avocado oil
1 teaspoon dried cilantro	¼ cup of water

Directions:
Mix minced garlic with grinded cod, dried cilantro, and cornflour.   Make the small balls.   After this, heat the avocado oil in the skillet well.   Add the fish balls and roast them on high heat for 2 minutes per side.   Transfer the fish balls in the Crock Pot.   Add water and cook them on High for 2 hours.
Nutrition Info: Per Serving: 83 calories, 14.4g protein, 4g carbohydrates, 1.1g fat, 0.4g fiber, 39mg cholesterol, 50mg sodium, 23mg potassium

493.   Shrimps Boil

Servings: 2   Cooking Time: 45 Minutes
Ingredients:

½ cup of water	1 tablespoon butter
1 tablespoon piri piri sauce	7 oz shrimps, peeled

Directions:
Pour water in the Crock Pot.   Add shrimps and cook them on high for 45 minutes.   Then drain water and transfer shrimps in the skillet.   Add butter and piri piri sauce.   Roast the shrimps for 2-3 minutes on medium heat.
Nutrition Info: Per Serving: 174 calories, 22.7g protein, 1.8g carbohydrates, 7.8g fat, 0.1g fiber, 224mg cholesterol, 285mg sodium, 170mg potassium

494. Mussels And Sausage Mix

Servings: 4   Cooking Time: 2 Hours

Ingredients:

- 2 pounds mussels, scrubbed and debearded
- 12 ounces amber beer
- 1 tablespoon olive oil
- 1 yellow onion, chopped
- 8 ounces spicy sausage
- 1 tablespoon paprika

Directions:

Grease your Crock Pot with the oil, add onion, paprika, sausage, mussels and beer, cover and cook on High for 2 hours.   Discard unopened mussels, divide the rest between bowls and serve.

Nutrition Info: calories 124, fat 3, fiber 1, carbs 7, protein 12

495. Coriander Salmon Mix

Servings: 2   Cooking Time: 3 Hours

Ingredients:

- 1 pound salmon fillets, boneless and roughly cubed
- 1 tablespoon coriander, chopped
- ½ teaspoon chili powder
- ¼ cup chicken stock
- 3 scallions, chopped
- Juice of 1 lime
- 2 teaspoons avocado oil
- A pinch of salt and black pepper

Directions:

In your Crock Pot, mix the salmon with the coriander, chili powder and the other ingredients, toss gently, put the lid on and cook on High for 3 hours.   Divide the mix between plates and serve.

Nutrition Info: calories 232, fat 10, fiber 4, carbs 6, protein 9

496. Curry Clams

Servings: 4   Cooking Time: 1.5 Hour

Ingredients:

- 1-pound clams
- 1 teaspoon curry paste
- ¼ cup of coconut milk
- 1 cup of water

Directions:

Mix coconut milk with curry paste and water and pour it in the Crock Pot.   Add clams and close the lid.   Cook the meal on High for 1.5 hours or until the clams are opened.

Nutrition Info: Per Serving: 97 calories, 1.1g protein, 13.6g carbohydrates, 4.5g fat, 0.8g fiber, 0mg cholesterol, 415mg sodium, 141mg potassium.

497. Herbed Octopus Mix

Servings: 6   Cooking Time: 3 Hrs.

Ingredients:

- 1 octopus, cleaned and prepared
- 2 rosemary springs
- 2 tsp oregano, dried
- ½ yellow onion, roughly chopped
- 4 thyme sprigs
- ½ lemon
- For the marinade:
- ¼ cup extra virgin olive oil
- Juice of ½ lemon
- 4 garlic cloves, minced
- 2 thyme sprigs
- 1 rosemary spring
- Salt and black pepper to the taste

Directions:

Place the octopus in the insert of the Crock Pot. Add rosemary springs, salt, peppercorns, lemon, onion, oregano, 3 tbsp olive oil, and 4 thyme springs.   Put the cooker's lid on and set the cooking time to 2 hours on High settings. Transfer the cooked octopus to a cutting board and dice it.   Put the diced octopus in a suitable bowl then add ¼ cup olive oil, and remaining ingredients.   Mix well then transfer the octopus along with marinade to the Crock Pot.   Put the cooker's lid on and set the cooking time to 1 hour on High settings.   Serve warm.

Nutrition Info: Per Serving: Calories: 200, Total Fat: 4g, Fiber: 3g, Total Carbs: 10g, Protein: 11g

498. Thyme And Sesame Halibut

Servings: 2   Cooking Time: 4 Hours

Ingredients:

- 1 tablespoon lemon juice
- 1 teaspoon thyme
- Salt and pepper to taste
- 8 ounces halibut or mahi-mahi, cut into 2 portions
- 1 tablespoons sesame seeds, toasted

Directions:

Line the bottom of the crockpot with a foil.   Mix lemon juice, thyme, salt and pepper in a shallow dish.   Place the fish and allow to marinate for 2 hours in the fish.   Sprinkle the fish with toasted sesame seeds.   Arrange the fish in the foil-lined crockpot.   Close the lid and cook on high for 2 hours or on low for 4 hours.

Nutrition Info: Calories per serving: 238; Carbohydrates: 3.9g; Protein: 23.1g; Fat: 14.9g; Sugar: 0.5g; Sodium:313 mg; Fiber:1.6 g

499. Mackerel Stuffed Tacos

Servings: 6   Cooking Time: 2 Hrs.

Ingredients:

- 9 oz mackerel fillet
- 1 tsp salt
- ¼ cup fish stock
- 1 tsp butter
- ½ tsp ground white pepper
- 1 tsp paprika
- 6 corn tortillas
- ¼ cup of salsa
- 1 tsp minced garlic
- ½ tsp mayo

Directions:

Whisk mayo with butter, garlic, white pepper, salt, and paprika in a small bowl.   Rub the mackerel fillet with the mayo garlic mixture.   Place this fish in the insert of Crock Pot and pour in fish stock.   Put the cooker's lid on and set the cooking time to 2 hours on Low settings.   Meanwhile, layer the corn tortilla with salad evenly.   Shred the cooked mackerel fillet and mix it with 2 tsp cooking liquid.   Divide the fish shreds on the corn tortillas and wrap them.   Serve warm.

Nutrition Info: Per Serving: Calories: 120, Total Fat: 2.4g, Fiber: 3g, Total Carbs: 14.37g, Protein: 11g

500. Tomato Seabass

Servings: 4   Cooking Time: 2.5 Hours
Ingredients:

1-pound seabass, cleaned, trimmed	1 cup tomatoes, chopped
1 tablespoon tomato paste	½ cup of water
1 tablespoon avocado oil	1 teaspoon cayenne pepper

Directions:
Mix water with tomato paste and pour it in the Crock Pot.   Add cayenne pepper, seabass, and chopped tomatoes.   Close the lid and cook the seabass on High for 2.5 hours.   Then transfer the seabass in the serving bowls and sprinkle with avocado oil.
Nutrition Info: Per Serving: 157 calories, 11.3g protein, 9.6g carbohydrates, 9.1g fat, 1.9g fiber, 0mg cholesterol, 696mg sodium, 168mg potassium

501. Chives Mackerel

Servings: 2   Cooking Time: 4 Hours
Ingredients:

1 pound mackerel fillets, boneless	1 tablespoon avocado oil
½ teaspoon cumin, ground	1 tablespoon lime juice
½ teaspoon coriander, ground	A pinch of salt and black pepper
2 garlic cloves, minced	2 tablespoons chives, chopped
½ cup chicken stock	

Directions:
In your Crock Pot, mix the mackerel with the cumin, coriander and the other ingredients, put the lid on and cook on Low for 4 hours.   Divide the mix between plates and serve with a side salad.
Nutrition Info: calories 613, fat 41.6, fiber 0.5, carbs 2, protein 54.7

502. Trout Cakes

Servings: 2   Cooking Time: 2 Hours
Ingredients:

7 oz trout fillet, diced	1 tablespoon semolina
1 teaspoon dried oregano	1 teaspoon cornflour
¼ teaspoon ground black pepper	1 egg, beaten
	1/3 cup water
	1 teaspoon sesame oil

Directions:
In the bowl mix diced trout, semolina, dried oregano, ground black pepper, and cornflour. Then add egg and carefully mix the mixture. Heat the sesame oil well.   Then make the fish cakes and put them in the hot oil.   Roast them for 1 minute per side and transfer in the Crock Pot.

Add water and cook the trout cakes for 2 hours on High.
Nutrition Info: Per Serving: 266 calories, 30g protein, 5.6g carbohydrates, 13.1g fat, 0.7g fiber, 155mg cholesterol, 99mg sodium, 519mg potassium.

503. Thai Salmon Cakes

Servings: 10   Cooking Time: 6 Hrs.
Ingredients:

6 oz squid, minced	1 egg yolk
10 oz salmon fillet, minced	1 tsp oyster sauce
2 tbsp chili paste	1 tsp salt
1 tsp cayenne pepper	½ tsp ground coriander
2 oz lemon leaves	1 tsp sugar
3 tbsp green peas, mashed	2 tbsp butter
2 tsp fish sauce	¼ cup cream
2 egg white	3 tbsp almond flour

Directions:
Mix seafood with chili paste, cayenne pepper, lemon leaves, mashed green peas, fish sauce, whisked egg yolk and egg whites in a bowl.   Stir in sugar, salt, oyster sauce, sugar, almond flour, and ground coriander.   Mix well, then make small-sized fish cakes out of this mixture.   Add cream and butter to the insert of the Crock Pot. Place the fish cakes in the butter and cream.   Put the cooker's lid on and set the cooking time to 5 hours on Low settings.   Serve warm with cream mixture.
Nutrition Info: Per Serving: Calories: 112, Total Fat: 6.7g, Fiber: 1g, Total Carbs: 2.95g, Protein: 10g

504. Mussels And Sausage Satay

Servings: 4   Cooking Time: 2 Hrs.
Ingredients:

2 lbs. mussels, scrubbed and debearded	1 yellow onion, chopped
12 oz. amber beer	8 oz. spicy sausage
1 tbsp olive oil	1 tbsp paprika

Directions:
Grease the insert of your Crock Pot with oil.   Toss in mussels, beer, onion, sausage, and paprika. Put the cooker's lid on and set the cooking time to 2 hours on High settings.   Discard all the unopened mussels, if any.   Serve the rest and enjoy it.
Nutrition Info: Per Serving: Calories: 124, Total Fat: 3g, Fiber: 1g, Total Carbs: 7g, Protein: 12g

505. Chili Tamarind Mackerel

Servings: 4   Cooking Time: 2 Hrs.
Ingredients:

18 oz. mackerel, cut into pieces	1 small piece of ginger, chopped
3 garlic cloves, minced	6 stalks laksa leaves
8 shallots, chopped	3 and ½ oz. water

1 tsp dried shrimp powder
1 tsp turmeric powder
1 tbsp chili paste
2 lemongrass sticks, cut into halves

5 tbsp vegetable oil
1 tbsp tamarind paste mixed with 3 oz. water
Salt to the taste
1 tbsp sugar

Directions:
Add shallots, garlic, chili paste, shrimp powder, and turmeric powder to a blender jug.   Blend it well then add the shallots mixture to the insert of the Crock Pot.   Now add fish and all other ingredients to the cooker.   Put the cooker's lid on and set the cooking time to 2 hours on High settings.   Serve warm.
Nutrition Info: Per Serving: Calories: 200, Total Fat: 3g, Fiber: 1g, Total Carbs: 20g, Protein: 22g

506.   Fish Corners

Servings: 4   Cooking Time: 3.5 Hours
Ingredients:

7 oz salmon, canned, shredded
¼ onion, diced
1 teaspoon dried basil

1 egg, beaten
1 teaspoon sesame oil
¼ teaspoon chili powder
4 oz puff pastry

Directions:
Roll up the puff pastry and cut it into squares. After this, mix canned salmon with onion, basil, egg, and chili powder.   Put the salmon mixture in the center of every puff pastry square and roll into the shape of corners.   Then brush the fish corners with sesame oil and put in the Crock Pot. Cook the meal on High for 3.hours.
Nutrition Info: Per Serving: 251 calories, 13.2g protein, 13.6g carbohydrates, 16.1g fat, 0.6g fiber, 63mg cholesterol, 110mg sodium, 236mg potassium

507.   Butter Tilapia

Servings: 4   Cooking Time: 6 Hours
Ingredients:

4 tilapia fillets
½ cup butter
1 teaspoon dried dill

½ teaspoon ground black pepper

Directions:
Sprinkle the tilapia fillets with dried dill and ground black pepper. Put them in the Crock Pot. Add butter.   Cook the tilapia on Low for 6 hours.

Nutrition Info: Per Serving: 298 calories, 21.3g protein, 0.3g carbohydrates, 24.1g fat, 0.1g fiber, 116mg cholesterol, 204mg sodium, 18mg potassium

508.   Moroccan Fish

Servings: 9   Cooking Time: 3 Hours 20 Minutes
Ingredients:

1 teaspoon tea seed oil
1 teaspoon red pepper flakes, crushed
3 pounds salmon fillets
2 garlic cloves, crushed

1 pound cherry tomatoes, crushed slightly
Salt, to taste
1 tablespoon fresh basil leaves, torn
1 teaspoon dried oregano, crushed

Directions:
Put the tea seed oil and salmon fillets in the crock pot and cover the lid.   Cook on LOW for about hours and add cherry tomatoes, garlic, oregano, salt and red pepper flakes.   Cook on HIGH for about 1 hour and garnish with basil leaves to serve.
Nutrition Info: Calories:243 Fat:11.3g Carbohydrates:2.7g

509.   Lamb Potato Stew

Servings: 4   Cooking Time: 8 Hrs
Ingredients:

1 and ½ lbs. lamb meat, cubed
¼ cup flour
Salt and black pepper to the taste
2 tbsp olive oil
1 tsp rosemary, dried

1 onion, sliced
½ tsp thyme, dried
2 cups of water
1 cup baby carrots
2 cups sweet potatoes, chopped

Directions:
First, mix the lamb with flour in a bowl.   Take oil in a non-stick pan and place it over medium-high heat.   Stir in meat and sauté until brown. Transfer the sauteed meat to the Crock Pot along with the rest of the ingredients.   Put the cooker's lid on and set the cooking time to 8 hours on Low settings.   Serve warm.
Nutrition Info: Per Serving: Calories 350, Total Fat 8g, Fiber 3g, Total Carbs 20g, Protein 16g

Poultry Recipes

---

510. Chicken Pocket

Servings: 4   Cooking Time: 4 Hours

Ingredients:

1-pound chicken fillet, skinless, boneless	3 oz prunes, chopped
	1 tablespoon olive oil
	1 teaspoon salt
1 teaspoon dried cilantro	½ cup of water

Directions:

Make the horizontal cut in the chicken fillet and fill it with prunes.   Then secure the cut and rub the chicken fillet with dried cilantro and salt. Sprinkle the chicken with olive oil and transfer in the Crock Pot.   Add water and close the lid. Cook the chicken on High for 4 hours.   Drain water and remove the toothpicks.   Cut the cooked meal into 4 servings.

Nutrition Info: Per Serving: 297 calories, 33.3g protein, 13.6g carbohydrates, 12g fat, 1.5g fiber, 101mg cholesterol, 680mg sodium, 432mg potassium.

---

511. Chicken With Basil And Tomatoes

Servings: 4   Cooking Time: 8 Hours

Ingredients:

¾ cup balsamic vinegar	8 plum tomatoes, sliced
¼ cup fresh basil leaves	4 boneless chicken breasts, bone and skin removed
2 tablespoons olive oil	

Directions:

Place balsamic vinegar, basil leaves, olive oil and tomatoes in a blender. Season with salt and pepper to taste. Pulse until fine.   Arrange the chicken pieces in the crockpot.   Pour over the sauce. Close the lid and cook on low for 8 hours or on high for 6 hours.

Nutrition Info: Calories per serving: 177; Carbohydrates:4 g; Protein:24 g; Fat: 115g; Sugar: 0g; Sodium: 171mg; Fiber: 3.5g

---

512. Chicken Potato Sandwich

Servings: 4   Cooking Time: 8 Hrs

Ingredients:

7 oz. chicken fillet	4 slices French bread, toasted
1 tsp cayenne pepper	
5 oz. mashed potato, cooked	2 tsp mayo
	1 cup of water
6 tbsp chicken gravy	

Directions:

Place the chicken fillet in the Crock Pot and add chicken gravy, water, and cayenne pepper on top. Put the cooker's lid on and set the cooking time to 8 hours on Low settings.   Layer the French bread with mashed potato mixture.   Slice the cooked chicken into strips and return to its gravy.   Mix well, then serve the chicken over the mashed potato.   Serve warm.

Nutrition Info: Per Serving: Calories 314, Total Fat 9.7g, Fiber 3g, Total Carbs 45.01g, Protein 12g

---

513. Chicken Soufflé

Servings: 6   Cooking Time: 3.5 Hours

Ingredients:

1-pound ground chicken	1 teaspoon dried sage
	1 teaspoon salt
1 teaspoon dried oregano	½ cup cream
1 teaspoon butter, softened	4 eggs, beaten
	2 oz provolone cheese, shredded

Directions:

Mix ground chicken with dried oregano, sage, butter, and salt.   Then mix the ground mixture with eggs and transfer in the ramekins.   Add cream and cheese.   Cover the ramekins with foil and transfer in the Crock Pot.   Cook the soufflé on High for 3.hours.

Nutrition Info: Per Serving: 238 calories, 28.2g protein, 1.3g carbohydrates, 12.8g fat, 0.2g fiber, 188mg cholesterol, 587mg sodium, 249mg potassium.

---

514. Curried Chicken Strips

Servings: 6   Cooking Time: 4 Hrs

Ingredients:

1 tbsp curry paste	2 tbsp maple syrup
11 oz. chicken fillet, cut into strips	1 tsp olive oil
	3 tbsp sour cream
1 tsp salt	½ cup fresh dill
	1 tbsp ground paprika

Directions:

Add chicken strips and all other ingredients in a Crock Pot.   Mix the chicken strips to coat well. Put the cooker's lid on and set the cooking time to hours on High settings.   Serve warm.

Nutrition Info: Per Serving: Calories: 177, Total Fat: 9.1g, Fiber: 2g, Total Carbs: 18.11g, Protein: 6g

---

515. Cyprus Chicken

Servings: 4   Cooking Time: 4.5 Hours

Ingredients:

1 tablespoon sesame seeds	1-pound chicken breast, skinless, boneless
½ cup black olives, pitted and halved	
	1 teaspoon cumin seeds
½ cup pearl onions, peeled	1 cup of water

Directions:

Chop the chicken breast roughly and put it in the Crock Pot.   Add sesame seeds, black olives, onions, cumin seeds, and water.   Close the lid and cook the meal on high for 4.5 hours.

Nutrition Info:Per Serving: 169 calories, 24.8g protein, 3.2g carbohydrates, 5.9g fat, 1.2g fiber, 73mg cholesterol, 208mg sodium, 463mg potassium.

516. Chili Chicken

Servings: 4   Cooking Time: 7 Hours

Ingredients:

1 teaspoon chili powder	½ teaspoon ground turmeric
1 tablespoon hot sauce	1 teaspoon garlic, minced
1 tablespoon coconut oil, melted	½ cup of water
	1-pound chicken wings

Directions:

Rub the chicken wings with hot sauce, chili powder, ground turmeric, garlic, and coconut oil.   Then pour water in the Crock Pot and add prepared chicken wings.   Cook the chicken on low for 7 hours.

Nutrition Info:Per Serving: 249 calories, 33g protein, 0.8g carbohydrates, 12g fat, 0.3g fiber, 101mg cholesterol, 200mg sodium, 303mg potassium.

517. Mexican Chicken "bake"

Servings: 6   Cooking Time: 8 Hours

Ingredients:

6 roma tomatoes, cut into quarters	1 jalapeno, seeded
1 cup cilantro leaves	2 pounds chicken breasts, bones and skin removed
1 yellow onion, quartered	½ cup queso quesadilla cheese, shredded
1 teaspoon cumin	
3 cloves of garlic, peeled	1-ounce black olives, pitted and sliced
Salt and pepper to taste	

Directions:

Place the tomatoes, cilantro, onion, cumin, jalapeno, and garlic in a food processor. Season with salt and pepper to taste. Pulse until smooth. Place the chicken breasts in the CrockPot and pour over the salsa sauce.   Top with cheese and olives. Close the lid and cook on high for 6 hours and on high for 8 hours.   Garnish with sour cream, avocado slices, or cilantro.

Nutrition Info:Calories per serving: 203; Carbohydrates: 5g; Protein: 18g; Fat: 11g; Sugar: 0g; Sodium:637 mg; Fiber: 1g

518. Sun-dried Tomato Chicken

Servings: 10   Cooking Time: 8 Hours

Ingredients:

1 tablespoon butter	1 cup sun-dried tomatoes in vinaigrette
3 cloves of garlic, minced	
4 pounds whole	Salt and pepper to taste

chicken, cut into pieces

Directions:

In a skillet, melt the butter and sauté the garlic until lightly browned.   Add the chicken pieces and cook for 3 minutes until slightly browned. Transfer to the crockpot and stir in the sun-dried tomatoes including the vinaigrette.   Season with salt and pepper to taste.   Close the lid and cook on low for 8 hours or on high for 6 hours.

Nutrition Info:Calories per serving: 397; Carbohydrates:9.4 g; Protein: 30.26g; Fat:14.1 g; Sugar: 0.4g; Sodium: 472mg; Fiber: 5.8g

519. Coriander Turkey Mix

Servings: 2   Cooking Time: 6 Hours

Ingredients:

1 pound turkey breasts, skinless, boneless and cubed	1 cup chicken stock
	1 teaspoon sweet paprika
1 tablespoon olive oil	1 tablespoon coriander, chopped
3 scallions, chopped	

Directions:

In your Crock Pot, mix the turkey with the oil, scallions and the other ingredients, toss, put the lid on and cook Low for 6 hours.   Divide the mix into bowls and serve.

Nutrition Info:calories 311, fat 11.2, fiber 2.1, carbs 12.2, protein 39.6

520. Crockpot Caesar Chicken

Servings: 4   Cooking Time: 8 Hours

Ingredients:

½ cup cashew nuts, soaked in water overnight	2 tablespoon Dijon mustard
	Salt and pepper to taste
4 boneless chicken breasts, skin and bones removed	¼ cup parmesan cheese, divided

Directions:

In a blender, place the cashew nuts and Dijon mustard. Season with salt and pepper to taste. Blend until smooth. Set aside.   Season the chicken breasts with salt and pepper to taste. Place in the crockpot and add half of the parmesan cheese.   Pour over the sauce and mix until well combined.   Sprinkle the remaining parmesan cheese.   Close the lid and cook on low for 8 hours or on high for hours.

Nutrition Info:Calories per serving: 320; Carbohydrates:4.2 g; Protein: 38g; Fat: 12g; Sugar: 1g; Sodium: 530mg; Fiber: 3g

521. Duck And Mushrooms

Servings: 2   Cooking Time: 6 Hours

Ingredients:

1 pound duck leg, skinless, boneless and sliced	1 cup chicken stock
	½ teaspoon cumin, ground
1 cup white	

mushrooms, sliced
½ teaspoon rosemary, dried

½ cup heavy cream
1 tablespoon olive oil
¼ cup chives, chopped

Directions:
In your Crock Pot, mix the duck with the stock, mushrooms and the other ingredients, toss, put the lid on and cook on Low for 6 hours.   Divide everything between plates and serve.
Nutrition Info:calories 262, fat 16, fiber 2, carbs 8, protein 16

---

522.   Pesto Chicken Mix

Servings: 2   Cooking Time: 6 Hours And 10 Minutes
Ingredients:

1 pound chicken breast, skinless, boneless and cut into strips
1 tablespoon basil pesto
1 tablespoon olive oil
4 scallions, chopped

½ cup kalamata olives, pitted and halved
1 cup chicken stock
1 tablespoon cilantro, chopped
A pinch of salt and black pepper

Directions:
Heat up a pan with the oil over medium-high heat, add the scallions and the meat, brown for minutes, transfer to the Crock Pot and mix with the remaining ingredients.   Toss, put the lid on, cook on Low for 6 hours, divide the mix between plates and serve.
Nutrition Info:calories 263, fat 14, fiber 1, carbs 8, protein 12

---

523.   Chicken With Figs

Servings: 4   Cooking Time: 7 Hours
Ingredients:

5 oz fresh figs, chopped
14 oz chicken fillet, chopped
1 cup of water

1 teaspoon peppercorns
1 tablespoon dried dill

Directions:
Put all ingredients in the Crock Pot.   Close the lid and cook the meal on Low for 7 hours.
Nutrition Info: Per Serving: 280 calories, 30.1g protein, 23.4g carbohydrates, 7.7g fat, 3.7g fiber, 88mg cholesterol, 93mg sodium, 515mg potassium.

---

524.   Turkey With Zucchini

Servings: 4   Cooking Time: 8 Hours
Ingredients:

1-pound ground turkey
2 red peppers cut into strips
Salt and pepper to taste

2 green onions, sliced
1 large zucchini, sliced

Directions:
Place the ground turkey and red peppers in the crockpot.   Season with salt and pepper to taste. Close the lid and cook on low for 8 hours or on high for 6 hours.   An hour before the cooking time is done, stir in the green onions and zucchini.   Cook further until the vegetables are soft.
Nutrition Info: Calories per serving: 195; Carbohydrates: 5.7g; Protein: 23.9g; Fat: 9.01g; Sugar: 0.4g; Sodium: 542mg; Fiber: 2.5g

---

525.   Curry Drumsticks

Servings: 4   Cooking Time: 3 Hours
Ingredients:

8 chicken drumsticks
1 teaspoon curry paste

1 cup cream
1 teaspoon olive oil

Directions:
Mix the curry paste with cream and pour the liquid in the Crock Pot.   Add olive oil and chicken drumsticks.   Close the lid and cook the chicken on High for hours.
Nutrition Info: Per Serving: 212 calories, 25.8g protein, 2.2g carbohydrates, 10.5g fat, 0g fiber, 92mg cholesterol, 93mg sodium, 205mg potassium.

---

526.   Chicken With Lentils

Servings: 4   Cooking Time: 4 Hrs
Ingredients:

8 oz. bacon, cooked and chopped
2 tbsp olive oil
1 cup yellow onion, chopped
8 oz. lentils, dried
12 parsley springs, chopped

2 carrots, chopped
Salt and black pepper to the taste
2 bay leaves
2 ½ lbs. of chicken pieces
1-quart chicken stock
2 tsp sherry vinegar

Directions:
Add oil, onions, bacon, lentils, carrots, parsley, stock, bay leaves, chicken pieces, salt, and black pepper to the Crock Pot.   Put the cooker's lid on and set the cooking time to 4 hours on High settings.   Transfer the slow-cooked chicken to a cutting board and remove the meat from the bones. Shred the meat and return to the Crock Pot   Mix well and vinegar.   Serve warm.
Nutrition Info: Per Serving: Calories: 321, Total Fat: 3g, Fiber: 12g, Total Carbs: 29g, Protein: 16g

---

527.   Paella

Servings: 6   Cooking Time: 4 Hours
Ingredients:

12 oz chicken fillet, chopped
4 oz chorizo, chopped
½ cup white rice
1 teaspoon garlic, diced

2 cups chicken stock
1 teaspoon dried cilantro
1 teaspoon chili flakes
Cooking spray

Directions:

Spray the skillet with cooking spray and put the chorizo inside.   Roast the chorizo for minutes per side and transfer in the Crock Pot.   Then put rice in the Crock Pot.   Then add all remaining ingredients and carefully stir the paella mixture. Cook it on High for 4 hours.
Nutrition Info: Per Serving: 254 calories, 22.3g protein, 13.1g carbohydrates, 11.7g fat, 0.2g fiber, 67mg cholesterol, 538mg sodium, 238mg potassium.

---

528.   Almond-stuffed Chicken

Servings: 6   Cooking Time: 8 Hours
Ingredients:

1/3 cup Boursin cheese or any herbed cheese of your choice	1 ½ teaspoons butter
¼ cup slivered almonds, toasted and chopped	4 boneless chicken breasts, halved
	Salt and pepper to taste

Directions:
Line the bottom of the crockpot with foil.   Grease the foil with butter.   In a mixing bowl, mix together the cheese and almonds.   Cut a slit through the chicken breasts to create a pocket. Season the chicken with salt and pepper to taste. Spoon the cheese mixture into the slit on the chicken. Secure the slit with toothpicks.   Place the chicken in the foil-lined crockpot.   Cover with lid and cook on low for hours or on high for 6 hours.
Nutrition Info: Calories per serving: 249; Carbohydrates: 0.9g; Protein: 42.1g; Fat: 10g; Sugar: 0g; Sodium:592 mg; Fiber:0.4 g

---

529.   Cardamom Chicken In Coconut Milk

Servings: 4   Cooking Time: 3 Hours
Ingredients:

12 oz chicken fillet, chopped	1 cup of coconut milk
1 onion, diced	1 teaspoon ground ginger
1 teaspoon ground cardamom	3 garlic cloves, diced
1 teaspoon chili pepper	1 tablespoon coconut oil

Directions:
Melt the coconut oil in the skillet.   Add diced onion, ground cardamom, chili pepper, ground ginger, and garlic.   Roast the mixture for 1 minute.   Then transfer it in the Crock Pot.   Add chicken fillet and coconut milk. Stir the mixture and close the lid.   Cook the chicken on high for 3 hours.
Nutrition Info: Per Serving: 347 calories, 26.5g protein, 7.4g carbohydrates, 24.1g fat, 2.2g fiber, 76mg cholesterol, 84mg sodium, 429mg potassium.

---

530.   Braised Chicken With Bay Leaf

Servings: 4   Cooking Time: 8 Hours
Ingredients:

1-pound chicken breast, skinless	1 teaspoon garlic powder
1 teaspoon salt	3 cups of water
4 bay leaves	

Directions:
Put all ingredients in the Crock Pot and close the lid.   Cook the chicken on low for 8 hours.   Then chop the chicken and transfer in the bowls.   Add chicken liquid from the Crock Pot.
Nutrition Info: Per Serving: 135 calories, 24.2g protein, 1.3g carbohydrates, 2.9g fat, 0.3g fiber, 73mg cholesterol, 645mg sodium, 434mg potassium.

---

531.   Chicken With Vegetables

Servings: 4   Cooking Time: 4 Hours
Ingredients:

1-pound chicken fillet, cut into slices	½ cup corn kernels, frozen
1 cup broccoli, chopped	1 cup of water
½ cup green peas, frozen	1 teaspoon dried rosemary
	½ teaspoon peppercorns

Directions:
Put all ingredients in the Crock Pot.   Close the lid and cook the meal on High for 4 hours.
Nutrition Info: Per Serving: 256 calories, 35.1g protein, 8.1g carbohydrates, 8.8g fat, 2.2g fiber, 101mg cholesterol, 111mg sodium, 451mg potassium.

---

532.   Coca Cola Dipped Chicken

Servings: 4   Cooking Time: 4 Hrs
Ingredients:

1 yellow onion, minced	4 chicken drumsticks
1 tbsp balsamic vinegar	15 oz. coca cola
1 chili pepper, chopped	Salt and black pepper to the taste
	2 tbsp olive oil

Directions:
Add chicken to a pan greased with oil and sear it until golden brown from both the sides.   Transfer the chicken to the Crock Pot.   Stir in coca-cola, chili, onion, vinegar, black pepper, and salt to the cooker.   Put the cooker's lid on and set the cooking time to hours on High settings.   Serve warm.
Nutrition Info: Per Serving: Calories: 372, Total Fat: 14g, Fiber: 3g, Total Carbs: 20g, Protein: 15g

---

533.   Crockpot Chicken Curry

Servings: 6   Cooking Time: 8 Hours
Ingredients:

2 pounds chicken breasts, bones removed
1 can coconut milk
1 onion, chopped

4 tablespoons curry powder
Salt and pepper to taste

Directions:
Place all ingredients in the crockpot.   Give a good stir to incorporate everything.   Close the lid and cook on low for 8 hours or 6 hours on high.
Nutrition Info: Calories per serving:468; Carbohydrates: 9g; Protein: 34.5g; Fat: 33.7g; Sugar: 1.2g; Sodium:646 mg; Fiber: 1.6g

534.   Crockpot Yellow Chicken Curry

Servings: 5   Cooking Time: 8 Hours
Ingredients:

1 ½ pounds boneless chicken breasts, cut into chunks
6 cups vegetable broth (made from boiling onions, broccoli, bell pepper, and carrots in 7 cups water)
1 cup coconut milk, unsweetened
1 cup tomatoes, crushed

1 tablespoon cumin
2 teaspoons ground coriander
1 teaspoon turmeric powder
1 thumb-size ginger, sliced
4 cloves of garlic, minced
1 teaspoon cinnamon
½ teaspoon cayenne pepper
Salt to taste

Directions:
Place all ingredients in the CrockPot.   Close the lid and cook on high for 6 hours or on low for 8 hours.
Nutrition Info: Calories per serving: 291; Carbohydrates: 6.1g; Protein: 32.5g; Fat: 15.4g; Sugar: 0.3g; Sodium: 527mg; Fiber: 2.8g

535.   Chicken Wings And Mint Sauce

Servings: 6   Cooking Time: 4 Hours
Ingredients:

18 chicken wings, cut into halves
1 tablespoon turmeric
1 tablespoon cumin, ground
1 tablespoon ginger, grated
1 tablespoon coriander, ground
1 tablespoon paprika
A pinch of cayenne pepper
Salt and black pepper to the taste

2 tablespoons olive oil
For the sauce:
Juice of ½ lime
1 cup mint leaves
1 small ginger piece, chopped
¾ cup cilantro
1 tablespoon olive oil
1 tablespoon water
Salt and black pepper to the taste
1 Serrano pepper

Directions:
In a bowl, mix tablespoon ginger with cumin, coriander, paprika, turmeric, salt, pepper, cayenne and 2 tablespoons oil and stir well.   Add chicken wings pieces to this mix, toss to coat well and keep in the fridge for   minutes.   Add marinated wings to your Crock Pot, cook on High for 4 hours and transfer to a bowl.   In your blender, mix mint with cilantro, 1 small ginger pieces, juice of ½ lime, 1 tablespoon olive oil, salt, pepper, water and Serrano pepper and blend very well.   Serve your chicken wings with this sauce on the side.
Nutrition Info:calories 230, fat 5, fiber 1, carbs 12, protein 9

536.   Chicken And Sour Cream

Servings: 4   Cooking Time: 4 Hours
Ingredients:

Salt and black pepper to the taste
1 teaspoon onion powder

4 chicken thighs
¼ cup sour cream
2 tablespoons sweet paprika

Directions:
In a bowl, mix paprika with salt, pepper and onion powder and stir.   Season chicken pieces with this paprika mix, place them in your Crock Pot, add sour cream, toss, cover and cook on High for 4 hours.   Divide everything between plates and serve.
Nutrition Info:calories 384, fat 31, fiber 2, carbs 11, protein 33

537.   Chipotle Chicken Enchilada Stew

Servings: 5   Cooking Time: 8 Hours
Ingredients:

1 ½ pounds chicken breasts, bones and skin removed
1 onion, chopped
1 green pepper, chopped
1 yellow pepper, chopped
3 jalapeno peppers, chopped
2 cups homemade chicken stock

1 cup tomatoes, diced
2 cups ground chicken
4 cloves of garlic, minced
1 tablespoon cumin
1 tablespoon chili powder
1 tablespoon chipotle pepper, chopped
1 teaspoon oregano
Salt and pepper to taste

Directions:
Place all ingredients in the CrockPot.   Close the lid and cook on high for 6 hours or on low for 8 hours.   Serve with avocado slices and cilantro.
Nutrition Info: Calories per serving: 708; Carbohydrates: 9.2g; Protein: 108.4g; Fat: 23.6g; Sugar: 0.8g; Sodium: 989mg; Fiber: 3.7g

538.   Chicken And Chickpeas

Servings: 4   Cooking Time: 4 Hours
Ingredients:

1 yellow onion, chopped
4 garlic cloves, minced

2 tablespoons butter
A pinch of cayenne pepper
15 ounces canned

1 tablespoon ginger, grated
1 and ½ teaspoon paprika
1 tablespoon cumin, ground
1 and ½ teaspoons coriander, ground
1 teaspoon turmeric, ground
Salt and black pepper to the taste

tomatoes, crushed
¼ cup lemon juice
1 pound spinach, chopped
3 pounds chicken drumsticks and thighs
½ cup cilantro, chopped
½ cup chicken stock
15 ounces canned chickpeas, drained
½ cup heavy cream

Directions:
Grease your Crock Pot with the butter, add onion, garlic, ginger, paprika, cumin, coriander, turmeric, salt, pepper, cayenne, tomatoes, lemon juice, spinach, chicken, stock, chickpeas and heavy cream, cover and cook on High for 4 hours.   Add cilantro, stir everything, divide between plates and serve.
Nutrition Info:calories 300, fat 4, fiber 6, carbs 30, protein 17

539.   Ginger Turkey

Servings: 4   Cooking Time: 5 Hours
Ingredients:
3 oz. fresh ginger, peeled and grated
9 oz. turkey fillet
1 tbsp maple syrup
1 tsp brown sugar
¼ cup thyme leaves

1 tsp thyme
½ tsp ground celery
1 tsp salt
1 tsp sesame oil
1 tsp ground ginger
¼ cup heavy cream

Directions:
Blend heavy cream with the ginger ground, sesame oil, salt, ground celery, thyme, and thyme leaves in a blender.   Add maple syrup and brown sugar then mix well.   Rub the turkey with ginger and place it in the Crock Pot.   Pour the cream-thyme mixture over this turkey.   Put the cooker's lid on and set the cooking time to hours on High settings. Slice and serve
Nutrition Info: Per Serving: Calories: 390, Total Fat: 33.6g, Fiber: 1g, Total Carbs: 8.96g, Protein: 13g

540.   Crockpot Cheesy Buttermilk Drumsticks

Servings: 8   Cooking Time: 8 Hours
Ingredients:
2 tablespoons butter, melted
Salt and pepper to taste

8 chicken drumsticks
¾ cup buttermilk
1/3 cup grated parmesan cheese

Directions:
Pour melted butter in the crockpot.   Season the chicken drumsticks with salt and pepper to taste.

Place in the crockpot and pour the buttermilk. Top with parmesan cheese.   Close the lid and cook on low for 8 hours and on high for 6 hours.
Nutrition Info: Calories per serving: 264; Carbohydrates:2.3 g; Protein: 25.6g; Fat: 16.8g; Sugar: 0.4g; Sodium: 783mg; Fiber:0 g

541.   Bourbon Chicken Cubes

Servings: 4   Cooking Time: 4 Hours
Ingredients:
½ cup bourbon
1 teaspoon liquid honey
1 tablespoon BBQ sauce

1 white onion, diced
1 teaspoon garlic powder
1-pound chicken fillet, cubed

Directions:
Put all ingredients in the Crock Pot.   Mix the mixture until liquid honey is dissolved.   Then close the lid and cook the meal on high for 4 hours.
Nutrition Info: Per Serving: 304 calories, 33.2g protein, 5.9g carbohydrates, 8.5g fat, 0.7g fiber, 101mg cholesterol, 143mg sodium, 333mg potassium.

542.   Chicken Chickpeas

Servings: 4   Cooking Time: 4 Hrs
Ingredients:
1 yellow onion, chopped
2 tbsp butter
4 garlic cloves, minced
1 tbsp ginger, grated
1 and ½ tsp paprika
1 and ½ tsp coriander, ground
1 tsp turmeric, ground
Salt and black pepper to the taste
A pinch of cayenne pepper

1 tbsp cumin, ground
15 oz. canned tomatoes, crushed
¼ cup lemon juice
1 lb. spinach, chopped
3 lbs. chicken drumsticks and thighs
½ cup cilantro, chopped
½ cup chicken stock
15 oz. canned chickpeas, drained
½ cup heavy cream

Directions:
Grease the base of the Crock Pot with butter.   Stir in chicken, chickpeas, and all other ingredients to the Crock Pot.   Put the cooker's lid on and set the cooking time to 4 hours on High settings.   Serve warm.
Nutrition Info: Per Serving: Calories: 300, Total Fat: 4g, Fiber: 6g, Total Carbs: 30g, Protein: 17g

543.   Chicken Stuffed With Plums

Servings: 6   Cooking Time: 4 Hours
Ingredients:
6 chicken fillets
1 cup plums, pitted, sliced
1 cup of water

1 teaspoon salt
1 teaspoon white pepper

Directions:

Beat the chicken fillets gently and rub with salt and white pepper. Then put the sliced plums on the chicken fillets and roll them. Secure the chicken rolls with toothpicks and put in the Crock Pot. Add water and close the lid. Cook the meal on High for 4 hours. Then remove the chicken from the Crock Pot, remove the toothpicks and transfer in the serving plates.

Nutrition Info: Per Serving: 283 calories, 42.4g protein, 1.6g carbohydrates, 10.9g fat, 0.2g fiber, 130mg cholesterol, 514mg sodium, 377mg potassium.

544.	Chicken Vegetable Curry

Servings: 6   Cooking Time: 8 Hours

Ingredients:

1-pound chicken breasts, bones removed	1 tablespoon butter
	1 cup water
1 package frozen vegetable mix	2 tablespoons curry powder

Directions:
Place all ingredients in the crockpot. Stir to combine everything. Close the lid and cook on low for 8 hours or on high for 6 hours.

Nutrition Info: Calories per serving: 273; Carbohydrates: 6.1g; Protein:21 g; Fat: 10g; Sugar: 0.1g; Sodium: 311mg; Fiber: 4g

545.	Cilantro Chicken And Eggplant Mix

Servings: 2   Cooking Time: 7 Hours

Ingredients:

1 pound chicken breasts, skinless, boneless and sliced	3 scallions, chopped
	A pinch of salt and black pepper
2 eggplants, roughly cubed	1 teaspoon chili powder
½ cup chicken stock	1 tablespoon cilantro, chopped
½ cup tomato sauce	

Directions:
In your Crock Pot, mix the chicken with the eggplant, stock and the other ingredients, toss, put the lid on, cook on Low for 7 hours, divide the mix between plates and serve.

Nutrition Info:calories 223, fat 9, fiber 2, carbs 4, protein 11

546.	Mediterranean Chicken

Servings: 4   Cooking Time: 4 Hours

Ingredients:

1 and ½ pounds chicken breast, skinless and boneless	¼ cup olive oil
	1 cucumber, chopped
Juice of 2 lemons	1 cup kalamata olives, pitted and sliced
1 rosemary spring, chopped	
3 garlic cloves, minced	¼ cup red onions, chopped
A pinch of salt and black pepper	2 tablespoons red vinegar

Directions:
In your Crock Pot, mix chicken with lemon juice, rosemary, oil, garlic, salt and pepper, stir, cover and cook on High for 4 hours. Transfer chicken to a cutting board, shred with forks, transfer to a bowl, add cucumber, olives, onion and vinegar, toss, divide between plates and serve.

Nutrition Info:calories 240, fat 3, fiber 3, carbs 12, protein 3

547.	Crockpot Rosemary Lemon Chicken

Servings: 6   Cooking Time: 8 Hours

Ingredients:

1 tablespoon butter	½ cup lemon juice, freshly squeezed
4 pounds chicken breasts, bones and skin removed	
	¾ cup homemade chicken broth
3 onions, chopped	1 tablespoon lemon zest
6 cloves of garlic, minced	
3 sprigs of fresh rosemary	Salt and pepper to taste

Directions:
Place all ingredients in the CrockPot. Close the lid and cook on high for 6 hours or on low for 8 hours. Garnish with parsley.

Nutrition Info: Calories per serving: 573; Carbohydrates: 4.8g; Protein: 64.3g; Fat: 30.1g; Sugar: 1.2g; Sodium: 837mg; Fiber: 2.7g

548.	Rosemary Chicken

Servings: 2   Cooking Time: 7 Hours

Ingredients:

1 pound chicken thighs, boneless, skinless and sliced	1 tablespoon rosemary, chopped
	1 cup chicken stock
1 tablespoon avocado oil	A pinch of salt and black pepper
1 teaspoon cumin, ground	1 tablespoon chives, chopped

Directions:
In your Crock Pot, mix the chicken with the oil, cumin and the other ingredients, toss, put the lid on and cook on Low for 7 hours. Divide the mix between plates and serve.

Nutrition Info:calories 273, fat 13, fiber 3, carbs 7, protein 17

549.	Turkey Gumbo

Servings: 4   Cooking Time: 7 Hours

Ingredients:

1 pound turkey wings	5 ounces water
Salt and black pepper to the taste	2 tablespoons chili powder
1 yellow onion, chopped	
	1 and ½ teaspoons cumin, ground
1 yellow bell pepper, chopped	A pinch of cayenne pepper
3 garlic cloves, chopped	2 cups veggies stock

Directions:
In your Crock Pot, mix turkey with salt, pepper, onion, bell pepper, garlic, chili powder, cumin, cayenne and stock, stir, cover and cook on Low for 7 hours.   Divide everything between plates and serve.
Nutrition Info:calories 232, fat 4, fiber 7, carbs 17, protein 20

---

550.   Crockpot Salsa Chicken

Servings: 4   Cooking Time: 7 Hours
Ingredients:

6 roma tomatoes, cut into quarters	4 chicken breasts, skin and bones removed
1 jalapeno, seeded	2 tablespoons oil
1 yellow onion, quartered	Salt and pepper to taste
3 cloves of garlic, peeled	2 tablespoon lime juice, freshly squeezed
1 cup cilantro leaves	
1 teaspoon cumin	

Directions:
Place in a food processor tomatoes, jalapeno, onion, garlic, cilantro, and cumin. Pulse until smooth.   Place the chicken breasts in the CrockPot. Add in the oil and season with salt and pepper to taste.   Pour the homemade salsa and add in the lime juice.   Close the lid and cook on high for 5 hours or on low for 6 hours.
Nutrition Info: Calories per serving: 598; Carbohydrates: 8.1g; Protein: g62.9; Fat: 34.2g; Sugar: 2.1g; Sodium: 1204mg; Fiber: 3.9g

---

551.Curry Chicken Wings

Servings: 4   Cooking Time: 7 Hours
Ingredients:

1-pound chicken wings	½ cup heavy cream
1 teaspoon curry paste	½ teaspoon ground nutmeg
1 teaspoon minced garlic	½ cup of water

Directions:
In the bowl mix curry paste, heavy cream, minced garlic, and ground nutmeg.   Add chicken wings and stir.   Then pour water in the Crock Pot. Add chicken wings with all remaining curry paste mixture and close the lid.   Cook the chicken wings on Low for 7 hours.
Nutrition Info: Per Serving: 278 calories, 33.2g protein, 1.1g carbohydrates, 14.8g fat, 0.1g fiber, 121mg cholesterol, 104mg sodium, 291mg potassium.

---

552.   Green Chicken Salad

Servings: 4   Cooking Time: 3.5 Hours
Ingredients:

1 cup celery stalk, chopped	1 tablespoon mayonnaise
10 oz chicken fillet	1 teaspoon lemon juice
1 teaspoon salt	

1 teaspoon ground black pepper	1 cup arugula, chopped
1 cup of water	1 cup of green grapes
1 tablespoon mustard	

Directions:
Put the chicken in the Crock Pot.   Add salt and ground black pepper. Add water.   Cook the chicken in high for 5 hours.   Meanwhile, put green grapes, arugula, and celery stalk in the bowl. Then chopped the cooked chicken and add it in the arugula mixture.   In the shallow bowl, mix mustard with lemon juice, and mayonnaise.   Add the mixture in the salad and shake it well.
Nutrition Info: Per Serving: 184 calories, 21.7g protein, 7.1g carbohydrates, 7.5g fat, 1.3g fiber, 64mg cholesterol, 693mg sodium, 329mg potassium.

---

553.   Buffalo Chicken

Servings: 12   Cooking Time: 4 Hours
Ingredients:

2 pounds chicken breasts, skinless and boneless	1 cup cayenne sauce
	½ cup chicken stock
Salt and black pepper to the taste	½ packet ranch seasoning mix
2 garlic cloves, minced	1 tablespoon brown sugar

Directions:
In your Crock Pot, mix chicken with salt, pepper, garlic, cayenne sauce, stock, seasoning and sugar, toss, cover and cook on High for 4 hours.   Divide between plates and serve.
Nutrition Info:calories 273, fat 6, fiber 7, carbs 17, protein 2

---

554.   Mexican Black Beans Salad

Servings: 10   Cooking Time: 10 Hrs
Ingredients:

1 cup black beans	7 oz. chicken fillet
1 cup sweet corn, frozen	5 oz. Cheddar cheese
3 tomatoes, chopped	4 tbsp mayonnaise
½ cup fresh dill, chopped	1 tsp minced garlic
	1 cup lettuce, chopped
1 chili pepper, chopped	5 cups chicken stock
	1 cucumber, chopped

Directions:
Add stock, chicken fillet, black beans, and corn to the Crock Pot.   Put the cooker's lid on and set the cooking time to 10 hours on Low settings.   Now shred the cooked chicken with the help of two forks.   Add chicken shred, beans and all other ingredients in a salad bowl.   Toss them well and serve.
Nutrition Info: Per Serving: Calories 182, Total Fat 7.8g, Fiber 2g, Total Carbs 19.6g, Protein 9g

---

555.   Curry-glazed Chicken

Servings: 12   Cooking Time: 9 Hours
Ingredients:

¼ cup butter, melted
¼ cup yellow mustard
Salt and pepper to taste

2 tablespoons curry powder
1 whole chicken, cut up into pieces

Directions:
Place all ingredients in the crockpot.   Mix everything to combine.   Close the lid and cook on low for 9 hours or on high for 7 hours.
Nutrition Info: Calories per serving: 119; Carbohydrates:3.5 g; Protein: 10.5g; Fat: 8.5g; Sugar: 0g; Sodium: 325mg; Fiber: 1.6g

---

556.   Mediterranean Stuffed Chicken

Servings: 4   Cooking Time: 8 Hours
Ingredients:

Salt and pepper to taste
1 cup feta cheese, crumbled
1/3 cup sun-dried tomatoes, chopped

4 chicken breasts, bones and skin removed
2 tablespoons olive oil

Directions:
Create a slit in the chicken breasts to thin out the meat. Season with salt and pepper to taste   In a mixing bowl, combine the feta cheese and sun-dried tomatoes.   Spoon the feta cheese mixture into the slit created into the chicken.   Close the slit using toothpicks.   Brush the chicken with olive oil.   Place in the crockpot and cook on high for hours or on low for 8 hours.
Nutrition Info: Calories per serving: 332; Carbohydrates: 3g; Protein:40 g; Fat: 17g; Sugar: 0g; Sodium: 621mg; Fiber:2.4 g

---

557.   Chicken Chowder

Servings: 4   Cooking Time: 6 Hours
Ingredients:

3 chicken breasts, skinless and boneless and cubed
4 cups chicken stock
8 ounces canned green chilies, chopped
1 yellow onion, chopped
15 ounces coconut cream

1 sweet potato, cubed
1 teaspoon garlic powder
4 bacon strips, cooked and crumbled
A pinch of salt and black pepper
1 tablespoon parsley, chopped

Directions:
In your Crock Pot, mix chicken with stock, sweet potato, green chilies, onion, garlic powder, salt and pepper, stir, cover and cook on Low for 5 hours and 40 minutes.   Add coconut cream and parsley, stir, cover and cook on Low for   minutes more. Ladle chowder into bowls, sprinkle bacon on top and serve.
Nutrition Info: calories 232, fat 3, fiber 7, carbs 14, protein 7

---

558.   Garlic Pulled Chicken

Servings: 4   Cooking Time: 4 Hours
Ingredients:

1-pound chicken breast, skinless, boneless
2 cups of water

1 tablespoon minced garlic
½ cup plain yogurt

Directions:
Put the chicken breast in the Crock Pot.   Add minced garlic and water.   Close the lid and cook the chicken on High for 4 hours.   Then drain water and shred the chicken breast.   Add plain yogurt and stir the pulled chicken well.
Nutrition Info: Per Serving: 154 calories, 25.9g protein, 2.9g carbohydrates, 3.2g fat, 0g fiber, 74mg cholesterol, 83mg sodium, 501mg potassium.

---

559.   Chicken Breasts

Servings: 4   Cooking Time: 6 Hours
Ingredients:

2 red bell peppers, chopped
2 pounds chicken breasts, skinless and boneless
4 garlic cloves, minced
2 teaspoons paprika

1 yellow onion, chopped
1 cup low sodium chicken stock
2 teaspoons cinnamon powder
¼ teaspoon nutmeg, ground

Directions:
In a bowl, mix bell peppers with chicken breasts, garlic, onion, paprika, cinnamon and nutmeg, toss to coat, transfer everything to your Crock Pot, add stock, cover and cook on Low for 6 hours.   Divide chicken and veggies between plates and serve.
Nutrition Info: calories 250, fat 3, fiber 5, carbs 12, protein 10

---

560.   Bali Style Chicken

Servings: 4   Cooking Time: 4 Hours
Ingredients:

4 chicken drumsticks
1 teaspoon chili powder
1 teaspoon allspices
1 teaspoon minced garlic

2 tablespoons olive oil
½ cup tomato juice
1 jalapeno pepper, chopped

Directions:
Mix chili powder, allspices, minced garlic, olive oil, jalapeno pepper, and tomato juice in the bowl. Add chicken drumsticks and mix the mixture. Marinate the chicken for 30 minutes.   Then transfer the chicken with tomato juice mixture in the Crock Pot and close the lid.   Cook the chicken on High for hours.
Nutrition Info: Per Serving: 148 calories, 13.1g protein, 2.4g carbohydrates, 9.8g fat, 0.6g fiber, 40mg cholesterol, 126mg sodium, 189mg potassium.

561. Hot Chicken And Zucchinis

Servings: 2   Cooking Time: 6 Hours

Ingredients:

1 pound chicken breasts, skinless, boneless and cubed	1 red onion, chopped
1 zucchini, cubed	2 tablespoons olive oil
2 garlic cloves, minced	A pinch of salt and black pepper
1 red chili, minced	1 cup chicken stock
½ teaspoon hot paprika	1 tablespoon chives, chopped
	,

Directions:

In your Crock Pot, mix the chicken with the zucchini, garlic, chili pepper and the other ingredients, toss, put the lid on and cook on Low for 6 hours.   Divide everything between plates and serve.

Nutrition Info:calories 221, fat 12, fiber 2, carbs 5, protein 17

562. Dill Turkey And Peas

Servings: 2   Cooking Time: 5 Hours

Ingredients:

1 pound turkey breast, skinless, boneless and sliced	A pinch of salt and black pepper
1 cup green peas	1 cup chicken stock
½ cup tomato sauce	1 teaspoon garam masala
½ cup scallions, chopped	1 tablespoon dill, chopped

Directions:

In your Crock Pot, mix the turkey with the peas, tomato sauce and the other ingredients, toss, put the lid on and cook on High for 5 hours.   Divide the mix into bowls and serve right away.

Nutrition Info:calories 326, fat 4.6, fiber 6.6, carbs 26.7, protein 44.6

563. Horseradish Mixed Chicken

Servings: 9   Cooking Time: 11 Hours

Ingredients:

3 tbsp horseradish, grated	1/3 cup beef broth
1 tbsp mustard	6 oz. carrot, grated
1 tsp salt	1 zucchini, sliced
1 tbsp mayonnaise	1 lb. chicken breast
3 tbsp sour cream	1 tsp olive oil

Directions:

Add chicken, zucchini, and all other ingredients to the Crock Pot.   Put the cooker's lid on and set the cooking time to 11 hours on Low settings.   Serve warm.

Nutrition Info: Per Serving: Calories: 203, Total Fat: 11.3g, Fiber: 2g, Total Carbs: 4.67g, Protein: 20g

564. Fennel And Chicken Saute

Servings: 4   Cooking Time: 7 Hours

Ingredients:

1 cup fennel, peeled, chopped	1 cup of water
10 oz chicken fillet, chopped	1 teaspoon ground black pepper
1 tablespoon tomato paste	1 teaspoon olive oil
	½ teaspoon fennel seeds

Directions:

Heat the olive oil in the skillet.   Add fennel seeds and roast them until you get saturated fennel smell. Transfer the seeds in the Crock Pot.   Add fennel, chicken fillet, tomato paste, water, and ground black pepper.   Close the lid and cook the meal on Low for 7 hours.

Nutrition Info: Per Serving: 157 calories, 28.1g protein, 2.8g carbohydrates, 6.5g fat, 1.1g fiber, 63mg cholesterol, 78mg sodium, 314mg potassium.

565. Corn And Chicken Saute

Servings: 4   Cooking Time: 8 Hours

Ingredients:

1 cup carrot, chopped	1 cup of water
2 corn on cobs, roughly chopped	1 teaspoon Italian seasonings
1-pound chicken fillet, chopped	1 teaspoon salt

Directions:

Put all ingredients from the list above in the Crock Pot.   Close the lid and cook the meal on Low for 8 hours.

Nutrition Info: Per Serving: 308 calories, 35.3g protein, 18.8g carbohydrates, 10.5g fat, 0.7g fiber, 105mg cholesterol, 714mg sodium, 544mg potassium.

566. Curry Chicken Strips

Servings: 6   Cooking Time: 3.5 Hours

Ingredients:

1 tablespoon curry paste	1 teaspoon liquid honey
1-pound chicken fillet, cut into strips	1 tablespoon cream cheese
1 teaspoon olive oil	1/3 cup water

Directions:

Mix curry paste with honey, olive oil, and cream cheese,   Then mix the curry mixture with chicken strips and carefully mix.   Put the chicken strips in the Crock Pot, add water, and close the lid.   Cook the meal in High for 3.5 hours.

Nutrition Info: Per Serving: 176 calories, 22.1g protein, 1.7g carbohydrates, 8.4g fat, 0g fiber, 69mg cholesterol, 70mg sodium, 186mg potassium.

567. Cinnamon And Cumin Chicken Drumsticks

Servings: 4   Cooking Time: 6 Hours

Ingredients:

8 chicken drumsticks	1 onion, peeled, chopped
1 teaspoon cumin seeds	1 teaspoon salt
	2 cups of water

1 teaspoon ground cinnamon
Directions:
Put all ingredients in the Crock Pot and carefully mix.   Close the lid and cook the chicken on low for 6 hours.
Nutrition Info: Per Serving: 170 calories, 25.g protein, 3.3g carbohydrates, 5.4g fat, 1g fiber, 81mg cholesterol, 661mg sodium, 237mg potassium.

568.   Fanta Chicken

Servings: 4   Cooking Time: 4.5 Hours
Ingredients:

1 cup Fanta	1 teaspoon ground
1-pound chicken	cumin
breast, skinless,	1 teaspoon ground
boneless, chopped	nutmeg

Directions:
Mix chicken breast with cumin and ground nutmeg and transfer in the Crock Pot.   Add Fanta and close the lid.   Cook the meal on high for 4.5 hours.
Nutrition Info: Per Serving: 162 calories, 24.2g protein, 9.3g carbohydrates, 3.2g fat, 0.2g fiber, 73mg cholesterol, 68mg sodium, 431mg potassium.

569.   Butter Chicken

Servings: 4   Cooking Time: 4 Hours
Ingredients:

12 oz chicken fillet	
1 teaspoon garlic	½ cup butter
powder	1 teaspoon salt

Directions:
Put all ingredients in the Crock Pot.   Cook them on High for 4 hours.   Then shred the chicken and transfer in the plates.   Sprinkle the chicken with fragrant butter from the Crock Pot.
Nutrition Info: Per Serving: 367 calories, 25g protein, 0.5g carbohydrates, 29.3g fat, 0.1g fiber, 137mg cholesterol, 818mg sodium, 221mg potassium.

570.   Lemongrass Chicken Thighs

Servings: 6   Cooking Time: 4 Hours
Ingredients:

6 chicken thighs	1 teaspoon salt
1 tablespoon dried	2 tablespoons sesame
sage	oil
1 teaspoon ground	1 cup of water
paprika	

Directions:
Mix dried sage with salt, and ground paprika. Then rub the chicken thighs with the sage mixture and transfer in the Crock Pot.   Sprinkle the chicken with sesame oil and water.   Close the chicken on High for hours.
Nutrition Info: Per Serving: 320 calories, 42.3g protein, 0.4g carbohydrates, 15.4g fat, 0.3g fiber, 130mg cholesterol, 514mg sodium, 367mg potassium.

571.Saffron Chicken Thighs

Servings: 6   Cooking Time: 6 Hrs
Ingredients:

2 and ½ lbs. chicken thighs, skinless and boneless	¼ tsp allspice, ground
1 and ½ tbsp olive oil	Salt and black pepper to the taste
2 yellow onions, chopped	A pinch of saffron
1 tsp cinnamon powder	To serve:
¼ tsp cloves, ground	A handful pine nuts
	A handful mint, chopped

Directions:
Add chicken, onions and rest of the ingredients to the Crock Pot.   Put the cooker's lid on and set the cooking time to 6 hours on Low settings.
Garnish with pine nuts and mint.   Serve.
Nutrition Info: Per Serving: Calories 223, Total Fat 3g, Fiber 2g, Total Carbs 6g, Protein 13g

572.   Cuban Chicken

Servings: 4   Cooking Time: 4 Hours
Ingredients:

4 gold potatoes, cut into medium chunks	1 chicken, cut into 8 pieces
1 yellow onion, thinly sliced	Salt and black pepper to the taste
4 big tomatoes, cut into medium chunks	Salt and black pepper to the taste
2 bay leaves	

Directions:
In your instant Crock Pot, mix potatoes with onion, chicken, tomato, bay leaves, salt and pepper, stir well, cover and cook on High for 4 hours.   Add more salt and pepper, discard bay leaves, divide chicken mix between plates and serve.
Nutrition Info:calories 263, fat 2, fiber 1, carbs 27, protein 14

573.   Grape Chicken Saute

Servings: 6   Cooking Time: 7 Hours
Ingredients:

1-pound chicken	1 teaspoon cayenne pepper
1 cup tomato, chopped	½ teaspoon dried
2 cups green grapes, chopped	sage
1 cup of water	1 teaspoon butter

Directions:
Put all ingredients in the Crock Pot.   Close the lid and cook the saute on Low for 7 hours.
Nutrition Info: Per Serving: 147 calories, 22.4g protein, 6.6g carbohydrates, 3.2g fat, 0.7g fiber, 60mg cholesterol, 55mg sodium, 278mg potassium.

574.   Party Chicken Wings

Servings: 4   Cooking Time: 4 Hours
Ingredients:

1-pound chicken wings

3 tablespoons hot sauce

2 tablespoons butter

¼ cup of soy sauce

Directions:
Put all ingredients in the Crock Pot and close the lid.   Cook the chicken wings on High for 4 hours. Then transfer the chicken wings in the big bowl and sprinkle with hot sauce gravy from the Crock Pot.
Nutrition Info: Per Serving: 276 calories, 33.9g protein, 1.4g carbohydrates, 14.2g fat, 0.2g fiber, 116mg cholesterol, 1322mg sodium, 327mg potassium.

575.   Chicken Thighs And Romano Cheese Mix

Servings: 4   Cooking Time: 4 Hours
Ingredients:

6 chicken things, boneless and skinless and cut into medium chunks

Salt and black pepper to the taste

½ cup white flour

2 tablespoons olive oil

10 ounces tomato sauce

1 teaspoon white wine vinegar

4 ounces mushrooms, sliced

1 tablespoon sugar

1 tablespoon oregano, dried

1 teaspoon garlic, minced

1 teaspoon basil, dried

1 yellow onion, chopped

1 cup Romano cheese, grated

Directions:
Grease your Crock Pot with the oil, add chicken pieces, onion, garlic, salt, pepper and flour and toss.   Add tomato sauce, vinegar, mushrooms, sugar, oregano, basil and cheese, cover and cook on High for 4 hours.   Divide between plates and serve.
Nutrition Info:calories 430, fat 12, fiber 6, carbs 25, protein 60

576.   Coriander And Turmeric Chicken

Servings: 2   Cooking Time: 6 Hours
Ingredients:

1 pound chicken breasts, skinless, boneless and cubed

1 tablespoon coriander, chopped

½ teaspoon turmeric powder

2 scallions, minced

1 tablespoon olive oil

1 tablespoon lime zest, grated

1 cup lime juice

1 tablespoon chives, chopped

¼ cup tomato sauce

Directions:
In your Crock Pot, mix the chicken with the coriander, turmeric, scallions and the other ingredients, toss, put the lid on and cook on Low for 6 hours.   Divide the mix between plates and serve right away.
Nutrition Info:calories 200, fat 7, fiber 1, carbs 5, protein 12

577.   Cannellini Chicken

Servings: 4   Cooking Time: 3 Hours
Ingredients:

1 cup cannellini beans, canned

12 oz chicken fillet, chopped

1 teaspoon lemon zest, grated

1 teaspoon salt

1 teaspoon dried oregano

1 cup of water

1 tablespoon butter

1 garlic clove, chopped

Directions:
Put the chopped chicken in the Crock Pot.   Add lemon zest, salt, water, butter, and garlic.   Close the lid and cook the chicken on high for 2 hours. Then add cannellini beans and stir the chicken well. Close the lid and cook the chicken on High for 1 hour.
Nutrition Info: Per Serving: 343 calories, 35.6g protein, 28.2g carbohydrates, 9.6g fat, 11.7g fiber, 83mg cholesterol, 688mg sodium, 866mg potassium.

578.   Basil Chicken

Servings: 4   Cooking Time: 7 Hours
Ingredients:

2 tablespoons balsamic vinegar

1 cup of water

1 teaspoon dried basil

1 teaspoon dried oregano

1-pound chicken fillet, sliced

1 teaspoon mustard

Directions:
Mix chicken fillet with mustard and balsamic vinegar.   Add dried basil, oregano, and transfer in the Crock Pot.   Add water and close the lid. Cook the chicken on low for 7 hours.
Nutrition Info: Per Serving: 222 calories, 33.1g protein, 0.6g carbohydrates, 8.7g fat, 0.3g fiber, 101mg cholesterol, 100mg sodium, 294mg potassium.

579.   Creamy Bacon Chicken

Servings: 4   Cooking Time: 12 Hours
Ingredients:

5 oz. bacon, cooked

8 oz. chicken breast

1 garlic clove, peeled and chopped

½ carrot, peeled and chopped

1 cup heavy cream

1 egg, beaten

1 tbsp paprika

1 tsp curry

3 tbsp chives, chopped

3 oz. scallions, chopped

Directions:
Carve a cut in the chicken breasts from sideways. Stuff the chicken with garlic clove and carrot. Place the stuffed chicken in the Crock Pot.   Mix egg with cream, paprika, curry, scallions, and paprika in a bowl.   Pour this curry mixture over the chicken and top it with chives and bacon. Add the remaining ingredients to the cooker.   Put the cooker's lid on and set the cooking time to 12 hours on Low settings.   Shred the slow-cooked

chicken and return to the cooker.   Mix well and serve.

Nutrition Info: Per Serving: Calories: 362, Total Fat: 29.6g, Fiber: 3g, Total Carbs: 7.17g, Protein: 19g

580.   Italian Turkey

Servings: 2   Cooking Time: 6 Hours

Ingredients:

1 pound turkey breasts, skinless, boneless and roughly cubed
1 tablespoon olive oil
½ cup black olives, pitted and halved

½ cup pearl onions, peeled
1 cup chicken stock
1 tablespoon Italian seasoning
A pinch of salt and black pepper

Directions:

In your Crock Pot, mix the turkey with the olives, onions and the other ingredients, toss, put the lid on and coo on Low for 6 hours.   Divide the mix between plates and serve.

Nutrition Info:calories 263, fat 14, fiber 4, carbs 6, protein 18

581.   Chicken Wings In Vodka Sauce

Servings: 4   Cooking Time: 6 Hours

Ingredients:

1-pound chicken wings
½ cup vodka sauce

1 tablespoon olive oil

Directions:

Put all ingredients in the Crock Pot and mix well. Close the lid and cook the meal on Low for 6 hours.

Nutrition Info: Per Serving: 273 calories, 34.1g protein, 2.8g carbohydrates, 13.2g fat, 0g fiber, 102mg cholesterol, 208mg sodium, 276mg potassium.

582.   African Chicken Meal

Servings: 6   Cooking Time: 8 Hrs

Ingredients:

13 oz. chicken breast
1 tsp peanut oil
1 tsp ground black pepper
1 tsp oregano
1 chili pepper
1 carrot

1 tbsp tomato sauce
1 cup tomatoes, canned
1 tbsp kosher salt
¼ tsp ground cardamom
½ tsp ground anise

Directions:

Rub the chicken breast with peanut oil then and sear for minute per side in the skillet.   Transfer the chicken to the Crock Pot.   Add tomato sauce, salt, and all other ingredients to the cooker.   Put the cooker's lid on and set the cooking time to 8 hours on Low settings.   Serve.

Nutrition Info: Per Serving: Calories: 131, Total Fat: 6.6g, Fiber: 1g, Total Carbs: 4.14g, Protein: 14g

583.   Buffalo Chicken Tenders

Servings: 4   Cooking Time: 3.5 Hours

Ingredients:

12 oz chicken fillet
3 tablespoons buffalo sauce

½ cup of coconut milk
1 jalapeno pepper, chopped

Directions:

Cut the chicken fillet into tenders and sprinkle the buffalo sauce.   Put the chicken tenders in the Crock Pot.   Add coconut milk and jalapeno pepper.   Close the lid and cook the meal on high for 3.5 hours.

Nutrition Info: Per Serving: 235 calories, 25.3g protein, 2.4g carbohydrates, 13.5g fat, 1g fiber, 76mg cholesterol, 318mg sodium, 293mg potassium.

584.   Chicken With Tomatoes And Eggplant Mix

Servings: 2   Cooking Time: 5 Hours And 10 Minutes.

Ingredients:

1 pound chicken breast, skinless, boneless and cubed
2 small eggplants, cubed
1 red onion, sliced
1 tablespoon olive oil
½ teaspoon cumin, ground
½ teaspoon sweet paprika

½ teaspoon red pepper flakes, crushed
½ cup canned tomatoes, crushed
1 cup chicken stock
1 teaspoon coriander, ground
A pinch of salt and black pepper
1 tablespoon oregano, chopped

Directions:

Heat up a pan with the oil over medium-high heat, add the chicken, onion and pepper flakes, stir, brown for   minutes and transfer to your Crock Pot. Add the rest of the ingredients, toss, put the lid on and cook on High for 5 hours.   Divide everything between plates and serve.

Nutrition Info:calories 252, fat 12, fiber 4, carbs 7, protein 13

585.   Sichuan Chicken

Servings: 4   Cooking Time: 4 Hours

Ingredients:

1 chili pepper, chopped
1 oz fresh ginger, chopped
1 onion, chopped
1-pound chicken fillet, chopped

3 oz scallions, chopped
1 garlic clove, chopped
2 tablespoons mustard
1 cup of water

Directions:

Mix mustard with chicken and leave for   minutes to marinate.   Meanwhile, put all remaining ingredients in the Crock Pot.   Add marinated

chicken and close the lid.   Cook the chicken on High for hours.
Nutrition Info: Per Serving: 286 calories, 36.5g protein, 11.5g carbohydrates, 10.5g fat, 2.9g fiber, 101mg cholesterol, 107mg sodium, 514mg potassium.

586.   Latin Chicken

Servings: 6   Cooking Time: 5 Hours
Ingredients:

6 oz. sweet pepper, julienned	½ cup salsa verde
1 tsp salt	¼ cup sweet corn, frozen
1 tsp chili flakes	
21 oz. chicken thighs	2 cups of water
1 onion, cut into petals	1 peach, pitted, chopped
1 tsp garlic powder	1 tsp canola oil

Directions:
Add chicken, salsa verde, and all other ingredients to the Crock Pot.   Put the cooker's lid on and set the cooking time to 5 hours on High settings. Serve warm.
Nutrition Info: Per Serving: Calories: 182, Total Fat: 9.2g, Fiber: 1g, Total Carbs: 7.35g, Protein: 18g

587.   Paprika Chicken And Artichokes

Servings: 2   Cooking Time: 7 Hours And 10 Minutes
Ingredients:

1 pound chicken breast, skinless, boneless and cut into strips	3 scallions, chopped
	1 tablespoon olive oil
	1 tablespoon sweet paprika
1 cup canned artichoke hearts, drained and halved	1 cup chicken stock
	½ cup parsley, chopped
2 garlic cloves, minced	

Directions:
Heat up a pan with the oil over medium-high heat, add the scallions, garlic and the chicken, brown for minutes and transfer to the Crock Pot.   Add the rest of the ingredients, toss, put the lid on and cook on Low for 7 hours.   Divide everything between plates and serve.
Nutrition Info: calories 350, fat 13.6, fiber 2.4, carbs 5.9, protein 50

588.   Mexican Style Chicken Wings

Servings: 4   Cooking Time: 3 Hours
Ingredients:

1 tablespoon Mexican seasonings	1-pound chicken wings, boneless, skinless
2 tablespoon sesame oil	1 teaspoon tomato paste
1 tablespoon mayonnaise	½ cup of water

Directions:

Mix sesame oil with mayonnaise, tomato paste, and Mexican seasonings.   Rub the chicken wings with Mexican seasonings mixture and leave for 10-15 minutes to marinate.   Transfer the marinated chicken wings and all remaining Mexican seasonings mixture in the Crock Pot.   Add water and close the lid.   Cook the chicken wings on High for 3 hours.
Nutrition Info: Per Serving: 297 calories, 33.1g protein, 2.3g carbohydrates, 16.4g fat, 0.1g fiber, 102mg cholesterol, 242mg sodium, 290mg potassium.

589.   Fennel Chicken

Servings: 8   Cooking Time: 9 Hours
Ingredients:

8 oz. fennel bulb, chopped	½ cup white wine
1 tbsp kosher salt	¼ tsp curry powder
1 large white onion, peeled and diced	17 oz. chicken drumsticks
1 cup cherry tomatoes, halved	1 oz. fennels seeds
1 tsp ground black pepper	1 tbsp smoked paprika
	1 cup of water
	1 cup chicken stock

Directions:
Mix white wine with black pepper, fennel seeds, smoked paprika, and curry powder in the bowl. Add chicken drumsticks, onions, and fennel bulbs to the Crock Pot.   Pour in white wine mixture, chicken stock, and water.   Put the cooker's lid on and set the cooking time to 9 hours on Low settings.   Serve warm.
Nutrition Info: Per Serving: Calories: 143, Total Fat: 6.6g, Fiber: 3g, Total Carbs: 8.15g, Protein: 13g

590.   Duck Saute

Servings: 3   Cooking Time: 5 Hours
Ingredients:

8 oz duck fillet, sliced	1 teaspoon salt
1 cup of water	1 teaspoon ground black pepper
1 cup mushrooms, sliced	1 tablespoon olive oil

Directions:
Heat the olive oil in the skillet well.   Add mushrooms and roast them for 3-5 minutes on medium heat.   Transfer the roasted mushrooms in the Crock Pot.   Add duck fillet, and all remaining ingredients.   Close the lid and cook saute for hours on High.
Nutrition Info: Per Serving: 141 calories, 23.1g protein, 1.2g carbohydrates, 5.2g fat, 0.4g fiber, 0mg cholesterol, 893mg sodium, 131mg potassium.

591.   Turkey And Plums Mix

Servings: 2   Cooking Time: 7 Hours
Ingredients:

1 pound turkey breast, skinless, boneless and sliced	½ teaspoon turmeric powder

1 cup plums, pitted and halved
½ cup chicken stock
½ teaspoon chili powder
½ teaspoon cumin, ground
1 tablespoon rosemary, chopped
A pinch of salt and black pepper

Directions:
In your Crock Pot, mix the turkey with the plums, stock and the other ingredients, toss, put the lid on and cook on Low for 7 hours.   Divide the mix between plates and serve right away.
Nutrition Info:calories 253, fat 13, fiber 2, carbs 7, protein 16

592.   Chives Duck

Servings: 4   Cooking Time: 20 Minutes
Ingredients:
1 pound duck breasts, boneless, skinless and sliced
1 tablespoon olive oil
1 red bell pepper, cut into strips
1 cup chicken stock
1 yellow onion, chopped
½ cup heavy cream
A pinch of salt and black pepper
1 tablespoon chives, chopped

Directions:
Set the instant pot on Sauté mode, add the oil, heat it up, add the onion and the bell pepper and sauté for 5 minutes.   Add the duck and the rest of the ingredients except the chives, put the lid on and cook on High for 15 minutes.   Release the pressure naturally for 10 minutes, divide everything between plates, sprinkle the chives on top and serve.
Nutrition Info:calories 293, fat 15, fiber 4, carbs 6, protein 14

593.   Cauliflower Chicken

Servings: 6   Cooking Time: 7 Hours
Ingredients:
2 cups cauliflower, chopped
1-pound ground chicken
1 teaspoon chili powder
1 teaspoon ground turmeric
1 teaspoon salt
1 cup of water
3 tablespoons plain yogurt

Directions:
Mix ground chicken with chili powder, ground turmeric, and salt.   Then mix the chicken mixture with cauliflower and transfer in the Crock Pot.   Add plain yogurt and water.   Close the lid and cook the meal on Low for 7 hours.
Nutrition Info: Per Serving: 160 calories, 23.1g protein, 2.8g carbohydrates, 5.8g fat, 1.1g fiber, 68mg cholesterol, 473mg sodium, 320mg potassium.

594.   Salsa Chicken Wings

Servings: 5   Cooking Time: 6 Hours
Ingredients:
2-pounds chicken wings
2 cups salsa
½ cup of water

Directions:
Put all ingredients in the Crock Pot.   Carefully mix the mixture and close the lid.   Cook the chicken wings on low for 6 hours.
Nutrition Info: Per Serving: 373 calories, 54.1g protein, 6.5g carbohydrates, 13.6g fat, 1.7g fiber, 161mg cholesterol, 781mg sodium, 750mg potassium.

595.   Lemon Chicken Thighs

Servings: 4   Cooking Time: 7 Hours
Ingredients:
4 chicken thighs, skinless, boneless
1 lemon, sliced
1 teaspoon ground black pepper
½ teaspoon ground nutmeg
1 teaspoon olive oil
1 cup of water

Directions:
Rub the chicken thighs with ground black pepper, nutmeg, and olive oil.   Then transfer the chicken in the Crock Pot.   Add lemon and water.   Close the lid and cook the meal on LOW for 7 hours.
Nutrition Info: Per Serving: 294 calories, 42.5g protein, 1.8g carbohydrates, 12.2g fat, 0.6g fiber, 130mg cholesterol, 128mg sodium, 383mg potassium.

596.   Easy Chicken Continental

Servings: 2   Cooking Time: 7 Hours
Ingredients:
2 oz dried beef
8 oz chicken breast, skinless, boneless, chopped
½ cup cream
½ can onion soup
1 tablespoon cornstarch

Directions:
Put oz of the dried beef in the Crock Pot in one layer.   Then add chicken breast and top it with remaining dried beef.   After this, mix cream cheese, onion, and cornstarch. Whisk the mixture and pour it over the chicken and dried beef. Cook the meal on Low for 7 hours.
Nutrition Info: Per Serving: 270 calories, 35.4g protein, 10.5g carbohydrates, 9g fat, 0.6g fiber, 109mg cholesterol, 737mg sodium, 598mg potassium.

597.   Mushrooms Stuffed With Chicken

Servings: 6   Cooking Time: 3 Hours
Ingredients:
16 ounces button mushroom caps
4 ounces cream cheese
1 teaspoon ranch seasoning mix
4 tablespoons hot
¼ cup carrot, chopped
¼ cup red onion, chopped
½ cup chicken meat, ground

sauce
¾ cup blue cheese, crumbled

Salt and black pepper to the taste
Cooking spray

Directions:
In a bowl, mix cream cheese with blue cheese, hot sauce, ranch seasoning, salt, pepper, chicken, carrot and red onion, stir and stuff mushrooms with this mix.   Grease your Crock Pot with cooking spray, add stuffed mushrooms, cover and cook on High for 3 hours.   Divide mushrooms between plates and serve.
Nutrition Info:calories 240, fat 4, fiber 1, carbs 12, protein 7

598.   Garlic Duck

Servings: 4   Cooking Time: 5 Hours
Ingredients:

1 tablespoon minced garlic
1 tablespoon butter, softened

1-pound duck fillet
1 teaspoon dried thyme
1/3 cup coconut cream

Directions:
Mix minced garlic with butter, and dried thyme. Then rub the suck fillet with garlic mixture and place it in the Crock Pot.   Add coconut cream and cook the duck on High for 5 hours.   Then slice the cooked duck fillet and sprinkle it with hot garlic coconut milk.
Nutrition Info: Per Serving: 216 calories, 34.1g protein, 2g carbohydrates, 8.4g fat, 0.6g fiber, 8mg cholesterol, 194mg sodium, 135mg potassium.

599.   Chicken Florentine

Servings: 4   Cooking Time: 8 Hours
Ingredients:

4 chicken breasts, bones and skin removed
Salt and pepper to taste

2 cups parmesan cheese, divided
½ cup heavy cream
1 cup baby spinach, rinsed

Directions:
Place the chicken in the crockpot. Season with salt and pepper to taste.   Stir in half of the parmesan cheese.   Close the lid and cook on low for 8 hours or on high for 6 hours.   Halfway through the cooking time, pour in the heavy cream.   Continue cooking.   An hour after the cooking time, add in the baby spinach.   Cook until the spinach has wilted.
Nutrition Info: Calories per serving: 553; Carbohydrates: 3g; Protein: 48g; Fat: 32g; Sugar:0 g; Sodium: 952mg; Fiber: 2.6g

600.   Lemon Garlic Dump Chicken

Servings: 6   Cooking Time: 8 Hours
Ingredients:

¼ cup olive oil
2 teaspoon garlic, minced

1 tablespoon parsley, chopped
2 tablespoons lemon

6 chicken breasts, bones removed

juice, freshly squeezed

Directions:
Heat oil in a skillet over medium flame.   Sauté the garlic until golden brown.   Arrange the chicken breasts in the crockpot.   Pour over the oil with garlic.   Add the parsley and lemon juice.   Add a little water.   Close the lid and cook on low for 8 hours or on high for hours.
Nutrition Info: Calories per serving: 581; Carbohydrates: 0.7g; Protein: 60.5g; Fat: 35.8g; Sugar: 0g; Sodium: 583mg; Fiber: 0.3g

601.   Stuffed Pasta

Servings: 6   Cooking Time: 4 Hours
Ingredients:

12 oz cannelloni
9 oz ground chicken
1 teaspoon Italian seasonings

2 oz Parmesan, grated
½ cup tomato juice
½ cup of water

Directions:
Mix the ground chicken with Italian seasonings and fill the cannelloni.   Put the stuffed cannelloni in the Crock Pot.   Add all remaining ingredients and close the lid.   Cook the meal on High for hours.
Nutrition Info: Per Serving: 250 calories, 21.5g protein, 14g carbohydrates, 12.1g fat, 0.8g fiber, 62mg cholesterol, 373mg sodium, 150mg potassium.

602.   Chicken Bowl

Servings: 6   Cooking Time: 4 Hours
Ingredients:

1-pound chicken breast, skinless, boneless, chopped
1 cup sweet corn, frozen
1 teaspoon ground paprika

1 teaspoon onion powder
1 cup tomatoes, chopped
1 cup of water
1 teaspoon olive oil

Directions:
Mix chopped chicken breast with ground paprika and onion powder. Transfer it in the Crock Pot. Add water and sweet corn. Cook the mixture on High for 4 hours.   Then drain the liquid and transfer the mixture in the bowl.   Add tomatoes and olive oil. Mix the meal.
Nutrition Info: Per Serving: 122 calories, 17.2g protein, 6.3g carbohydrates, 3g fat, 1.1g fiber, 48mg cholesterol, 45mg sodium, 424mg potassium.

603.   Apple Chicken Bombs

Servings: 7   Cooking Time: 4 Hrs
Ingredients:

2 green apples, peeled and grated
12 oz. ground chicken
1 tsp minced garlic
1 tsp turmeric

1 tsp onion powder
1 tsp chili flakes
½ tsp salt
1 tsp garlic powder

1 egg
1 tbsp flour

1 tsp butter
½ cup panko bread crumbs

Directions:
Mix garlic, flour, turmeric, chili flakes, onion powder, garlic powder, and salt in a bowl. Whisk in egg, ground chicken, and apple, then mix well. Make small meatballs out of this mixture and coat them with breadcrumbs. Grease the insert of the Crock Pot with butter. Add the coated meatballs to the greased cooker. Put the cooker's lid on and set the cooking time to 3 hours on High settings. Flip the chicken balls and cook for another 1 hour on High setting. Serve.
Nutrition Info: Per Serving: Calories: 136, Total Fat: 6.1g, Fiber: 2g, Total Carbs: 10.64g, Protein: 10g

604. Lime Chicken Mix

Servings: 2   Cooking Time: 7 Hours
Ingredients:

1 pound chicken thighs, boneless and skinless
1 tablespoon olive oil
Juice of 1 lime
Zest of 1 lime, grated

½ cup tomato sauce
2 spring onions, chopped
Salt and black pepper to the taste
1 tablespoon oregano, chopped

Directions:
In your Crock Pot, mix the chicken with the oil, lime juice and the other ingredients, toss, put the lid on and cook on Low for 7 hours. Divide the mix between plates and serve.
Nutrition Info:calories 192, fat 12, fiber 3, carbs 5, protein 12

605. Cinnamon Turkey

Servings: 5   Cooking Time: 6 Hours
Ingredients:

1 teaspoon ground cinnamon
1-pound turkey fillet, chopped

½ teaspoon dried thyme
1 teaspoon salt
½ cup cream

Directions:
Mix turkey with cinnamon, salt, and thyme. Transfer it in the Crock Pot. Add cream and cook the meal on Low for 6 hours.
Nutrition Info: Per Serving: 102 calories, 19g protein, 1.1g carbohydrates, 1.8g fat, 0.2g fiber, 52mg cholesterol, 678mg sodium, 11mg potassium.

606. Chicken And Creamy Mushroom Sauce

Servings: 4   Cooking Time: 4 Hours
Ingredients:

8 chicken thighs
Salt and black pepper to the taste
1 yellow onion,

4 garlic cloves, minced
10 ounces cremini mushrooms, halved

chopped
1 tablespoon olive oil
4 bacon strips, cooked and chopped

2 cups white chardonnay wine
1 cup whipping cream
A handful parsley, chopped

Directions:
Heat up a pan with the oil over medium heat, add chicken pieces, season them with salt and pepper, cook until they brown and also transfer to your Crock Pot. Add onions, garlic, bacon, mushrooms, wine, parsley and cream, stir, cover and cook on High for 4 hours. Divide between plates and serve.
Nutrition Info:calories 340, fat 10, fiber 7, carbs 14, protein 24

607. Chicken Thighs Delight

Servings: 6   Cooking Time: 6 Hours
Ingredients:

2 pounds chicken thighs, boneless and skinless
1 yellow onion, chopped
1/3 cup prunes, dried and halved
3 garlic cloves, minced
½ cup green olives, pitted
2 teaspoon sweet paprika

3 carrots, chopped
1 teaspoon cinnamon, ground
2 teaspoons cumin, ground
2 teaspoons ginger, grated
1 cup chicken stock
A pinch of salt and black pepper
1 tablespoon cilantro, chopped

Directions:
In your Crock Pot, mix chicken with onion, carrots, prunes, garlic, olives, paprika, cinnamon, cumin, ginger, stock, salt and pepper, stir, cover and cook on Low for 6 hours. Divide between plates, sprinkle cilantro on top and serve.
Nutrition Info:calories 384, fat 12, fiber 4, carbs 20, protein 34

608. Chicken Enchilada

Servings: 10   Cooking Time: 8 Hours
Ingredients:

4 ½ cups shredded chicken
1 ¼ cup sour cream
1 can sugar-free green enchilada sauce

4 cups Monterey jack cheese
½ cup cilantro, chopped

Directions:
Place the shredded chicken in the crockpot. Add in the sour cream and enchilada sauce. Sprinkle with Monterey jack cheese. Close the lid and cook on low for 8 hours or on high for 6 hours. An hour before the cooking time ends, sprinkle with cilantro.
Nutrition Info: Calories per serving: 469; Carbohydrates: 5g; Protein: 34g; Fat:29 g; Sugar:2.2 g; Sodium: 977mg; Fiber: 1g

609.   Turkey Curry

Servings: 4   Cooking Time: 4 Hours

Ingredients:

- 18 ounces turkey meat, minced
- 3 ounces spinach
- 20 ounces canned tomatoes, chopped
- 2 tablespoons coconut oil
- 2 tablespoons coconut cream
- 1 tablespoon coriander, ground
- 2 tablespoons ginger, grated
- 1 tablespoons turmeric powder
- 1 tablespoon cumin, ground
- Salt and black pepper
- 2 garlic cloves, minced
- 2 yellow onions, sliced
- to the taste
- 2 tablespoons chili powder

Directions:

In your Crock Pot, mix turkey with spinach, tomatoes, oil, cream, garlic, onion, coriander, ginger, turmeric, cumin, chili, salt and pepper, stir, cover and cook on High for 4 hours.   Divide into bowls and serve.

Nutrition Info:calories 240, fat 4, fiber 3, carbs 13, protein 12

Soups & Stews Recipes

610. Ham White Bean Soup

Servings: 6   Cooking Time: 2 1/4 Hours

Ingredients:

1 tablespoon olive oil	4 oz. ham, diced
1 sweet onion, chopped	1 carrot, diced
2 garlic cloves, chopped	1 cup diced tomatoes
1 yellow bell pepper, cored and diced	1 can (15 oz.) white beans, drained
1 red bell pepper, cored and diced	2 cups chicken stock
	3 cups water
	Salt and pepper to taste

Directions:

Heat the oil in a skillet and add the ham. Cook for 2 minutes then stir in the onion and garlic. Sauté for 2 additional minutes.   Transfer the mixture in your Crock Pot and stir in the remaining ingredients.   Adjust the taste with salt and pepper and cook on high settings for 2 hours. Serve the soup warm or chilled.

611. Chicken Sweet Potato Soup

Servings: 6   Cooking Time: 6 1/4 Hours

Ingredients:

2 chicken breasts, cubed	2 shallots, chopped
2 tablespoons olive oil	1 cup chicken stock
1 celery stalk, sliced	4 cups water
1 can fire roasted tomatoes	Salt and pepper to taste
1 1/2 pounds sweet potatoes, peeled and cubed	1/2 teaspoon cumin seeds
	1/4 teaspoon caraway seeds
	1 thyme sprig

Directions:

Heat the oil in a skillet and stir in the chicken, shallots and celery. Sauté for a few minutes until softened then transfer in your Crock Pot.   Add the remaining ingredients and season with salt and pepper.   Cook on low settings for 6 hours.   The soup is best served warm.

612. Mexican Beef Soup

Servings: 6   Cooking Time: 8 1/4 Hours

Ingredients:

1 pound ground beef	2 cups beef stock
2 tablespoons canola oil	1 can (15 oz.) black beans, drained
2 red bell peppers, cored and diced	3 cups water
1 sweet onion, chopped	1/2 cup red salsa
1 can (15 oz.) diced tomatoes	1 chipotle pepper, chopped
	Salt and pepper to taste

Directions:

Heat the oil in a skillet and stir in the beef. Cook for 5 minutes, stirring often, then transfer the beef in your Crock Pot.   Add the remaining ingredients and adjust the taste with salt and pepper.   Cook on low settings for 8 hours.   Serve the soup warm or chilled.

613. Herbed Chickpea Soup

Servings: 6   Cooking Time: 6 1/4 Hours

Ingredients:

1 cup dried chickpeas	2 tablespoons tomato paste
1 shallot, chopped	2 tablespoons chopped parsley
1 carrot, diced	2 tablespoons chopped cilantro
1 red bell pepper, cored and diced	1 tablespoon chopped dill
1 celery stalk, sliced	Salt and pepper to taste
1 small fennel bulb, chopped	
2 cups chicken stock	
4 cups water	

Directions:

Combine the chickpeas, shallot, carrot, bell pepper, celery, fennel, tomato paste, stock and water in your Crock Pot.   Add salt and pepper to taste and cook on low settings for 6 hours.   When done, stir in the chopped herbs and serve the soup warm and fresh.

614. Spiced Lasagna Soup

Servings: 6   Cooking Time: 6 Hours

Ingredients:

2 sheets of lasagna noodles, crushed	2 cups ground beef
1 oz Parmesan, grated	6 cups beef broth
1 teaspoon ground turmeric	1/2 cup tomatoes, chopped
1 yellow onion, diced	1 tablespoon dried basil

Directions:

Roast the ground beef in the hot skillet for 4 minutes. Stir it constantly and transfer in the Crock Pot.   Add turmeric, onion, tomatoes, basil, and beef broth.   Stir the soup, add lasagna noodles, and close the lid.   Cook the soup on High for 6 hours.   Top the cooked soup with Parmesan.

Nutrition Info: Per Serving: 208 calories, 17.8g protein, 14.6g carbohydrates, 8.3g fat, 0.7g fiber, 40mg cholesterol, 840mg sodium, 390mg potassium.

615. Beef Vegetable Soup

Servings: 8   Cooking Time: 7 1/4 Hours

Ingredients:

1 pound beef roast, cubed	1/2 head cauliflower, cut into florets
2 tablespoons canola oil	2 large potatoes, peeled and cubed
1 celery stalk, sliced	1 cup diced tomatoes
1 sweet onion, chopped	1/2 teaspoon dried basil
1 carrot, sliced	2 cups beef stock

1 garlic clove,
chopped

4 cups water
Salt and pepper to
taste

Directions:
Heat the oil in a skillet and add the beef. Cook on all sides for a few minutes then transfer the beef in your Crock Pot.   Add the remaining ingredients and season with salt and pepper.   Cover and cook on low settings for 7 hours.   The soup is delicious either warm or chilled.

616.   Two-fish Soup

Servings: 8   Cooking Time: 6 1/4 Hours
Ingredients:

1 tablespoon canola oil
1 sweet onion, chopped
1 red bell pepper, cored and diced
1 chipotle pepper, chopped
1 carrot, diced
1 celery stalk, diced

1 cup diced tomatoes
1 lemon, juiced
3 salmon fillets, cubed
3 cod fillets, cubed
2 tablespoons chopped parsley
Salt and pepper to taste

Directions:
Heat the canola oil in a skillet and add the onion. Sauté for 2 minutes until softened.   Transfer the onion in a Crock Pot and stir in the remaining ingredients.   Add salt and pepper to taste and cook on low settings for 6 hours.   Serve the soup warm.

617.Three Bean Quinoa Soup

Servings: 10   Cooking Time: 7 1/2 Hours
Ingredients:

2 tablespoons olive oil
2 sweet onions, chopped
2 garlic cloves, chopped
1 celery stalk, sliced
1/2 cup dried black beans
1/4 cup dried kidney beans
1/4 cup cannellini beans

2 carrots, diced
1/2 teaspoon cumin seeds
1/2 teaspoon chili powder
4 cups chicken stock
4 cups water
1 rosemary sprig
1 thyme sprig
1/4 cup red quinoa, rinsed
1/2 cup tomato sauce
Salt and pepper to taste

Directions:
Heat the oil in a skillet and stir in the onion and garlic. Cook for 2 minutes until softened then transfer in your Crock Pot.   Add the celery, carrots, beans, cumin seeds, chili powder, stock, water and herbs.   Stir in the quinoa and tomato sauce and season with salt and pepper.   Cook on low settings for 7 hours and serve the soup warm.

618.   Salmon Fennel Soup

Servings: 6   Cooking Time: 5 1/4 Hours
Ingredients:

1 shallot, chopped
1 garlic clove, sliced
1 fennel bulb, sliced
1 carrot, diced
1 celery stalk, sliced

3 salmon fillets, cubed
1 lemon, juiced
1 bay leaf
Salt and pepper to taste

Directions:
Combine the shallot, garlic, fennel, carrot, celery, fish, lemon juice and bay leaf in your Crock Pot. Add salt and pepper to taste and cook on low settings for 5 hours.   Serve the soup warm.

619.   Vegetable Chicken Soup

Servings: 8   Cooking Time: 7 1/2 Hours
Ingredients:

2 chicken breasts, cubed
1 sweet onion, chopped
1 garlic clove, chopped
2 carrots, diced
1 parsnip, diced
1 celery stalk, diced
1 red bell pepper, cored and diced

1 cup diced tomatoes
Salt and pepper to taste
1 cup chicken stock
4 cups water
1 can condensed cream of chicken soup
1 lemon, juiced
1 tablespoon chopped parsley

Directions:
Combine the chicken and the remaining ingredients in your Crock Pot.   Add salt and pepper as needed and cook on low settings for 7 hours.   The soup is best served warm, but it can also be re-heated.

620.   Comforting Chicken Soup

Servings: 8   Cooking Time: 8 1/2 Hours
Ingredients:

1 whole chicken, cut into pieces
2 carrots, cut into sticks
1 celery stalk, sliced
4 potatoes, peeled and cubed

8 cups water
6 oz. egg noodles
2 garlic cloves, chopped
Salt and pepper to taste
1 whole onion
1 bay leaf

Directions:
Combine all the ingredients in your Crock Pot. Add salt and pepper to taste and cook on low settings for 8 hours.   Serve the soup warm.

621.   Snow Peas Soup

Servings: 4   Cooking Time: 3.5 Hours
Ingredients:

1 tablespoon chives, chopped
1 teaspoon ground ginger
8 oz salmon fillet, chopped

5 oz bamboo shoots, canned, chopped
2 cups snow peas
1 teaspoon hot sauce
5 cups of water

Directions:
Put bamboo shoots in the Crock Pot.   Add ground ginger, salmon, snow peas, and water.

Close the lid and cook the soup for hours on high. Then add hot sauce and chives. Stir the soup carefully and cook for 30 minutes on high.
Nutrition Info: Per Serving: 120 calories, 14.6g protein, 7.9g carbohydrates, 3.8g fat, 3.1g fiber, 25mg cholesterol, 70mg sodium, 612mg potassium

---

622. Creamy Noodle Soup

Servings: 8   Cooking Time: 8 1/4 Hours
Ingredients:

2 chicken breasts, cubed	2 shallots, chopped
2 tablespoons all-purpose flour	2 cups water
1 celery stalk, sliced	2 cups chicken stock
1 can condensed chicken soup	Salt and pepper to taste
	1 cup green peas
	6 oz. egg noodles

Directions:
Sprinkle the chicken with salt, pepper and flour and place it in your Crock Pot.   Add the remaining ingredients and season with salt and pepper.   Cover and cook on low settings for 8 hours.   This soup is best served warm.

---

623. Yogurt Soup

Servings: 4   Cooking Time: 5 Hours
Ingredients:

1 cup Greek yogurt	1 tablespoon coconut oil
½ teaspoon dried mint	3 cups chicken stock
½ teaspoon ground black pepper	7 oz chicken fillet, chopped
1 onion, diced	

Directions:
Melt the coconut oil in the skillet.   Add onion and roast it until light brown.   After this, transfer the roasted onion in the Crock Pot.   Add dried mint, ground black pepper, chicken stock, and chicken fillet.   Add Greek yogurt and carefully mix the soup ingredients.   Close the lid and cook the soup on High for 5 hours.
Nutrition Info: Per Serving: 180 calories, 20.2g protein, 5.3g carbohydrates, 8.6g fat, 0.7g fiber, 47mg cholesterol, 633mg sodium, 247mg potassium.

---

624. Corn And Red Pepper Chowder

Servings: 8   Cooking Time: 8 1/4 Hours
Ingredients:

2 tablespoons olive oil	2 cups chicken stock
1 shallot, chopped	2 cups water
1 red bell pepper, cored and diced	1/4 teaspoon smoked paprika
2 large potatoes, peeled and cubed	1/4 teaspoon cumin powder
2 cups frozen sweet corn	Salt and pepper to taste

Directions:

Heat the oil in a skillet and stir in the shallot. Sauté until softened then transfer in your Crock Pot. Add the remaining ingredients and adjust the taste with salt and pepper.   Cook on low settings for 8 hours.   When done, puree the soup in a blender and serve it warm.

---

625. Beef Cabbage Soup

Servings: 8   Cooking Time: 7 1/2 Hours
Ingredients:

1 pound beef roast, cubed	1 can (15 oz.) diced tomatoes
2 tablespoons olive oil	2 cups beef stock
1 sweet onion, chopped	2 cups water
1 carrot, grated	1/2 teaspoon cumin seeds
1 small cabbage head, shredded	Salt and pepper to taste

Directions:
Heat the oil in a skillet and add the beef roast. Cook for 5-6 minutes on all sides then transfer the meat in your Crock Pot.   Add the remaining ingredients and season with salt and pepper.   Cook on low settings for 7 hours.   Serve the cabbage soup warm.

---

626. Chicken Gnocchi Soup

Servings: 8   Cooking Time: 6 1/4 Hours
Ingredients:

1 sweet onion, chopped	2 carrots, sliced
1 garlic clove, chopped	8 oz. gnocchi
8 chicken thighs, without skin	1 can condensed cream of mushroom soup
1 celery stalk, sliced	2 cups chicken stock
1 cup frozen green peas	3 cups water
	1 thyme sprig
	1 rosemary sprig
	Salt and pepper to taste

Directions:
Combine the onion, garlic, chicken thighs, carrots, celery, peas and gnocchi in your Crock Pot.   Add the mushroom soup, stock, water, thyme and rosemary and season with salt and pepper.   Cook on low settings for 6 hours.   The soup is best served warm.

---

627. Hot And Sour Soup

Servings: 8   Cooking Time: 7 1/2 Hours
Ingredients:

2 oz. dried shiitake mushrooms	1 teaspoon grated ginger
1 pound fresh mushrooms, sliced	1/2 teaspoon chili flakes
1 can (8 oz.) bamboo shoots, drained	2 cups chicken stock
2 carrots, sliced	5 cups water
1 sweet onion, chopped	2 tablespoons soy sauce
	2 tablespoons rice

14 oz. tofu, cubed

1/2 head green cabbage, shredded

vinegar

2 green onions, sliced

Directions:
Place the shiitake mushrooms in a bowl and cover them with boiling water. Allow to rehydrate for minutes then chop and place in your Crock Pot. Add the remaining ingredients, except the green onions and cook on low settings for 7 hours. When done, stir in the green onions and serve right away.

628. Hungarian Borscht

Servings: 8   Cooking Time: 8 1/4 Hours

Ingredients:

1 pound beef roast, cubed	Salt and pepper to taste
2 tablespoons canola oil	4 cups water
4 medium size beets, peeled and cubed	1 cup vegetable stock
1 can diced tomatoes	1/2 teaspoon cumin seeds
2 potatoes, peeled and cubed	1 teaspoon red wine vinegar
1 sweet onion, chopped	1 teaspoon honey
2 tablespoons tomato paste	1/2 teaspoon dried dill
	1 teaspoon dried parsley

Directions:
Heat the oil in a skillet and stir in the beef. Cook for a few minutes on all sides until golden.   Transfer the meat in your Crock Pot and add the beets, tomatoes, potatoes, onion and tomato paste. Add salt and pepper, as well as the remaining ingredients and cook on low settings for 8 hours. Serve the soup warm or chilled.

629. Black Bean Soup

Servings: 8   Cooking Time: 7 1/4 Hours

Ingredients:

1/2 pound black beans, rinsed	2 tomatoes, diced
2 cups chicken stock	1/2 teaspoon cumin powder
5 cups water	1/4 teaspoon chili powder
1 sweet onion, chopped	1 bay leaf
2 carrots, diced	Salt and pepper to taste
1 parsnip, diced	2 tablespoons chopped cilantro for serving
1 celery stalk, diced	
1 red bell peppers, cored and diced	
2 tablespoons tomato paste	1/2 cup sour cream for serving

Directions:
Combine the black beans, chicken stock, water and vegetables in your Crock Pot.   Add the cumin powder, chili powder, bay leaf, salt and pepper and cook the soup on low settings for 7 hours.   When done, stir in the cilantro. Pour the soup in bowls and top with sour cream just before serving.

630. Crock-pot Low-carb Taco Soup

Servings: 8   Cooking Time: 4 Hours

Ingredients:

2 lbs. ground pork, beef or sausage	2 tablespoons cilantro, fresh or dried
2 8-ounce packages of cream cheese	1 can corn kernels, drained
2 10-ounce cans of Rotel	½ cup cheddar cheese, shredded for garnish (optional)
2 tablespoons of taco seasoning	
4 cups chicken broth	

Directions:
Brown the ground meat until fully cooked over medium-high heat in a pan.   While the meat is browning, place cream cheese, Rotel, corn and taco seasoning in Crock-Pot.   Drain grease off meat and place meat in Crock-Pot.   Stir and combine.   Pour chicken broth over mixture, cover and cook on LOW for 4 hours.   Just before serving, add in cilantro and garnish with shredded cheddar cheese.

Nutrition Info: Calories: 547, Total Fat: 43 g, Saturated Fat: 20 g, Carbohydrates: 5 g, Sugar: 4 g Sodium: 1174 mg, Fiber: 1 g, Cholesterol: 168 mg, Protein: 33 g

631. Leek Potato Soup

Servings: 8   Cooking Time: 6 1/2 Hours

Ingredients:

4 leeks, sliced	3 cups water
1 tablespoon olive oil	1 bay leaf
4 bacon slices, chopped	Salt and pepper to taste
1 celery stalk, sliced	1/4 teaspoon cayenne pepper
4 large potatoes, peeled and cubed	1/4 teaspoon smoked paprika
2 cups chicken stock	1 thyme sprig
	1 rosemary sprig

Directions:
Heat the oil in a skillet and add the bacon. Cook until crisp then stir in the leeks.   Sauté for 5 minutes until softened then transfer in your Crock Pot.   Add the remaining ingredients and cook on low settings for about 6 hours.   Serve the soup warm.

632. Lentil Stew

Servings: 4   Cooking Time: 6 Hours

Ingredients:

2 cups chicken stock	1 eggplant, chopped
½ cup red lentils	1 cup of water
1 tablespoon tomato paste	1 teaspoon Italian seasonings

Directions:
Mix chicken stock with red lentils and tomato paste.   Pour the mixture in the Crock Pot.   Add eggplants and Italian seasonings.   Cook the stew on low for 6 hours.

Nutrition Info: Per Serving: 125 calories, 7.8g protein, 22.4g carbohydrates, 1.1g fat, 11.5g fiber, 1mg cholesterol, 392mg sodium, 540mg potassium.

---

633.   Provencal Beef Soup

Servings: 8   Cooking Time: 7 1/4 Hours
Ingredients:

2 tablespoons olive oil	2 carrots, sliced
1 pound beef roast, cubed	1 can diced tomatoes
1 sweet onion, chopped	1 cup beef stock
1 garlic clove, chopped	1 cup red wine
1 celery stalk, sliced	4 cups water
	1/2 teaspoon dried thyme
	1 bay leaf
	Salt and pepper to taste

Directions:
Heat the oil in a skillet and stir in the beef roast. Cook on all sides for a few minutes then transfer the beef in a Crock Pot.   Add the remaining ingredients and adjust the taste with salt and pepper.   Cook on low settings for 7 hours. Serve the soup warm or chilled.

---

634.   Crock-pot Clam Chowder

Servings: 8   Cooking Time: 6 Hours
Ingredients:

1 cup chopped onion	2 cups chicken broth
13 slices thick cut bacon	1 teaspoon thyme, ground
1 cup celery, chopped	1 teaspoon sea salt
2 cups heavy whipping cream	1 teaspoon pepper

Directions:
Cook the bacon until crispy and reserve the bacon grease in pan. Chop celery and onion. Place celery and onion in bacon grease and cook until soft; add grease to Crock-Pot along with veggies. Once veggies are soft, add them to the Crock-Pot and all other ingredients. Cover and cook on LOW for 6 hours.
Nutrition Info: Calories: 427, Total Fat: 33 g, Cholesterol: 252 mg, Sodium: 1636 mg, Potassium: 107 mg, Carbohydrates: 5 g, Dietary Fiber: 0 g, Sugars: 0 g, Protein: 27 g

---

635.   Hearty Turkey Chili

Servings: 5   Cooking Time: 8 Hours 15 Minutes
Ingredients:

1/4 cup olive oil	1 green pepper, chopped
1 pound ground turkey breast	1 can diced tomatoes
1/2 teaspoon salt	2 tablespoons chili powder
1 can white beans, drained and rinsed	4 garlic cloves, minced
2 teaspoons dried marjoram	1 can no-salt-added tomatoes
1 large onion, chopped	

Directions:

Put olive oil, green peppers, onions and garlic in the crock pot and sauté for about 3 minutes.   Add rest of the ingredients and cover the lid.   Cook on LOW for about 8 hours and dish out in a bowl to serve hot.
Nutrition Info: Calories:350 Fat: 17.6g Carbohydrates:18.1g

---

636.   Meatball Tortellini Soup

Servings: 6   Cooking Time: 6 1/2 Hours
Ingredients:

1/2 pound ground chicken	1 celery stalk, sliced
1/4 cup white rice	1 carrot, sliced
1 garlic clove, chopped	1 shallot, chopped
1 tablespoon chopped parsley	6 oz. spinach tortellini
2 cups chicken stock	Salt and pepper to taste
4 cups water	

Directions:
Mix the chicken, rice, garlic, parsley, salt and pepper in a bowl.   Combine the stock, water, celery, carrot, shallot, salt and pepper in your Crock Pot.   Form small meatballs and drop them in the liquid.   Add the tortellini as well and cook on low settings for 6 hours.   Serve the soup warm and fresh.

---

637.   Cheesy Meatball Soup

Servings: 6   Cooking Time: 8 Hours 20 Minutes
Ingredients:

For stock	1 pound ground beef
1/2 green bell pepper, finely chopped	1/4 cup ground flax seed meal
1/2 cup purple onion, chopped	1 teaspoon oregano
2 cups organic beef broth	1 tablespoons parsley
1/2 red bell pepper, finely chopped	1/2 teaspoon pepper
1 celery stalk, chopped	1 teaspoon salt
5 large mushrooms, chopped	1/2 teaspoon garlic powder
5 strips bacon	For cheese sauce
For meatballs	4 tablespoons heavy white cream
1 egg	8 slices American cheese
	4 tablespoons water
	4 tablespoons butter

Directions:
For meatballs: Mix together the ingredients and roll into medium sized meatballs.   Put this mixture in the crock pot along with the ingredients for stock and thoroughly stir.   Cover and cook on LOW for about 8 hours.   For cheese sauce: Put all the ingredients in a microwave safe dish and microwave for about 3 minutes.   Add this cheese sauce to the soup, gently stirring.   Dish out and serve hot.
Nutrition Info: Calories:419 Fat:32g Carbohydrates:3.7g

638. Roasted Chicken Stock

Servings: 10   Cooking Time: 9 Hours

Ingredients:

1 whole chicken, cut into smaller pieces	2 onions, halved
2 carrots, cut in half	10 cups water
1 parsnip	1 bay leaf
1 celery root, peeled and sliced	1 rosemary sprig
	1 thyme sprig
	Salt and pepper to taste

Directions:

Season the chicken with salt and pepper and place it in a baking tray. Roast in the preheated oven at 400F for 40 minutes.   Transfer the chicken in your Crock Pot and add the remaining ingredients. Season with salt and pepper and cook on low settings for 8 hours.   Use the stock right away or store in the fridge or freezer.

639. Shrimp Soup

Servings: 6   Cooking Time: 6 1/4 Hours

Ingredients:

2 tablespoons olive oil	1 pinch chili powder
1 large sweet onion, chopped	4 medium size tomatoes, peeled and diced
1 fennel bulb, sliced	1 bay leaf
4 garlic cloves, chopped	1/2 pound cod fillets, cubed
1 cup dry white wine	1/2 pound fresh shrimps, peeled and deveined
1/2 cup tomato sauce	
2 cup water	Salt and pepper to taste
1 teaspoon dried oregano	1 lime, juiced
1 teaspoon dried basil	

Directions:

Heat the oil in a skillet and stir in the onion, fennel and garlic. Sauté for 5 minutes until softened. Transfer the mixture in your Crock Pot and stir in the wine, tomato sauce, water, oregano, basil, chili powder, tomatoes and bay leaf.   Cook on high settings for 1 hour then add the cod and shrimps, as well as lime juice, salt and pepper and continue cooking on low settings for 5 additional hours. Serve the soup warm or chilled.

640. French Soup

Servings: 5   Cooking Time: 7 Hours

Ingredients:

5 oz Gruyere cheese, shredded	2 cups chicken stock
2 cups of water	½ teaspoon cayenne pepper
2 cups white onion, diced	½ cup heavy cream

Directions:

Pour chicken stock, water, and heavy cream in the Crock Pot.   Add onion, cayenne pepper, and close the lid.   Cook the ingredients on high for 4 hours. When the time is finished, open the lid, stir the

mixture, and add cheese.   Carefully mix the soup and cook it on Low for 3 hours.

Nutrition Info: Per Serving: 181 calories, 9.5g protein, 5.1g carbohydrates, 13.9g fat, 1g fiber, 48mg cholesterol, 410mg sodium, 110mg potassium.

641. Creamy Bacon Soup

Servings: 6   Cooking Time: 1 3/4 Hours

Ingredients:

1 tablespoon olive oil	1 sweet onion, chopped
6 bacon slices, chopped	1/2 celery root, cubed
1 1/2 pounds potatoes, peeled and cubed	2 cups chicken stock
	3 cups water
1 parsnip, diced	Salt and pepper to taste

Directions:

Heat the oil in a skillet and add the bacon. Cook until crisp then remove the bacon on a plate. Pour the fat of the bacon in your Crock Pot and add the remaining ingredients.   Adjust the taste with salt and pepper and cook on high settings for 1 1/2 hours.   When done, puree the soup with an immersion blender until smooth.   Pour the soup in a bowl and top with bacon.   Serve right away.

642. Lasagna Soup

Servings: 8   Cooking Time: 8 1/2 Hours

Ingredients:

2 tablespoons olive oil	1 pound ground beef
	1 cup diced tomatoes
1 large sweet onion, chopped	2 cups beef stock
	6 cups water
2 garlic cloves, chopped	1 1/2 cups uncooked pasta shells
1 teaspoon dried oregano	Salt and pepper to taste
1 1/2 cups tomato sauce	Grated Cheddar for serving

Directions:

Heat the oil in a skillet and add the ground beef. Cook for 5 minutes then transfer in your Crock Pot. Add the remaining ingredients and season with salt and pepper.   Cook on low settings for 8 hours. When done, pour into serving bowls and top with cheese.   Serve the soup warm and fresh.

643. Roasted Bell Pepper Quinoa Soup

Servings: 6   Cooking Time: 6 1/2 Hours

Ingredients:

1 shallot, chopped	1 cup water
1 garlic clove, chopped	1/2 teaspoon dried oregano
4 roasted red bell peppers, chopped	1/2 teaspoon dried basil
1/2 cup tomato paste	1 pinch cayenne pepper
2 cups vegetable stock	Salt and pepper to taste

1/2 cup red quinoa,
rinsed
Directions:
Combine the shallot, garlic, bell peppers, tomato paste, stock and water in your Crock Pot.   Add the quinoa, herbs and spices, as well as salt and pepper to taste and cover with a lid.   Cook on low settings for 6 hours.   Serve the soup warm or chilled.

---

644.   Spicy White Chicken Soup

Servings: 8   Cooking Time: 6 1/4 Hours
Ingredients:

2 chicken breasts, cubed	1/4 teaspoon cayenne pepper
2 tablespoons olive oil	1/2 teaspoon dried oregano
1 large onion, chopped	1/2 teaspoon dried basil
2 garlic cloves, chopped	2 cans (15 oz.) white beans, drained
2 cups chicken stock	5 cups water
1 parsnip, diced	1 bay leaf
1/2 teaspoon cumin seeds	Salt and pepper to taste

Directions:
Heat the oil in a skillet and add the chicken. Cook on all sides until golden then transfer in your Crock Pot.   Add the onion, garlic, stock, parsnip, cumin seeds, cayenne pepper, oregano, basil, beans, water and bay leaf.   Adjust the taste with salt and pepper and cook on low settings for 6 hours. Serve the soup warm and fresh.

---

645.   Chicken Sausage Rice Soup

Servings: 6   Cooking Time: 6 1/4 Hours
Ingredients:

2 fresh chicken sausages, sliced	1 cup diced tomatoes
1 shallot, chopped	2 large potatoes, peeled and cubed
1 carrot, sliced	1/4 cup jasmine rice
1 celery stalk, sliced	2 cups chicken stock
1 yellow bell pepper, cored and diced	4 cups water
	Salt and pepper to taste

Directions:
Combine the chicken, shallot and the rest of the ingredients in your Crock Pot.   Add salt and pepper to taste and cook on low settings for 6 hours.   The soup is best served warm.

---

646.   Herbed Spinach Lentil Soup

Servings: 8   Cooking Time: 3 1/4 Hours
Ingredients:

1 cup green lentils, rinsed	2 cups chicken stock
	6 cups water
1 celery stalk, sliced	1 bay leaf
1 carrot, sliced	1 thyme sprig
1 sweet onion, chopped	Salt and pepper to taste

2 sweet potatoes, peeled and cubed   4 cups fresh spinach, shredded
Directions:
Combine the lentils, celery, carrot, onion, potatoes, stock and water in your Crock Pot.   Add the bay leaf and thyme and season with salt and pepper. Cook on high settings for 2 hours then add the spinach and cook one more hour.   Serve the soup warm or chilled.

---

647.   Ground Beef Stew

Servings: 5   Cooking Time: 7 Hours
Ingredients:

1 cup bell pepper, diced	2 cups ground beef
1 teaspoon minced garlic	1 cup tomatoes, chopped
1 teaspoon dried rosemary	1 teaspoon salt
	3 cups of water

Directions:
Put all ingredients in the Crock Pot and stir them. Close the lid and cook the stew on Low for 7 hours.
Nutrition Info: Per Serving: 135 calories, 18.6g protein, 3.5g carbohydrates, 4.8g fat, 0.9g fiber, 55mg cholesterol, 524mg sodium, 419mg potassium.

---

648.   Stroganoff Soup

Servings: 8   Cooking Time: 8 1/4 Hours
Ingredients:

2 pound beef roast, cubed	1 can condensed cream of mushroom soup
2 tablespoons all-purpose flour	2 cups chicken stock
2 tablespoons canola oil	1 cup water
	1/2 cup sour cream
1 sweet onion, chopped	Salt and pepper to taste

Directions:
Season the beef with salt and pepper and sprinkle with flour.   Heat the oil in a skillet and stir in the beef. Cook for a few minutes on all sides then transfer the beef in your Crock Pot.   Add the onion, soup, stock, water and sour cream. Season with salt and pepper and cook on low settings for 8 hours.   Serve the soup warm.

---

649.   Russet Potato Soup

Servings: 6   Cooking Time: 7 Hours
Ingredients:

1 cup onion, diced	5 cups of water
2 cups russet potatoes, chopped	1 garlic clove
	1/2 cup carrot, grated
1 teaspoon dried parsley	1 oz Parmesan, grated
	1 cup heavy cream

Directions:
Put the onion in the Crock Pot.   Add water, potatoes, parsley, peeled garlic clove, carrot, and heavy cream.   Close the lid and cook the soup on low for 7 hours.   When the time is finished, mash

the soup gently with the help of the potato mash. Add Parmesan and stir the soup.

Nutrition Info: Per Serving: 131 calories, 3.1g protein, 11.5g carbohydrates, 8.5g fat, 1.9g fiber, 31mg cholesterol, 68mg sodium, 281mg potassium.

---

650.   Chicken Pearl Barley Soup

Servings: 8   Cooking Time: 6 1/2 Hours

Ingredients:

3 chicken breasts, cubed	2 tomatoes, peeled and diced
2 tablespoons olive oil	2 potatoes, peeled and cubed
1 teaspoon dried oregano	1/2 cup pearl barley
1/2 teaspoon paprika	2 cups chicken stock
1 large sweet onion, chopped	4 cups water
2 carrots, sliced	Salt and pepper to taste
2 celery stalks, sliced	2 tablespoons chopped parsley

Directions:
Heat the oil in a skillet and add the chicken. Cook on all sides for a few minutes until golden then transfer in your Crock Pot.   Add the oregano, paprika, onion, carrots, celery, tomatoes, potatoes, pearl barley, water, chicken stock, salt and pepper. Cook on low settings for 6 hours.   When done, stir in the parsley and serve the soup warm.

---

651.   Creamy Cauliflower Soup

Servings: 6   Cooking Time: 3 1/4 Hours

Ingredients:

1 tablespoon canola oil	1 head cauliflower, cut into florets
1 sweet onion, chopped	1 can condensed cream of chicken soup
2 garlic cloves, chopped	Salt and pepper to taste
2 medium size potatoes, peeled and cubed	1/2 cup water
	1/2 cup grated Parmesan cheese

Directions:
Heat the oil in a skillet and add the onion. Cook for 2 minutes then transfer the onion in your Crock Pot.   Add the remaining ingredients, except the cheese, and season with salt and pepper.   Cook on high settings for hours.   When done, puree the soup with an immersion blender.   Serve the soup warm.

---

652.   Creamy Carrot Lentil Soup

Servings: 6   Cooking Time: 2 1/4 Hours

Ingredients:

2 tablespoons olive oil	2 cups water
4 carrots, sliced	1/4 teaspoon cumin powder
1 shallot, chopped	Salt and pepper to taste
1 small fennel bulb, sliced	1 thyme sprig
	1 rosemary sprig
1/2 cup red lentils	
2 cups chicken stock	

Directions:
Heat the oil in a skillet and add the shallot and carrots. Sauté for 5 minutes then transfer the mixture in your Crock Pot.   Add the remaining ingredients and cook on high settings for hours. When done, remove the thyme and rosemary and puree the soup with an immersion blender. Serve the soup warm.

---

653.   Fennel Stew

Servings: 6   Cooking Time: 5 Hours

Ingredients:

1-pound beef sirloin, chopped	1 yellow onion, chopped
1 cup fennel bulb, chopped	1 tablespoon dried dill
3 cups of water	1 teaspoon olive oil

Directions:
Roast beef sirloin in the skillet for 2 minutes per side.   Then transfer the meat in the Crock Pot. Add olive oil, a fennel bulb, water, onion, and dried dill.   Close the lid and cook the stew on high for 5 hours.

Nutrition Info: Per Serving: 160 calories, 23.4g protein, 3.1g carbohydrates, 5.6g fat, 0.9g fiber, 68mg cholesterol, 63mg sodium, 410mg potassium.

---

654.   Red Kidney Beans Soup

Servings: 6   Cooking Time: 5 Hours

Ingredients:

2 cups red kidney beans, canned	1 cup carrot, diced
1 cup cauliflower, chopped	1 teaspoon Italian seasonings
1 teaspoon chili powder	1 cup tomatoes, canned
	4 cups chicken stock

Directions:
Put all ingredients except red kidney beans in the Crock Pot.   Close the lid and cook the soup on High for 4 hours.   Then add red kidney beans and stir the soup carefully with the help of the spoon.   Close the lid and cook it on high for 1 hour more.

Nutrition Info: Per Serving: 234 calories, 15.1g protein, 42.3g carbohydrates, 1.4g fat, 10.7g fiber, 1mg cholesterol, 540mg sodium, 1032mg potassium.

---

655.   Simple Chicken Noodle Soup

Servings: 8   Cooking Time: 8 1/4 Hours

Ingredients:

1 1/2 pounds chicken breasts, cubed	2 cups chicken stock
2 large carrots, sliced	5 cups water
2 celery stalks, sliced	1 thyme sprig
1 onion, chopped	2 cups dried egg noodles
	Salt and pepper to taste

Directions:

Combine all the ingredients in your Crock Pot. Add salt and pepper and cook on low settings for 8 hours, mixing once during cooking. Serve the soup warm.

656. Thai Chicken Soup

Servings: 8   Cooking Time: 6 1/2 Hours

Ingredients:

8 chicken thighs	1 teaspoon fish sauce
2 celery stalks, sliced	1 lime, juiced
1 sweet onion, chopped	2 cups coconut milk
1 teaspoon grated ginger	2 cups chicken stock
2 tablespoons soy sauce	4 cups water
1 tablespoon brown sugar	1 lemongrass stalk, crushed
	1 cup green peas
	Salt and pepper to taste

Directions:

Combine the chicken, celery, onion, ginger, fish sauce, soy sauce, sugar and lime juice in your Crock Pot.   Add the remaining ingredients and season with salt and pepper if needed.   Cook the soup on low settings for 6 hours.   Serve the soup warm and fresh.

657. Hamburger Soup

Servings: 8   Cooking Time: 7 Hours 15 Minutes

Ingredients:

1 pound ground meat, cooked	1 can kidney beans
1 can diced tomatoes	1 can mixed vegetables
1 can lima beans	1½ teaspoons red chili powder
Salt, to taste	1 can beef broth
2 tablespoons olive oil	

Directions:

Put olive oil and ground meat in a crock pot and cook for about 5 minutes.   Transfer the remaining ingredients into the crock pot and cover the lid.   Cook on LOW for about 7 hours and ladle out into serving bowl to serve hot.

Nutrition Info: Calories:262 Fat:14.4g Carbohydrates:12.2g

658. Italian Barley Soup

Servings: 8   Cooking Time: 6 1/4 Hours

Ingredients:

2 tablespoons olive oil	1 celery stalk, diced
1 shallot, chopped	1 teaspoon dried oregano
1 garlic clove, chopped	1 teaspoon dried basil
1 carrot, diced	2/3 cup pearl barley
2 red bell peppers, cored and diced	3 cups water
2 tomatoes, peeled and diced	2 cups fresh spinach, chopped
2 cups vegetable stock	1 lemon, juiced
	Salt and pepper to taste

Directions:

Heat the oil in a skillet and stir in the shallot, garlic, carrot and celery, as well as bell peppers.   Cook for 5 minutes just until softened then transfer in your Crock Pot. You can skip this step, but sautéing the vegetables first improves the taste.   Add the remaining ingredients to the pot and season with salt and pepper.   Cook on low settings for 6 hours.   The soup is great served either warm or chilled.

659. Cajun Black Bean Soup

Servings: 8   Cooking Time: 6 1/4 Hours

Ingredients:

2 tablespoons olive oil	1/2 teaspoon dried basil
1 red onion, chopped	1/2 teaspoon dried oregano
1 garlic clove, chopped	1 teaspoon Cajun seasoning
1 parsnip, diced	4 cups chicken stock
1 celery stalk, sliced	1 cup tomato paste
1 red bell pepper, cored and diced	2 cups water
1 green bell pepper, cored and diced	2 cans (15 oz.) black beans, drained
2 jalapenos, chopped	Salt and pepper to taste
1 teaspoon dried thyme	2 tablespoons chopped cilantro for serving

Directions:

Heat the oil in a skillet and stir in the onion, garlic, parsnip and bell peppers. Cook for 5 minutes, stirring often, until softened.   Transfer the mixture in your Crock Pot and add the remaining ingredients.   Adjust the taste with salt and pepper as needed and cook on low settings for 6 hours.   When done, stir in the chopped cilantro and serve right away.

660. Lentil Soup With Garlic Topping

Servings: 8   Cooking Time: 6 1/2 Hours

Ingredients:

Soup:	2 cups chicken stock
1/2 cup red lentils, rinsed	Salt and pepper to taste
1/2 cup green lentils, rinsed	Topping:
1 shallot, chopped	3 garlic cloves, chopped
1 celery stalk, sliced	2 tablespoons chopped parsley
1 carrot, diced	2 tomatoes, peeled and diced
1 red bell pepper, cored and diced	Salt and pepper to taste
1/2 cup tomato sauce	1 tablespoon olive oil
1 bay leaf	
2 cups water	

Directions:

To make the soup, combine all the ingredients in your Crock Pot.   Add salt and pepper to taste and cook on low settings for 6 hours.   For the topping, mix the garlic, parsley, tomatoes, salt, pepper and olive oil in a bowl.   Pour the warm soup into serving bowls and top with the tomato and garlic topping.   Serve right away.

661.   Smoky Sweet Corn Soup

Servings: 6   Cooking Time: 5 1/2 Hours
Ingredients:

1 shallot, chopped	3 cups frozen corn
1 garlic clove, chopped	2 cups chicken stock
2 tablespoons olive oil	2 cups water
2 bacon slices, chopped	1/4 teaspoon chili powder
	Salt and pepper to taste

Directions:
Heat the oil in a skillet and add the garlic, shallot and bacon. Cook on all sides until golden then transfer in your Crock Pot.   Add the corn, stock, water and chili powder and season with salt and pepper.   Cook on low settings for 5 hours. When done, puree the soup with an immersion blender and serve it warm.

662.   Moroccan Lentil Soup

Servings: 6   Cooking Time: 6 1/4 Hours
Ingredients:

1 large sweet onion, chopped	1 parsnip, diced
2 garlic cloves, chopped	1/2 teaspoon ground coriander
2 tablespoons olive oil	2 cups water
2 carrots, diced	3 cups chicken stock
1 cup chopped cauliflower	1 cup red lentils
1/2 teaspoon cumin powder	2 tablespoons tomato paste
1/4 teaspoon turmeric powder	2 tablespoons lemon juice
	Salt and pepper to taste

Directions:
Heat the oil in a skillet and stir in the onion, garlic, carrots and parsnip. Cook for 5 minutes then transfer in your Crock Pot.   Stir in the cauliflower, cumin powder, turmeric and coriander, as well as water, stock, lentils and tomato paste. Add the lemon juice, salt and pepper and cook on low settings for 6 hours.   Serve the soup warm or chilled.

663.   Taco Spices Stew

Servings: 4   Cooking Time: 8 Hours
Ingredients:

1-pound beef sirloin	3 cups of water
1 teaspoon liquid honey	1 teaspoon salt
1 cup sweet potato, chopped	1 teaspoon taco seasonings

Directions:
Cut the beef sirloin into the strips and sprinkle with taco seasonings.   Then transfer the beef strips in the Crock Pot.   Add salt, sweet potato, water, and liquid honey.   Close the lid and cook the stew for 8 hours on Low.
Nutrition Info: Per Serving: 264 calories, 35.4g protein, 12.3g carbohydrates, 7.2g fat, 1.7g fiber, 101mg cholesterol, 732mg sodium, 697mg potassium.

664.   Turmeric Squash Soup

Servings: 6   Cooking Time: 9 Hours
Ingredients:

3 chicken thighs, skinless, boneless, chopped	1 teaspoon ground turmeric
3 cups butternut squash, chopped	1 oz green chilies, chopped, canned
1 onion, sliced	6 cups of water

Directions:
Put chicken thighs in the bottom of the Crock Pot and top them with green chilies.   Then add the ground turmeric, butternut squash, and water. Add sliced onion and close the lid.   Cook the soup on low for 9 Hours.
Nutrition Info: Per Serving: 194 calories, 22.6g protein, 13.4g carbohydrates, 5.8g fat, 3.2g fiber, 65mg cholesterol, 78mg sodium, 551mg potassium.

665.   Beef Tortellini Soup

Servings: 8   Cooking Time: 8 1/2 Hours
Ingredients:

1 pound beef roast, cubed	1/2 teaspoon dried basil
2 tablespoons olive oil	8 oz. cheese tortellini
1 large onion, chopped	1/4 cup dried kidney beans, rinsed
1 carrot, sliced	2 cups beef stock
1 celery stalk, sliced	1/2 cup dark beer
2 garlic cloves, chopped	4 cups water
1 cup diced tomatoes	1 bay leaf
	Salt and pepper to taste

Directions:
Heat the oil in a skillet and add the beef. Cook on all sides until golden brown, for about 5 minutes, then transfer in your Crock Pot.   Add the remaining ingredients and season with salt and pepper.   Cook on low settings for 8 hours. Serve the soup warm.

666.   Cabbage Stew

Servings: 2   Cooking Time: 3 Hours
Ingredients:

2 cups white cabbage, shredded	1 cup cauliflower, chopped
½ cup tomato juice	½ cup potato, chopped
1 teaspoon ground white pepper	1 cup of water

Directions:
Put cabbage, potato, and cauliflower in the Crock Pot.   Add tomato juice, ground white pepper, and

water. Stir the stew ingredients and close the lid. Cook the stew on high for hours.

Nutrition Info: Per Serving: 57 calories, 2.8g protein, 13.3g carbohydrates, 0.2g fat, 3.9g fiber, 0mg cholesterol, 196mg sodium, 503mg potassium.

667. Chicken Sausage Soup

Servings: 8   Cooking Time: 6 1/2 Hours

Ingredients:

1 pound Italian sausages, sliced	1 can diced tomatoes
1 sweet onion, chopped	1 can cannellini beans
2 garlic cloves, chopped	1/4 cup dry white wine
1 red bell pepper, cored and diced	2 cups chicken stock
1 carrot, diced	3 cups water
1/2 teaspoon dried oregano	1/2 cup short pasta
1/2 teaspoon dried basil	Salt and pepper to taste
	2 tablespoons chopped parsley

Directions:
Combine the sausages, onion, garlic, bell pepper, carrot, oregano, basil, tomatoes, beans, wine, stock and water in a Crock Pot.   Cook on high settings for 1 hour then add the pasta and continue cooking for 5 hours.   Serve the soup warm, topped with freshly chopped parsley.

668. Quick Lentil Ham Soup

Servings: 6   Cooking Time: 1 3/4 Hours

Ingredients:

1 tablespoon olive oil	1 shallot, chopped
4 oz. ham, diced	1 cup dried lentils, rinsed
1 carrot, diced	2 cups water
1 celery stalk, sliced	1/2 cup tomato sauce
1/2 teaspoon dried oregano	1 1/2 cups chicken stock
1/2 teaspoon dried basil	Salt and pepper to taste

Directions:
Combine the olive oil, ham, carrot, celery, shallot, oregano, basil, lentils, water, tomato sauce and stock.   Add salt and pepper to taste and cook on high settings for 1 1/hours.   The soup can be served both warm and chilled.

669. Cheesy Broccoli Soup

Servings: 8   Cooking Time: 4 1/4 Hours

Ingredients:

1 shallot, chopped	1 can condensed chicken soup
2 garlic cloves, chopped	2 cups water1/2 teaspoon dried oregano
2 tablespoons olive oil	1 cup grated Cheddar soup
1 head broccoli, cut into florets	Salt and pepper to taste
1 large potato, peeled and cubed	

Directions:
Heat the olive oil in a skillet and stir in the shallot and garlic. Cook for 2 minutes until softened. Transfer the shallot and garlic in your Crock Pot and add the remaining ingredients.   Cook on low settings for 4 hours then puree the soup with an immersion blender.   Serve the soup warm.

670. Spicy Chili Soup With Tomatillos

Servings: 8   Cooking Time: 8 1/2 Hours

Ingredients:

1/2 pound beef roast, cubed	1 can fire roasted tomatoes
10 oz. canned tomatillos, rinsed, drained and chopped	1 cup beef stock
1 dried ancho chili, seeded and chopped	4 cups water
1 jalapeno pepper, chopped	Salt and pepper to taste
1 can (15 oz.) black beans, drained	1 bay leaf
	1 thyme sprig
	Chopped cilantro and sour cream for serving

Directions:
Combine the beef roast, tomatillos, ancho chili, jalapeno pepper and black beans in your Crock Pot. Add the tomatoes, beef stock, water, salt and pepper, as well as bay leaf and thyme sprig.   Cook on low settings for 8 hours.   The soup is best served warm, topped with chopped cilantro and a dollop of sour cream.

671.Chicken Bacon Orzo Soup

Servings: 6 (1.7 Ounces Per Serving)   Cooking Time: 5 Hours

Ingredients:

5 slices of bacon	½ cup orzo
2 cups yellow onion, diced	1 ½ teaspoons sea salt
2 cloves garlic, minced	½ teaspoon fresh ground pepper
1 cup carrots, diced	Parsley, fresh, chopped to taste
1 cup celery, diced	
6 cups chicken stock	

Directions:
Cook bacon in pan over medium-high heat until crisp. Place bacon on plate lined with paper towels. Save 2 tablespoons of fat from pan. Add the garlic, celery, carrots, onions to the pan with a pinch of salt. Cook the veggies over medium heat for several minutes, stirring periodically. Place chicken breasts in Crock-Pot and cover with veggies and chicken stock. Cover and cook over LOW heat for 5 hours. Halfway through cooking time, take out chicken, shred it up, and then place back in Crock-Pot along with orzo. Garnish each bowl of soup with diced bacon and fresh parsley. Serve hot.

Nutrition Info: Calories: 507, Total Fat: 7 g, Saturated Fat: 1 g, Sodium: 220 mg, Carbs: 87 g, Fiber: 23 g, Sugars: 10 g, Protein: 28.3 g

672.	Crock-pot Buffalo Chicken Soup

Servings: 5   Cooking Time: 6 Hours

Ingredients:

3 medium chicken thighs, deboned, sliced	½ teaspoon celery seed
1 teaspoon garlic powder	¼ cup butter
1 teaspoon onion powder	3 cups beef broth
½ cup Frank's hot sauce or to taste, depending on how hot you like it	1 cup heavy cream
	2 ounces cream cheese
	¼ teaspoon Xanthan gum
	Salt and pepper to taste

Directions:
Cut up chicken into chunks and place in Crock-Pot. Add all the other ingredients except the cream cheese and Xanthan gum. Set to Crock-Pot on LOW for 6 hours and allow to cook completely. Once cooking is done, remove the chicken from pot and shred with fork. Add the cream cheese and Xanthan gum to Crock-Pot. Using an immersion blender, emulsify all the liquids together. Add chicken back to Crock-Pot and stir. Season with salt and pepper to taste. Serve hot.

Nutrition Info: Calories: 523.2, Total Fats: 44.2 g, Carbs: 3.4 g, Fiber: 0 g, Net Carbs: 3.4 g, Protein: 20.8 g

673.	Asparagus Crab Soup

Servings: 6   Cooking Time: 2 1/4 Hours

Ingredients:

1 tablespoon olive oil	1 cup green peas
1 shallot, chopped	1 cup chicken stock
1 celery stalk, sliced	2 cups water
1 bunch asparagus, trimmed and chopped	Salt and pepper to taste
	1 can crab meat, drained

Directions:
Heat the oil in a skillet and add the shallot and celery. Sauté for 2 minutes until softened then transfer in your Crock Pot. Add the asparagus, green peas, stock and water and season with salt and pepper. Cook on high settings for 2 hours. When done, puree the soup with an immersion blender until creamy. Pour the soup into serving bowls and top with crab meat. Serve the soup right away.

674.	Roasted Tomato Soup

Servings: 6   Cooking Time: 5 Hours

Ingredients:

2 pounds heirloom tomatoes, halved	2 cups vegetable stock
2 red onions, halved	1 cup water
4 garlic cloves	1 carrot, sliced
1 teaspoon dried oregano	1/2 celery root, peeled and cubed
2 tablespoons olive oil	Salt and pepper to taste

Directions:
Combine the tomatoes, red onions, garlic and oregano in a baking tray lined with parchment paper. Season with salt and pepper and roast in the preheated oven at 400F for 30 minutes. Transfer the vegetables and juices in your Crock Pot. Add the remaining ingredients and cook on low settings for hours. When done, puree the soup with an immersion blender. The soup can be served warm or chilled.

675.	Summer Vegetable Soup

Servings: 8   Cooking Time: 6 1/2 Hours

Ingredients:

1 sweet onion, chopped	2 ripe tomatoes, peeled and cubed
1 garlic clove, chopped	1 carrot, sliced
2 tablespoons olive oil	1 celery stalk, sliced
1 zucchini, cubed	1/2 cup edamame
1 yellow squash, cubed	2 cups chicken stock
1/2 head cauliflower, cut into florets	5 cups water
1/2 head broccoli, cut into florets	Salt and pepper to taste
	1 lemon, juiced
	1 tablespoon chopped parsley

Directions:
Combine the onion, garlic, olive oil and the rest of the ingredients in your Crock Pot. Add salt and pepper to taste and cook on low settings for 6 hours. When done, stir in the lemon juice and parsley and serve the soup warm or chilled.

676.	Posole Soup

Servings: 8   Cooking Time: 6 1/4 Hours

Ingredients:

1 tablespoons canola oil	1/4 teaspoon chili powder
1 pound pork tenderloin, cubed	1 can (15 oz.) black beans, drained
1 sweet onion, chopped	1 can sweet corn, drained
2 garlic cloves, chopped	1 cup diced tomatoes
1/2 teaspoon cumin powder	2 jalapeno peppers, chopped
1/2 teaspoon dried oregano	4 cups chicken stock
1/2 teaspoon dried basil	2 cups water
	Salt and pepper to taste
	2 limes, juiced

Directions:

Heat the canola oil in a skillet and stir in the tenderloin. Cook for 5 minutes on all sides. Add the pork in your Crock Pot and stir in the remaining ingredients, except the lime juice. Add salt and pepper to taste and cook on low settings for 6 hours. When done, stir in the lime juice and serve the soup warm or chilled.

677. Ham Bone Cabbage Soup

Servings: 8   Cooking Time: 7 1/4 Hours
Ingredients:

1 ham bone	1 can diced tomatoes
1 sweet onion, chopped	2 cups beef stock
1 mediums size cabbage head, shredded	Salt and pepper to taste
	1 bay leaf
2 tablespoons tomato paste	1 thyme sprig
	1 lemon, juiced

Directions:
Combine the ham bone, onion, cabbage, tomato paste, tomatoes, stock, bay leaf and thyme sprig in your Crock Pot. Add salt and pepper to taste and cook on low settings for 7 hours. When done, stir in the lemon juice and serve the soup warm.

678. Potato Kielbasa Soup

Servings: 8   Cooking Time: 6 1/4 Hours
Ingredients:

1 pound kielbasa sausages, sliced	2 large potatoes, peeled and cubed
1 sweet onion, chopped	2 cups chicken stock
2 carrots, diced	3 cups water
1 parsnip, diced	1/2 pound fresh spinach, shredded
1 garlic clove, chopped	1 lemon, juiced
2 red bell peppers, cored and diced	Salt and pepper to taste

Directions:
Combine the sausages, onion, carrots, parsnip, garlic, potatoes and bell peppers in your Crock Pot. Stir in the stock, water, spinach and lemon juice then add salt and pepper to taste. Cook on low settings for 6 hours. Serve the soup warm or chilled.

679. Indian Cauliflower Creamy Soup

Servings: 8   Cooking Time: 6 1/2 Hours
Ingredients:

2 tablespoons olive oil	2 medium size potatoes, peeled and cubed
1 sweet onion, chopped	2 cups vegetable stock
1 celery stalk, sliced	2 cups water
2 garlic cloves, chopped	1/4 teaspoon cumin powder
1 tablespoon red curry paste	1 pinch red pepper flakes

1 cauliflower head, cut into florets — Salt and pepper to taste

Directions:
Heat the oil in a skillet and stir in the onion, celery and garlic. Sauté for 2 minutes until softened. Transfer the mix in your Crock Pot. Add the remaining ingredients and cook on low settings for 6 hours. When done, puree the soup with an immersion blender and serve it warm.

680. Mexican Chicken Stew

Servings: 6   Cooking Time: 9 Hours 20 Minutes
Ingredients:

3 chicken breasts, boneless and skinless	1 can corn
1 can black beans, not drained	½ cup sour cream
2 cans diced tomatoes and chilies	1 cup onions, optional
	½ cup Mexican cheese, shredded

Directions:
Place chicken breasts at the bottom of the crock pot and top with tomatoes, beans and corns. Cover and cook on LOW for about 9 hours. Dish out and serve hot.
Nutrition Info: Calories:286 Fat:12.7g
Carbohydrates:16.8g

681. Ham Potato Chowder

Servings: 8   Cooking Time: 4 1/4 Hours
Ingredients:

1 tablespoon olive oil	1 cup diced ham
1 sweet onion, chopped	1 cup sweet corn, drained
1 can condensed chicken soup	1/2 teaspoon celery seeds
2 cups water	1/2 teaspoon cumin seeds
4 potatoes, peeled and cubed	Salt and pepper to taste

Directions:
Mix the olive oil, onion, chicken soup, water, potatoes, ham and corn in your Crock Pot. Add the celery seeds and cumin seeds and season with salt and pepper. Cook on high settings for 4 hours. Serve the soup warm.

682. Rabbit Stew

Servings: 5   Cooking Time: 8 Hours 15 Minutes
Ingredients:

½ cup celery, diced	1 piece of bacon
1 sausage, cubed	½ cup apple cider vinegar
1 bay leaf	
1 garlic clove, diced	3 cups chicken broth
1 cup Swiss chards, stalks	½ cup olive oil
½ can water chestnuts, diced	1 pound rabbit, cubed
	Salt and black pepper, to taste

Directions:
Marinate rabbit in olive oil and apple cider vinegar and keep aside overnight. Put chicken broth in

the crock pot and warm it up. Meanwhile, sear bacon and sausage in a pan and transfer it to the crock pot. Stir in rest of the ingredients and cover the lid. Cook on LOW for about 8 hours and dish out to serve hot.
Nutrition Info: Calories:418 Fat:30.7g Carbohydrates:2.7g

683. Pork And Corn Soup

Servings: 8   Cooking Time: 8 1/4 Hours
Ingredients:

1 pound pork roast, cubed	2 carrots, sliced
1 sweet onion, chopped	2 cups frozen sweet corn
2 bacon slices, chopped	1/2 teaspoon cumin seeds
1 garlic clove, chopped	1/2 red chili, sliced
1 celery stalk, sliced	2 cups chicken stock
2 yellow bell peppers, cored and diced	4 cups water
	Salt and pepper to taste
	2 tablespoons chopped cilantro

Directions:
Combine the pork roast, sweet onion, bacon and garlic in a skillet and cook for 5 minutes, stirring all the time. Transfer in your Crock Pot and add the carrots, celery, bell peppers, sweet corn, cumin seeds, red chili, stock, water, salt and pepper. Cook on low settings for 8 hours. When done, add the chopped cilantro and serve the soup warm.

684. Spinach Sweet Potato Soup

Servings: 6   Cooking Time: 3 1/2 Hours
Ingredients:

1 shallot, chopped	4 cups water
1 garlic clove, chopped	Salt and pepper to taste
1/2 pound ground chicken	4 cups fresh spinach, shredded
2 tablespoons olive oil	1/2 teaspoon dried oregano
2 medium size sweet potatoes, peeled and cubed	1/2 teaspoon dried basil
2 cups chicken stock	1 tablespoon chopped parsley

Directions:
Heat the oil in a skillet and add the ground chicken, shallot and garlic. Cook for about 5 minutes, stirring often. Transfer the meat mix in your Crock Pot and add the potatoes, stock, water, salt and pepper. Cook on high settings for 2 hours then stir in the spinach, oregano, basil and parsley and cook one additional hour on high. Serve the soup warm.

685. Cheddar Garlic Soup

Servings: 6   Cooking Time: 2 1/4 Hours
Ingredients:

8 garlic cloves, chopped	2 tablespoons all-purpose flour
2 tablespoons olive oil	2 cups chicken stock
1 teaspoon cumin seeds	1/4 cup white wine
1 teaspoon mustard seeds	4 cups water
	3 cups grated Cheddar
	Salt and pepper to taste

Directions:
Heat the oil in a skillet and add the garlic. Sauté on low heat for 2 minutes then add the seeds and cook for minute to release flavor. Add the flour and cook for 1 hour then transfer the mix in your Crock Pot. Add the remaining ingredients and season with salt and pepper. Cook on high settings for 2 hours. The soup is best served warm.

686. Chorizo Soup

Servings: 6   Cooking Time: 5 Hours
Ingredients:

9 oz chorizo, chopped	1 zucchini, chopped
7 cups of water	½ cup spinach, chopped
1 cup potato, chopped	1 teaspoon salt
1 teaspoon minced garlic, chopped	

Directions:
Put the chorizo in the skillet and roast it for 2 minutes per side on high heat. Then transfer the chorizo in the Crock Pot. Add water, potato, minced garlic, zucchini, spinach, and salt. Close the lid and cook the soup on high for 5 hours. Then cool the soup to the room temperature.
Nutrition Info: Per Serving: 210 calories, 11g protein, 4.3g carbohydrates, 16.4g fat, 0.7g fiber, 37mg cholesterol, 927mg sodium, 326mg potassium.

687. Coconut Cod Stew

Servings: 6   Cooking Time: 6.5 Hours
Ingredients:

1-pound cod fillet, chopped	1 teaspoon curry powder
2 oz scallions, roughly chopped	1 teaspoon garlic, diced
1 cup coconut cream	

Directions:
Mix curry powder with coconut cream and garlic. Add scallions and gently stir the liquid. After this, pour it in the Crock Pot and add cod fillet. Stir the stew mixture gently and close the lid. Cook the stew on low for 6.hours.
Nutrition Info: Per Serving: 158 calories, 14.7g protein, 3.3g carbohydrates, 10.3g fat, 1.3g fiber, 37mg cholesterol, 55mg sodium, 138mg potassium.

688. Roasted Garlic Soup

Servings: 6   Cooking Time: 3 ½ Hours
Ingredients:

1 tablespoon extra-virgin olive oil	1 large head of cauliflower, chopped, about 5 cups
2 bulbs of garlic	
3 shallots, chopped	Fresh ground pepper

6 cups gluten-free vegetable broth

to taste
Sea salt to taste

Directions:

Preheat oven to 400°Fahrenheit. Peel the outer layers off garlic bulbs. Cut about 4 inch off the top of the bulbs, place into foil pan. Coat bulbs with olive oil, and cook in oven for 35 minutes. Once cooked, allow them to cool. Squeeze the garlic out of the bulbs into your food processor. Meanwhile, in a pan, sauté remaining olive oil and chopped shallots over medium-high heat for about 6 minutes. Add other ingredients to saucepan, cover and reduce heat to a simmer for 20 minutes or until the cauliflower is softened. Add the mixture to food processor and puree until smooth. Add mix to Crock Pot, cover with lid, and cook on LOW for 3 ½ hours. Serve hot.

Nutrition Info: Calories: 73, Total Fat: 2.4 g, Sodium: 1201 mg, Carbs: 11.3 g, Dietary Fiber: 2.1 g, Net Carbs: 2.1 g, Sugars: 4.1 g, Protein: 2.1 g

689.   Italian Veggie Pasta Soup

Servings: 10   Cooking Time: 8 1/2 Hours

Ingredients:

2 tablespoons olive oil	1 cup tomato sauce
1 sweet onion, chopped	2 cups chicken stock
2 garlic cloves, chopped	4 cups water
2 red bell peppers, cored and diced	1 bay leaf
2 zucchinis, sliced	1/2 teaspoon dried basil
1 can white beans, drained	1 teaspoon dried oregano
2 ripe tomatoes, peeled and diced	1/2 cup fusilli pasta
	1/4 cup short pasta of your choice
	Salt and pepper to taste

Directions:

Heat the oil in a skillet or saucepan and stir in the onion, garlic, bell peppers and zucchinis. Sauté for 5 minutes, stirring often, then transfer in your Crock Pot. Add the remaining ingredients and season with salt and pepper. Cook on low settings for 8 hours. The soup can be served both warm and chilled.

690.   Chinese Style Cod Stew

Servings: 2   Cooking Time: 5 Hours

Ingredients:

6 oz cod fillet	1 teaspoon olive oil
1 teaspoon sesame seeds	¼ cup of soy sauce
1 garlic clove, chopped	¼ cup fish stock
	4 oz fennel bulb, chopped

Directions:

Pour fish stock in the Crock Pot. Add soy sauce, olive oil, garlic, and sesame seeds. Then chop the fish roughly and add in the Crock Pot. Cook the meal on Low for 5 hours.

Nutrition Info: Per Serving: 139 calories, 18.9g protein, 7.4g carbohydrates, 4.2g fat, 2.2g fiber, 42mg cholesterol, 1926mg sodium, 359mg potassium.

691.   Broccoli Cheese Soup

Servings: 6   Cooking Time: 6 Hours 20 Minutes

Ingredients:

1½ cups heavy cream	¾ teaspoon salt
2½ cups water	2 tablespoons butter
½ cup red bell pepper, chopped	½ teaspoon dry mustard
2 cups broccoli, chopped, thawed and drained	8 ounces cheddar cheese, shredded
2 tablespoons chives, chopped	4 cups chicken broth
	¼ teaspoon cayenne pepper

Directions:

Put all the ingredients in a crockpot except chives and cheese and mix well. Cover and cook on LOW for about 6 hours. Sprinkle with cheese and cook on LOW for about   minutes. Garnish with chives and serve hot.

Nutrition Info: Calories:353 Fat:10g Carbohydrates:4g

692.   Mexican Style Stew

Servings: 6   Cooking Time: 6 Hours

Ingredients:

1 cup corn kernels	4 cups chicken stock
1 cup green peas	1 teaspoon dried cilantro
¼ cup white rice	1 tablespoon butter
1 teaspoon taco seasoning	

Directions:

Put butter and wild rice in the Crock Pot. Then add corn kernels, green peas, chicken stock, taco seasoning, and dried cilantro. Close the lid and cook the stew on Low for 6 hours.

Nutrition Info: Per Serving: 97 calories, 3.2g protein, 15.6g carbohydrates, 2.7g fat, 2g fiber, 5mg cholesterol, 599mg sodium, 148mg potassium.

693.   Beef Chili

Servings: 8   Cooking Time: 3 Hours 15 Minutes

Ingredients:

29 ounces canned diced tomatoes, not drained	1 jalapeno, minced
3 tablespoons chili powder	3 garlic cloves, minced
1 yellow onion, chopped	2 (16-ounce) cans red kidney beans, rinsed and drained
2 pounds lean ground beef	1 teaspoon Kosher salt
¼ cup tomato paste	1 teaspoon ground cumin
½ cup saltine cracker crumbs, finely ground	1 teaspoon black pepper

Directions:
Cook onions and beef over medium high heat in a pot until brown.   Transfer to the crock pot along with the rest of the ingredients.   Cover and cook on HIGH for about hours and dish out to serve.
Nutrition Info: Calories:638 Fat:9.1g Carbohydrates:78.9g

694.   Paprika Noddle Soup

Servings: 4   Cooking Time: 4 Hours
Ingredients:

3 oz egg noodles	1 teaspoon butter
3 cups chicken stock	½ teaspoon salt
1 teaspoon ground paprika	2 tablespoons fresh parsley, chopped

Directions:
Put egg noodles in the Crock Pot.   Add chicken stock, butter, ground paprika, and salt.   Close the lid and cook the soup on High for 4 hours.   Then open the lid, add parsley, and stir the soup.
Nutrition Info: Per Serving: 47 calories, 1.6g protein, 6.3g carbohydrates, 1.9g fat, 0.5g fiber, 9mg cholesterol, 873mg sodium, 42mg potassium.

695.   Beef Barley Soup

Servings: 8   Cooking Time: 14 Hours 20 Minutes
Ingredients:

2 tablespoons butter	1 cup celery, diced
¼ cup onions	¼ tablespoon dried basil
3 cups water	
16 oz round beef steak	¼ teaspoon savory, ground
½ cup barley	
½ teaspoon black pepper	1 cup carrots, chopped
2 cups beef broth	¾ fl oz red wine

Directions:
Put water, beef steaks, barley and beef broth in the one pot crock pot and cover the lid.   Cook on LOW for about 13 hours and add the remaining ingredients.   Cover and cook on LOW for 1 more hour.   Dish out to serve hot.
Nutrition Info: Calories:210 Fat:9g Carbohydrates:10.9g

696.   Creamy Potato Soup

Servings: 6   Cooking Time: 6 1/2 Hours
Ingredients:

6 bacon slices, chopped	1 can condensed chicken soup
1 sweet onion, chopped	Salt and pepper to taste
6 medium size potatoes, peeled and cubed	1 1/2 cups half and half
2 cups water	1 tablespoon chopped parsley

Directions:
Heat a skillet over medium flame and add the bacon. Cook until crisp then transfer the bacon and its fat in your Crock Pot.   Add the onion, chicken soup, potatoes, water, salt and pepper and cook on low settings for 4 hours.   Add the half and half and continue cooking for 2 additional hours. When done, stir in the chopped parsley and serve the soup warm.

697.   Tuscan White Bean Soup

Servings: 6   Cooking Time: 6 1/2 Hours
Ingredients:

1 cup dried white beans	1 bay leaf
2 cups chicken stock	2 cups spinach, shredded
4 cups water	Salt and pepper to taste
1 carrot, diced	1 teaspoon dried oregano
1 celery stalk, diced	
4 garlic cloves, chopped	1 teaspoon dried basil
2 tablespoons tomato paste	1/2 lemon, juiced

Directions:
Combine the beans, stock, water, carrot, celery, garlic and tomato paste in your Crock Pot.   Add the bay leaf, dried herbs and lemon juice, as well as salt and pepper.   Cook on low settings for 4 hours then add the spinach and cook for 2 additional hours on low settings.   Serve the soup warm or chilled.

698.   Chicken Chili

Servings: 4   Cooking Time: 5 Hours
Ingredients:

1 chili pepper, chopped	2 cups ground chicken
1 yellow onion, chopped	1 teaspoon dried basil
2 tablespoons tomato paste	½ teaspoon ground coriander
	3 cups of water

Directions:
Mix ground chicken with dried basil and ground coriander.   Then transfer the chicken in the Crock Pot.   Add onion, chili pepper, tomato paste, and water. Carefully stir the mixture and close the lid.   Cook the chili on high for 5 hours.
Nutrition Info: Per Serving: 151 calories, 20.9g protein, 4.2g carbohydrates, 5.3g fat, 1g fiber, 62mg cholesterol, 75mg sodium, 296mg potassium.

699.   Curried Lentil Soup

Servings: 8   Cooking Time: 4 1/4 Hours
Ingredients:

4 bacon slices, chopped	1 cup diced tomatoes
1 sweet onion, chopped	2 cups chicken stock
	4 cups water
2 garlic cloves, chopped	1 teaspoon curry powder
1 cup dried lentils, rinsed	1/4 teaspoon ground ginger
1 carrot, diced	Salt and pepper to taste
	1 lime, juiced

1 celery stalk, sliced 2 tablespoons
1 parsnip, diced chopped parsley

Directions:
Heat a skillet over medium flame and stir in the bacon. Cook for a few minutes until crisp. Transfer the bacon in a Crock Pot and stir in the onion, garlic, lentils, carrot, celery, parsnip, tomatoes, stock, water, curry powder and ginger. Add salt and pepper to taste and cook on low settings for 4 hours.   When done, stir in the lime juice and chopped parsley and serve the soup warm or chilled.

700.   Spiced Pork Soup

Servings: 8   Cooking Time: 7 1/4 Hours

Ingredients:

1 pound pork roast, cubed
1 tablespoon all-purpose flour
1 teaspoon dried oregano
1 teaspoon cumin powder
1/2 teaspoon smoked paprika
1/4 teaspoon cinnamon powder
4 bacon slices, chopped
2 carrots, diced

1 can fire roasted tomatoes
1 celery stalk, sliced
2 red bell peppers, cored and diced
2 large potatoes, peeled and cubed
1 large sweet potatoes, peeled and cubed
2 cups chicken stock
5 cups water
Salt and pepper to taste

Directions:
Season the pork with salt and pepper and sprinkle it with flour, oregano, cumin powder, paprika and cinnamon.   Heat a skillet in a skillet and add the bacon. Cook until crisp then add the pork and cook for a few minutes. Transfer the meat and bacon in your Crock Pot.   Add the remaining ingredients and cook on low settings for 7 hours.   Serve the soup warm.

701.   Red Chili Quinoa Soup

Servings: 8   Cooking Time: 3 1/4 Hours

Ingredients:

2 shallots, chopped
1 carrot, diced
1/2 celery root, peeled and diced
1 can diced tomatoes
1/2 cup quinoa, rinsed
1 can (15 oz.) red beans, drained
2 cups water

2 cups chicken stock
Salt and pepper to taste
1/2 teaspoon chili powder
2 tablespoons chopped cilantro for serving
Sour cream for serving

Directions:
Combine the shallots, carrot, celery and diced tomatoes in your Crock Pot.   Add the quinoa, water, stock and chili powder and season with salt and pepper.   Cook on high settings for hours. Serve the soup warm, topped with cilantro and sour cream.

702.   Orange Sweet Potato Soup

Servings: 8   Cooking Time: 3 1/2 Hours

Ingredients:

2 tablespoons olive oil
1 shallot, chopped
2 carrots, sliced
1/2 celery stalk
2 large sweet potatoes, peeled and cubed
1 teaspoon orange zest

2 oranges, juiced
2 cups chicken stick
1 bay leaf
1/2 cinnamon stalk
Salt and pepper to taste
1 teaspoon pumpkin seeds oil
2 tablespoons pumpkin seeds

Directions:
Heat the olive oil in a skillet and add the shallot and carrots. Sauté for 5 minutes then transfer in your Crock Pot.   Add the celery stalk, potatoes, orange juice, orange zest, stock, bay leaf, cinnamon, salt and pepper.   Cook the soup on high settings for 2 hours then on low settings for 1 additional hour.   When done, remove the bay leaf and cinnamon stick and puree the soup with an immersion blender.   To serve, pour the soup into bowls and top with pumpkin seeds drizzle of pumpkin seed oil. Serve right away.

703.   Creamy Mediterranean Soup

Servings: 6   Cooking Time: 4 1/4 Hours

Ingredients:

2 tablespoons olive oil
1 sweet onion, chopped
1 garlic clove, chopped
1/2 head cauliflower, cut into florets
1 head broccoli, cut into florets

1 teaspoon dried oregano
2 cups vegetable stock
2 cups water
2 tablespoons Italian pesto
Salt and pepper to taste

Directions:
Heat the oil in a skillet and add the onion and garlic. Sauté for 2 minutes until softened. Transfer in your Crock Pot and add the remaining ingredients.   Season with salt and pepper and cook on low settings for 4 hours.   When done, puree the soup with an immersion blender and serve the soup warm.

704.   Sausage Bean Soup

Servings: 8   Cooking Time: 3 1/4 Hours

Ingredients:

2 bacon slices, chopped
1 sweet onion, chopped
1 garlic clove, chopped
1/2 teaspoon dried rosemary
1/2 teaspoon dried thyme
4 pork sausages, sliced

1 carrot, diced
1 parsnip, diced
1 celery stalk, sliced
1 can diced tomatoes
1 can (15 oz.) white beans, drained
2 cups chicken stock
4 cups water
Salt and pepper to taste

Directions:
Heat a skillet over medium flame and stir in the bacon. Sauté for 2-3 minutes until crisp. Transfer the bacon in your Crock Pot.   Add the

remaining ingredients and season with salt and pepper.   Cook the soup on high settings for 3 hours.   The soup is best served warm, but it tastes great chilled as well.

705.   Mexican Style Soup

Servings: 6   Cooking Time: 5 Hours

Ingredients:

1-pound chicken fillet, cut into strips	6 cups chicken stock
2 tablespoons enchilada sauce	1 cup tomatoes, chopped
1 cup black beans, soaked	1 teaspoon garlic powder
	¼ cup fresh cilantro, chopped

Directions:
Put all ingredients in the Crock Pot and close the lid.   Cook the soup on high for 5 hours.   When the time is finished, open the lid and carefully mix the soup with the help of the ladle.
Nutrition Info: Per Serving: 276 calories, 30.1g protein, 23.8g carbohydrates, 6.8g fat, 5.9g fiber, 67mg cholesterol, 833mg sodium, 784mg potassium.

706.   Creamy Edamame Soup

Servings: 6   Cooking Time: 2 1/4 Hours

Ingredients:

1 tablespoon olive oil	2 shallots, chopped
2 garlic cloves, chopped	Salt and pepper to taste
1 large potato, peeled and cubed	2 cups chicken stock
1 celery root, peeled and cubed	1 cup water
1 pound frozen edamame	1/4 teaspoon dried oregano
	1/4 teaspoon dried marjoram

Directions:
Heat the oil in a skillet and stir in the shallots and garlic. Sauté for 2 minutes until softened then transfer in your Crock Pot.   Add the remaining ingredients and season with salt and pepper. Cook on high settings for 2 hours.   When done, puree the soup with an immersion blender until creamy.   Serve the soup right away.

707.   Tuscan Kale And White Bean Soup

Servings: 8   Cooking Time: 8 1/2 Hours

Ingredients:

1 1/2 cups dried white beans, rinsed	6 cups water
1 sweet onion, chopped	1 bay leaf
2 carrots, diced	1 teaspoon dried basil
1 celery stalk, sliced	1 bunch kale, shredded
1 teaspoon dried	Salt and pepper to

oregano	taste
2 cups chicken stock	1 lemon, juiced

Directions:
Combine the beans, onion, carrots, celery, dried herbs, stock and water in your Crock Pot.   Add salt and pepper to taste and throw in the bay leaf as well.   Cook on low settings for 4 hours then add the kale and lemon juice and cook for 4 additional hours.   Serve the soup warm or chilled.

708.   Vegan Grain-free Cream Of Mushroom Soup

Servings: 2   Cooking Time: 4 Hours

Ingredients:

2 cups cauliflower florets	1 2/3 cups unsweetened almond milk
1 teaspoon onion powder	¼ teaspoon
1 ½ cups white mushrooms, diced	Himalayan rock salt
	½ yellow onion, diced

Directions:
Place onion powder, milk, cauliflower, salt, and pepper in a pan, cover and bring to a boil over medium heat.   Reduce heat to low and simmer for 8 minutes or until cauliflower is softened.   Then, puree mixture in food processor.   In a pan, add oil, mushrooms, and onions, heat over high heat for about 8 minutes.   Add mushrooms and onion mix to cauliflower mixture in Crock-Pot.   Cover and cook on LOW for 4 hours. Serve hot.
Nutrition Info: Calories: 95, Total Fat: 4 g, Sodium: 475 mg, Carbs: 12.3 g, Dietary Fiber: 4.4 g, Net Carbs: 7.9 g, Sugars: 4.9 g, Protein: 4.9 g

709.   Portobello Mushroom Soup

Servings: 6   Cooking Time: 6 1/4 Hours

Ingredients:

4 Portobello mushrooms, sliced	2 cups chicken stock
1 shallot, chopped	Salt and pepper to taste
2 garlic cloves, chopped	1/2 teaspoon cumin seeds
1 cup diced tomatoes	1 tablespoon chopped parsley
1 tablespoon tomato paste	1 tablespoon chopped cilantro
1 can condensed cream of mushroom soup	

Directions:
Combine the mushrooms, shallot, garlic, tomatoes, tomato paste, stock and mushroom soup in your Crock Pot.   Add the cumin seeds then season with salt and pepper.   Cook on low settings for 6 hours.   When done, stir in the chopped parsley and cilantro.   Serve the soup warm.

Vegetable & Vegetarian Recipes

710.   Vegetable Korma
Servings: 6   Cooking Time: 6 Hours
Ingredients:

1 cup tomatoes, chopped	1 teaspoon curry powder
1 cup potatoes, chopped	1 teaspoon garam masala
1 cup green peas, frozen	6 oz green beans, chopped
2 cups of water	1 cup coconut cream

Directions:
Put all ingredients in the Crock Pot and gently stir with the help of the spoon.   Close the lid and cook korma on Low for 6 hours.
Nutrition Info: Per Serving: 144 calories, 3.5g protein, 13g carbohydrates, 9.8g fat, 4.1g fiber, omg cholesterol, 15mg sodium, 402mg potassium.

711. Dill Brussel Sprouts
Servings: 4   Cooking Time: 2 Hours
Ingredients:

4 cups Brussel sprouts, halved	1 tablespoon dried dill
2 tablespoons avocado oil	1 tablespoon vegan butter
½ teaspoon salt	2 cups of water

Directions:
Pour water in the Crock Pot. Add Brussel sprouts. Then close the lid and cook the vegetables on high for hours.   After this, drain water and transfer the vegetables in the hot skillet.   Sprinkle them with avocado oil, dried dill, salt, and vegan butter. Roast Brussel sprouts for 3-4 minutes on high heat.
Nutrition Info: Per Serving: 106 calories, 1g protein, 4.4g carbohydrates, 9.8g fat, 2g fiber, 8mg cholesterol, 362mg sodium, 298mg potassium.

712.Thyme Tomatoes
Servings: 4   Cooking Time: 5 Hours
Ingredients:

1-pound tomatoes, sliced	2 tablespoons olive oil
1 tablespoon dried thyme	1 tablespoon apple cider vinegar
1 teaspoon salt	½ cup of water

Directions:
Put all ingredients in the Crock Pot and close the lid.   Cook the tomatoes on Low for 5 hours.
Nutrition Info: Per Serving: 83 calories, 1.1g protein, 4.9g carbohydrates, 7.3g fat, 1.6g fiber, omg cholesterol, 588mg sodium, 277mg potassium

713.Creamy White Mushrooms
Servings: 4   Cooking Time: 8 Hours
Ingredients:

1-pound white mushrooms, chopped	1 teaspoon ground black pepper
1 cup cream	1 tablespoon dried parsley
1 teaspoon chili flakes	

Directions:
Put all ingredients in the Crock Pot.   Cook the mushrooms on low for 8 hours.   When the mushrooms are cooked, transfer them in the serving bowls and cool for 10-15 minutes.
Nutrition Info: Per Serving: 65 calories, 4.1g protein, 6g carbohydrates, 3.7g fat, 1.3g fiber, 11mg cholesterol, 27mg sodium, 396mg potassium.

714.Yam Fritters
Servings: 1   Cooking Time: 4 Hours
Ingredients:

1 yam, grated, boiled	1 egg, beaten
1 teaspoon dried parsley	1 teaspoon flour
¼ teaspoon chili powder	5 tablespoons coconut cream
¼ teaspoon salt	Cooking spray

Directions:
In the mixing bowl mix grated yams, dried parsley, chili powder, salt, egg, and flour.   Make the fritters from the yam mixture.   After this, spray the Crock Pot bottom with cooking spray.   Put the fritters inside in one layer.   Add coconut cream and cook the meal on Low for 4 hours.
Nutrition Info: Per Serving: 115 calories, 6.4g protein, 4.9g carbohydrates, 7.9g fat, 0.4g fiber, 175mg cholesterol, 670mg sodium, 110mg potassium.

715.Lentil Rice Salad
Servings: 5   Cooking Time: 7 Hrs
Ingredients:

¼ chili pepper, chopped	¼ tsp ground ginger
1 red onion, chopped	½ tsp ground thyme
½ cup lentils	1 tsp salt
¼ cup of rice	2 cups chicken stock
¼ tsp minced garlic	3 tbsp sour cream
1 tsp chili flakes	1 cup lettuce, torn

Directions:
Add lentils with all other ingredients to the Crock Pot except the lettuce and sour cream.   Put the cooker's lid on and set the cooking time to 7 hours on High settings.   Stir in torn lettuce leaves and mix gently.   Garnish with sour cream.   Serve warm.
Nutrition Info: Per Serving: Calories 84, Total Fat 3.3g, Fiber 2g, Total Carbs 11.29g, Protein 5g

716.Herbed Mushrooms
Servings: 4   Cooking Time: 4.5 Hours
Ingredients:

1-pound cremini mushrooms
1 teaspoon cumin seeds
1 teaspoon coriander seeds
2 cups of water
1 teaspoon fennel seeds
3 tablespoons sesame oil
1 teaspoon salt
3 tablespoons lime juice

Directions:
Pour water in the Crock Pot. Add mushrooms. Close the lid and cook them on High for 4.5 hours. Then drain water and transfer mushrooms in the big bowl.   Sprinkle them with cumin seeds, coriander seeds, fennel seeds, sesame oil, salt, and lime juice.   Carefully mix the mushrooms and leave them to marinate for 30 minutes.

Nutrition Info: Per Serving: 125 calories, 3g protein, 5.4g carbohydrates, 10.5g fat, 1g fiber, 0mg cholesterol, 594mg sodium, 531mg potassium.

717. Chorizo Cashew Salad

Servings: 6   Cooking Time: 4 Hours 30 Minutes

Ingredients:
8 oz. chorizo, chopped
1 tsp olive oil
1 tsp cayenne pepper
1 tsp chili flakes
1 tsp ground black pepper
1 tsp onion powder
2 garlic cloves
3 tomatoes, chopped
1 cup lettuce, torn
1 cup fresh dill
1 tsp oregano
3 tbsp crushed cashews

Directions:
Add chorizo sausage to the Crock Pot.   Put the cooker's lid on and set the cooking time to 4 hours on High settings.   Mix chili flakes, cayenne pepper, black pepper, and onion powder in a bowl. Now add tomatoes to the Crock Pot and cover again.   Crock Pot for another 30 minutes on High setting.   Stir in oregano and dill then mix well. Add sliced garlic and torn lettuce to the mixture. Garnish with cashews.   Serve.

Nutrition Info: Per Serving: Calories 249, Total Fat 19.8g, Fiber 2g, Total Carbs 7.69g, Protein 11g

718. Zucchini Basil Soup

Servings: 8   Cooking Time: 3 Hours

Ingredients:
9 cups zucchini, diced
2 cups white onions, chopped
4 cups vegetable broth
1 cup basil leaves
8 cloves of garlic, minced
4 tablespoons olive oil
Salt and pepper to taste

Directions:
Place the ingredients in the CrockPot.   Give a good stir.   Close the lid and cook on high for 2 hours or on low for hours.   Once cooked, transfer into a blender and pulse until smooth.

Nutrition Info: Calories per serving: 93; Carbohydrates: 5.4g; Protein: 1.3g; Fat: 11.6g; Sugar: 0g; Sodium: 322mg; Fiber: 4.2g

719. Arugula And Halloumi Salad

Servings: 4   Cooking Time: 30 Minutes

Ingredients:
1 tablespoon coconut oil
1 teaspoon smoked paprika
½ teaspoon ground turmeric
1 cup cherry tomatoes
½ teaspoon garlic powder
2 cups arugula, chopped
1 tablespoon olive oil
6 oz halloumi

Directions:
Slice the halloumi and sprinkle with melted coconut oil.   Put the cheese in the Crock Pot in one layer and cook on high for 15 minutes per side. Meanwhile, mix arugula with cherry tomatoes in the salad bowl.   Add cooked halloumi, smoked paprika, ground turmeric, garlic powder, and olive oil.   Shake the salad gently.

Nutrition Info: Per Serving: 210 calories, 9.9g protein, 4.4g carbohydrates, 17.8g fat, 1g fiber, 29mg cholesterol, 430mg sodium, 167mg potassium.

720. Garlic Gnocchi

Servings: 4   Cooking Time: 3 Hours

Ingredients:
2 cups mozzarella, shredded
1 teaspoon garlic, minced
3 egg yolks, beaten
½ cup heavy cream
Salt and pepper to taste

Directions:
In a mixing bowl, combine the mozzarella and egg yolks.   Form gnocchi balls and place in the fridge to set.   Boil a pot of water over high flame and drop the gnocchi balls for   seconds. Take them out and transfer to the crockpot.   Into the crockpot add the garlic and heavy cream.   Season with salt and pepper to taste.   Close the lid and cook on low for 3 hours or on high for 1 hour.

Nutrition Info: Calories per serving: 178; Carbohydrates: 4.1g; Protein:20.5 g; Fat: 8.9g; Sugar:0.3g; Sodium: 421mg; Fiber: 2.1g

721. White Beans Luncheon

Servings: 10   Cooking Time: 4 Hrs

Ingredients:
2 lbs. white beans
3 celery stalks, chopped
2 carrots, chopped
1 bay leaf
1 yellow onion, chopped
3 garlic cloves, minced
1 tsp rosemary, dried
1 tsp oregano, dried
1 tsp thyme, dried
10 cups water
Salt and black pepper to the taste
28 oz. canned tomatoes, chopped
6 cups chard, chopped

Directions:
Add beans, carrots, and all other ingredients to a Crock Pot.   Put the cooker's lid on and set the

cooking time to 4 hours on High settings.   Serve warm.
Nutrition Info: Per Serving: Calories 341, Total Fat 8, Fiber 12, Total Carbs 20, Protein 6

722.   Rice Cauliflower Casserole

Servings: 6   Cooking Time: 8 Hrs 10 Minutes
Ingredients:

1 cup white rice	1 cup chicken stock
5 oz. broccoli, chopped	1 tsp onion powder
4 oz. cauliflower, chopped	2 yellow onions, chopped
1 cup Greek Yogurt	1 tsp paprika
6 oz. Cheddar cheese, shredded	1 tbsp salt
	2 cups of water
	1 tsp butter

Directions:
Add cauliflower, broccoli, water, chicken stock, salt, paprika, rice, and onion powder to the Crock Pot. Top the broccoli-cauliflower mixture with onion slices.   Put the cooker's lid on and set the cooking time to 8 hours on Low settings.   Add butter and cheese on top of the casserole.   Put the cooker's lid on and set the cooking time to 10 minutes on High settings.   Serve warm.
Nutrition Info: Per Serving: Calories 229, Total Fat 4.2g, Fiber 3g, Total Carbs 36.27g, Protein 12g

723.   Sauteed Garlic

Servings: 4   Cooking Time: 6 Hours
Ingredients:

10 oz garlic cloves, peeled	1 teaspoon ground black pepper
2 tablespoons lemon juice	1 tablespoon vegan butter
1 cup of water	1 bay leaf

Directions:
Put all ingredients in the Crock Pot.   Close the lid and cook the garlic on Low for 6 hours.
Nutrition Info: Per Serving: 135 calories, 4.7g protein, 24.1g carbohydrates, 3.3g fat, 1.7g fiber, 8mg cholesterol, 36mg sodium, 303mg potassium

724.   Wild Rice Peppers

Servings: 5   Cooking Time: 7.5 Hrs
Ingredients:

1 tomato, chopped	1 tsp turmeric
1 cup wild rice, cooked	1 tsp curry powder
4 oz. ground chicken	1 cup chicken stock
2 oz. mushroom, sliced	2 tsp tomato paste
½ onion, sliced	1 oz. black olives
1 tsp salt	5 red sweet pepper, cut the top off and seeds removed

Directions:
Toss rice with salt, turmeric, olives, tomato, onion, chicken, mushrooms, curry powder in a bowl. Pour tomato paste and chicken stock into the Crock Pot.   Stuff the sweet peppers with chicken mixture.   Place the stuffed peppers in the cooker. Put the cooker's lid on and set the cooking time to 7

hours 30 minutes on Low settings.   Serve warm with tomato gravy.
Nutrition Info: Per Serving: Calories 232, Total Fat 3.7g, Fiber 5g, Total Carbs 41.11g, Protein 12g

725.   Turmeric Parsnip

Servings: 2   Cooking Time: 7 Hours
Ingredients:

10 oz parsnip, chopped	½ teaspoon onion powder
1 teaspoon ground turmeric	½ teaspoon salt
1 teaspoon chili flakes	1 cup of water
	1 teaspoon vegan butter

Directions:
Put parsnip in the Crock Pot,   Add chili flakes and ground turmeric.   Then add onion powder, salt, water, and butter.   Close the lid and cook the meal on Low for 7 hours.
Nutrition Info: Per Serving: 129 calories, 1.9g protein, 26.7g carbohydrates, 2.5g fat, 7.2g fiber, 5mg cholesterol, 614mg sodium, 569mg potassium.

726.   Cardamom Pumpkin Wedges

Servings: 4   Cooking Time: 6 Hours
Ingredients:

2-pound pumpkin, peeled	2 tablespoons lemon juice
1 teaspoon ground cardamom	1 teaspoon lemon zest, grated
2 tablespoons sugar	1 cup of water

Directions:
Cut the pumpkin into wedges and place them in the Crock Pot.   Add water.   Then sprinkle the pumpkin with ground cardamom, lemon juice, lemon zest, and sugar.   Close the lid and cook the pumpkin on Low for 6 hours.   Serve the pumpkin wedges with sweet liquid from the Crock Pot.
Nutrition Info: Per Serving: 103 calories, 2.6g protein, 25g carbohydrates, 0.7g fat, 6.8g fiber, 0mg cholesterol, 15mg sodium, 484mg potassium.

727.   Onion Chives Muffins

Servings: 7   Cooking Time: 8 Hrs
Ingredients:

1 egg	1 tsp cilantro
5 tbsp butter, melted	½ tsp sage
1 cup flour	1 tsp apple cider vinegar
½ cup milk	
1 tsp baking soda	1 tbsp chives
1 cup onion, chopped	1 tsp olive oil

Directions:
Whisk egg with melted butter, onion, milk, and all other ingredients to make a smooth dough. Grease a muffin tray with olive oil and divide the batter into its cups.   Pour 2 cups water into the Crock Pot and set the muffin tray in it.   Put the cooker's lid on and set the cooking time to 8 hours on Low settings.   Serve.

Nutrition Info: Per Serving: Calories 180, Total Fat 11g, Fiber 1g, Total Carbs 16.28g, Protein 4g

728. Tofu Kebabs

Servings: 4   Cooking Time: 2 Hours

Ingredients:

2 tablespoons lemon juice	1 teaspoon chili powder
1 teaspoon ground turmeric	¼ cup of water
2 tablespoons coconut cream	1 teaspoon avocado oil
	1-pound tofu, cubed

Directions:
Pour water in the Crock Pot.   After this, in the mixing bowl mix lemon juice, ground turmeric, coconut cream, chili powder, and avocado oil. Coat every tofu cube in the coconut cream mixture and string on the wooden skewers. Place them in the Crock Pot.   Cook the tofu kebabs on Low for 2 hours.
Nutrition Info: Per Serving: 104 calories, 9.7g protein, 3.3g carbohydrates, 6.9g fat, 1.6g fiber, 0mg cholesterol, 24mg sodium, 227mg potassium.

729. Potato Bake

Servings: 3   Cooking Time: 7 Hours

Ingredients:

2 cups potatoes, peeled, halved	1 tablespoon vegan butter, softened
4 oz vegan Provolone cheese, grated	½ cup vegetable stock
1 teaspoon dried dill	1 carrot, diced

Directions:
Grease the Crock Pot bottom with butter and put the halved potato inside.   Sprinkle it with dried dill and carrot.   Then add vegetable stock and Provolone cheese.   Cook the potato bake on low for 7 hours.
Nutrition Info: Per Serving: 185 calories, 8.8g protein, 14.1g carbohydrates, 10.6g fat, 2.2g fiber, 27mg cholesterol, 380mg sodium, 404mg potassium.

730. Creamy Puree

Servings: 4   Cooking Time: 4 Hours

Ingredients:

2 cups potatoes, chopped	3 cups of water
1 tablespoon vegan butter	¼ cup cream
	1 teaspoon salt

Directions:
Pour water in the Crock Pot.   Add potatoes and salt.   Cook the vegetables on high for 4 hours. Then drain water, add butter, and cream.   Mash the potatoes until smooth.
Nutrition Info: Per Serving: 87 calories, 1.4g protein, 12.3g carbohydrates, 3.8g fat, 1.8g fiber, 10mg cholesterol, 617mg sodium, 314mg potassium

731. Lentils Fritters

Servings: 6   Cooking Time: 1.5 Hours

Ingredients:

1 cup red lentils, cooked	1 tablespoon flour
1 teaspoon fresh cilantro, chopped	½ carrot, grated
	1 teaspoon flax meal
1 teaspoon scallions, chopped	1 tablespoon coconut oil
	¼ cup of water

Directions:
Pour water in the Crock Pot.   Add coconut oil. After this, in the mixing bowl mix all remaining ingredients. Make the small fritters and freeze them for 15-20 minutes in the freezer.   Put the fritters in the Crock Pot and close the lid.   Cook them on High for 1.hours.
Nutrition Info: Per Serving: 141 calories, 8.5g protein, 20.9g carbohydrates, 2.8g fat, 10g fiber, 0mg cholesterol, 6mg sodium, 328mg potassium.

732. Sugar Yams

Servings: 4   Cooking Time: 2 Hours

Ingredients:

4 yams, peeled	2 tablespoons vegan butter
1 cup of water	
1 tablespoon sugar	

Directions:
Cut the yams into halves and put them in the Crock Pot.   Add water and cook for hours on high. Then melt the butter in the skillet.   Add sugar and heat it until sugar is melted.   Then drain water from the yams.   Put the yams in the sugar butter and roast for 2 minutes per side.
Nutrition Info: Per Serving: 63 calories, 0.1g protein, 3.3g carbohydrates, 5.8g fat, 0g fiber, 15mg cholesterol, 43mg sodium, 9mg potassium.

733. Vegan Kofte

Servings: 4   Cooking Time: 4 Hours

Ingredients:

2 eggplants, peeled, boiled	½ cup chickpeas, canned
1 teaspoon minced garlic	3 tablespoons breadcrumbs
1 teaspoon ground cumin	1/3 cup water
¼ teaspoon minced ginger	1 tablespoon coconut oil

Directions:
Blend the eggplants until smooth.   Add minced garlic, ground cumin, minced ginger, chickpeas, and blend the mixture until smooth.   Transfer it in the mixing bowl. Add breadcrumbs.   Make the small koftes and put them in the Crock Pot.   Add coconut oil and close the lid.   Cook the meal on Low for 4 hours.
Nutrition Info: Per Serving: 212 calories, 8.3g protein, 35.5g carbohydrates, 5.8g fat, 14.3g fiber, 0mg cholesterol, 50mg sodium, 870mg potassium.

734. Marinated Onions

Servings: 4   Cooking Time: 330 Minutes

Ingredients:

- 1 cup of water
- ¼ cup sunflower oil
- 1 bay leaf
- 2 garlic cloves, peeled
- ¼ cup apple cider vinegar
- 1 teaspoon liquid honey
- 4 red onions, sliced

Directions:

Pour water in the Crock Pot.   Add the sunflower oil, bay leaf, garlic cloves, and apple cider vinegar. Cook the liquid on High for   minutes.   Then add onion and liquid honey. Stir the mixture and leave for 30 minutes to marinate.

Nutrition Info: Per Serving: 176 calories, 1.3g protein, 12.5g carbohydrates, 13.8g fat, 2.5g fiber, 0mg cholesterol, 7mg sodium, 180mg potassium.

735. Quinoa Avocado Salad(1)

Servings: 6   Cooking Time: 7 Hrs

Ingredients:

- ½ lemon, juiced
- 1 avocado, pitted, peeled and diced
- 1 red onion, diced
- 1 cup white quinoa
- 1 cup of water
- 1 tsp canola oil
- ½ cup fresh dill
- 1 cup green peas, frozen
- 1 tsp garlic powder

Directions:

Add quinoa, green peas and water to the Crock Pot. Put the cooker's lid on and set the cooking time to 7 hours on Low settings.   Transfer the cooked quinoa and peas to a salad bowl.   Stir in the remaining ingredients for the salad and toss well. Serve fresh.

Nutrition Info: Per Serving: Calories 195, Total Fat 7.7g, Fiber 6g, Total Carbs 26.77g, Protein 6g

736. Cauliflower Mac And Cheese

Servings: 6   Cooking Time: 4 Hours

Ingredients:

- 1 large cauliflower, cut into small florets
- 2 tablespoons butter
- 1 cup heavy cream
- 2 ounces grass-fed cream cheese
- 1 ½ teaspoons Dijon mustard
- 1 ½ cup organic sharp cheddar cheese
- 1 tablespoon garlic powder
- ½ cup nutritional yeast
- Salt and pepper to taste

Directions:

Place all ingredients in the CrockPot.   Give a good stir.   Close the lid and cook on high for   hours or on low for 4 hours.

Nutrition Info: Calories per serving:329; Carbohydrates: 10.8g; Protein: 16.1g; Fat: 25.5g; Sugar: 0g; Sodium: 824mg; Fiber: 5.8g

737. Vegetarian Keto Burgers

Servings: 4   Cooking Time: 4 Hours

Ingredients:

- 2 Portobello mushrooms, chopped
- 2 tablespoons basil, chopped
- 1 egg, beaten
- 1 clove of garlic, minced
- ½ cup boiled cauliflower, mashed

Directions:

Line the bottom of the crockpot with foil.   In a food processor, combine all ingredients.   Make 4 burger patties using your hands and place gently in the crockpot.   Close the lid and cook on low for   hours or on high for 3 hours.

Nutrition Info: Calories per serving: 134; Carbohydrates: 18g; Protein: 10g; Fat: 3.1g; Sugar:0.9g; Sodium:235mg; Fiber: 5g

738. Spicy Okra

Servings: 2   Cooking Time: 1.5 Hours

Ingredients:

- 2 cups okra, sliced
- ½ cup vegetable stock
- 1 teaspoon chili powder
- ½ teaspoon ground turmeric
- 1 teaspoon chili flakes
- 1 teaspoon dried oregano
- 1 tablespoon butter

Directions:

Put okra in the Crock Pot.   Add vegetable stock, chili powder, ground turmeric, chili flakes, and dried oregano.   Cook the okra on High for 1.5 hours.   Then add butter and stir the cooked okra well.

Nutrition Info: Per Serving: 102 calories, 2.5g protein, 9.2g carbohydrates, 6.4g fat, 4.1g fiber, 15mg cholesterol, 252mg sodium, 358mg potassium.

739. Cinnamon Banana Sandwiches

Servings: 4   Cooking Time: 2 Hrs

Ingredients:

- 2 bananas, peeled and sliced
- 8 oz. French toast slices, frozen
- 1 tbsp peanut butter
- ¼ tsp ground cinnamon
- 5 oz. Cheddar cheese, sliced
- ¼ tsp turmeric

Directions:

Layer half of the French toast slices with peanut butter.   Whisk cinnamon with turmeric and drizzle over the peanut butter layer.   Place the banana slice and cheese slices over the toasts. Now place the remaining French toast slices on top. Place these banana sandwiches in the Crock Pot. Put the cooker's lid on and set the cooking time to 2 hours on High settings.   Serve.

Nutrition Info: Per Serving: Calories 248, Total Fat 7.5g, Fiber 2g, Total Carbs 36.74g, Protein 10g

740. Jalapeno Corn

Servings: 4   Cooking Time: 5 Hours

Ingredients:

1 cup heavy cream
½ cup Monterey Jack cheese, shredded
1-pound corn kernels
3 jalapenos, minced

1 teaspoon vegan butter
1 tablespoon dried dill

Directions:
Pour heavy cream in the Crock Pot.   Add Monterey Jack cheese, corn kernels, minced jalapeno, butter, and dried dill.   Cook the corn on Low for 5 hours.
Nutrition Info: Per Serving: 203 calories, 5.6g protein, 9.3g carbohydrates, 16.9g fat, 1.5g fiber, 56mg cholesterol, 101mg sodium, 187mg potassium.

741.Crockpot Vindaloo Vegetables

Servings: 6   Cooking Time: 4 Hours
Ingredients:

3 cloves of garlic, minced
1 tablespoon ginger, chopped
1 ½ teaspoon coriander powder
1 ¼ teaspoon ground cumin
½ teaspoon dry mustard
½ teaspoon cayenne pepper

½ teaspoon cardamom
½ teaspoon turmeric powder
1 onion, chopped
4 cups cauliflower florets
1 red bell peppers, chopped
1 green bell peppers, chopped
Salt and pepper to taste

Directions:
Place all ingredients in the CrockPot.   Give a good stir.   Close the lid and cook on high for hours or on low for 4 hours.
Nutrition Info: Calories per serving: 159; Carbohydrates: 32.6g; Protein: 9g; Fat: 1g; Sugar:0.3g; Sodium: 464mg; Fiber: 25.3g

742.   Lazy Minestrone Soup

Servings: 4   Cooking Time: 3 Hours
Ingredients:

1 cup zucchini, sliced
1 package diced vegetables of your choice

2 cups chicken broth
2 tablespoons basil, chopped
½ cup diced celery

Directions:
Place all ingredients in the crockpot.   Season with salt and pepper to taste.   Close the lid and cook on low for hours or on high for 1 hour.
Nutrition Info: Calories per serving: 259; Carbohydrates: 13.5g; Protein:30.3 g; Fat: 8.3g; Sugar: 0.4g; Sodium: 643mg;Fiber: 4.2g

743.   Paprika Okra

Servings: 4   Cooking Time: 40 Minutes
Ingredients:

4 cups okra, sliced
1 tablespoon smoked

2 tablespoons coconut oil

paprika
1 teaspoon salt

1 cup organic almond milk

Directions:
Pour almond milk in the Crock Pot.   Add coconut oil, salt, and smoked paprika.   Then add sliced okra and gently mix the ingredients.   Cook the okra on High for   minutes. Then cooked okra should be tender but not soft.
Nutrition Info: Per Serving: 119 calories, 2.4g protein, 10.4g carbohydrates, 7.8g fat, 3.9g fiber, 0mg cholesterol, 624mg sodium, 340mg potassium.

744.   Green Peas Puree

Servings: 2   Cooking Time: 1 Hour
Ingredients:

2 cups green peas, frozen
1 tablespoon coconut oil

1 teaspoon smoked paprika
1 cup vegetable stock

Directions:
Put green peas, smoked paprika, and vegetable stock in the Crock Pot.   Cook the ingredients in high for 1 hour.   Then drain the liquid and mash the green peas with the help of the potato masher. Add coconut oil and carefully stir the cooked puree.
Nutrition Info: Per Serving: 184 calories, 8.4g protein, 21.9g carbohydrates, 7.8g fat, 7.8g fiber, 0mg cholesterol, 389mg sodium, 386mg potassium.

745.   Curried Vegetable Stew

Servings: 10   Cooking Time: 3 Hours
Ingredients:

1 teaspoon olive oil
2 tablespoon curry powder
1 tablespoon grated ginger
3 cloves of garlic, minced
1/8 teaspoon cayenne pepper
1 cup tomatoes, crushed

1 onion, diced
1 bag baby spinach
1 yellow bell pepper, chopped
1 red bell pepper, chopped
2 cups vegetable broth
1 cup coconut milk
Salt and pepper to taste

Directions:
Place all ingredients in the CrockPot.   Give a good stir.   Close the lid and cook on high for 2 hours or on low for hours.
Nutrition Info: Calories per serving: 88; Carbohydrates: 5.1g; Protein: 2.9g; Fat: 9.3g; Sugar: 0g; Sodium: 318mg; Fiber: 3.9g

746.   Broccoli And Cheese Casserole

Servings: 4   Cooking Time: 4 Hours
Ingredients:

¾ cup almond flour
1 head of broccoli, cut into florets
2 large eggs, beaten

Salt and pepper to taste

½ cup mozzarella cheese

Directions:
Place the almond flour and broccoli in the crockpot. Stir in the eggs and season with salt and pepper to taste.   Sprinkle with mozzarella cheese.   Close the lid and cook on low for hours or on high for 2 hours.
Nutrition Info: Calories per serving: 78; Carbohydrates: 4g; Protein: 8.2g; Fat:5.8 g; Sugar: 0g; Sodium: 231mg; Fiber:2.3 g

747.   Zucchini Soup With Rosemary And Parmesan

Servings: 6   Cooking Time: 3 Hours
Ingredients:

2 tablespoons olive oil	1 onion, chopped
1 tablespoon butter	2 pounds zucchini, chopped
1 teaspoon minced garlic	8 cups vegetable stock
1 teaspoon Italian seasoning	Salt and pepper to taste
4 teaspoons rosemary, chopped	1 cup grated parmesan cheese

Directions:
Place all ingredients except for the parmesan cheese in the CrockPot.   Give a good stir.   Close the lid and cook on high for hours or on low for 4 hours   Place inside a blender and pulse until smooth.   Serve with parmesan cheese on top.
Nutrition Info: Calories per serving: 172; Carbohydrates: 5.9g; Protein: 9.2g; Fat: 13.7g; Sugar: 0g; Sodium: 367mg; Fiber: 2.6g

748.   Rice Stuffed Eggplants

Servings: 4   Cooking Time: 8 Hrs
Ingredients:

4 medium eggplants	1 tsp paprika
1 cup rice, half-cooked	½ cup fresh cilantro
½ cup chicken stock	3 tbsp tomato sauce
1 tsp salt	1 tsp olive oil

Directions:
Slice the eggplants in half and scoop 2/3 of the flesh from the center to make boats.   Mix rice with tomato sauce, paprika, salt, and cilantro in a bowl.   Now divide this rice mixture into the eggplant boats.   Pour stock and oil into the Crock Pot and place the eggplants in it.   Put the cooker's lid on and set the cooking time to 8 hours on Low settings.   Serve warm.
Nutrition Info: Per Serving: Calories 277, Total Fat 9.1g, Fiber 24g, Total Carbs 51.92g, Protein 11g

749.   Corn Salad

Servings: 4   Cooking Time: 1.5 Hours
Ingredients:

2 cups corn kernels	1 cup of water
1 teaspoon vegan	1 teaspoon chili flakes
butter	1 teaspoon salt
1 cup lettuce, chopped	1 tablespoon sunflower oil
1 cup tomatoes, chopped	

Directions:
Pour water in the Crock Pot, add corn kernels and cook them on high for 5 hours.   Then drain water and transfer the corn kernels in the salad bowl.   Add lettuce, tomatoes, chili flakes, salt, and sunflower oil.   Shake the salad gently.
Nutrition Info: Per Serving: 116 calories, 3.1g protein, 16.5g carbohydrates, 5.5g fat, 2.8g fiber, 3mg cholesterol, 604mg sodium, 317mg potassium.

750.   Ranch Broccoli

Servings: 3   Cooking Time: 1.5 Hours
Ingredients:

3 cups broccoli	2 tablespoons ranch dressing
1 teaspoon chili flakes	2 cups of water

Directions:
Put the broccoli in the Crock Pot.   Add water and close the lid.   Cook the broccoli on high for 1.5 hours.   Then drain water and transfer the broccoli in the bowl.   Sprinkle it with chili flakes and ranch dressing. Shake the meal gently.
Nutrition Info: Per Serving: 34 calories, 2.7g protein, 6.6g carbohydrates, 0.3g fat, 2.4g fiber, 0mg cholesterol, 91mg sodium, 291mg potassium.

751.Pumpkin Hummus

Servings: 6   Cooking Time: 4 Hours
Ingredients:

1 cup chickpeas, canned	1 teaspoon harissa
1 tablespoon tahini paste	2 cups of water
1 cup pumpkin, chopped	2 tablespoons olive oil
	1 tablespoon lemon juice

Directions:
Pour water in the Crock Pot.   Add pumpkin and cook it for 4 hours on High or until the pumpkin is soft.   After this, drain water and transfer the pumpkin in the food processor.   Add all remaining ingredients and blend the mixture until smooth.   Add water from pumpkin if the cooked hummus is very thick.
Nutrition Info: Per Serving: 193 calories, 7.4g protein, 24.4g carbohydrates, 8.3g fat, 7.2g fiber, 0mg cholesterol, 26mg sodium, 390mg potassium.

752.   Saag Aloo

Servings: 6   Cooking Time: 6 Hours
Ingredients:

1 yellow onion, chopped	1 teaspoon ground cumin
1 cup potatoes, chopped	1 teaspoon garam masala
3 garlic cloves, diced	1 cup tomatoes, chopped
1 chili pepper,	

chopped
2 cups of water
1 cup spinach, chopped

Directions:
Put onion, potatoes, and chili pepper in the Crock Pot.   Add tomatoes and spinach.   After this, add sprinkle the ingredients with garam masala, ground cumin, and garlic.   Add water and close the lid.   Cook the meal on Low for 6 hours.
Nutrition Info: Per Serving: 35 calories, 1.2g protein, 7.g car7bohydrates, 0.2g fat, 1.6g fiber, 0mg cholesterol, 12mg sodium, 242mg potassium.

---

753.   Beet And Capers Salad

Servings: 4   Cooking Time: 4 Hours
Ingredients:

2 teaspoons capers
1 cup lettuce, chopped
2 oz walnuts, chopped
1 tablespoon lemon juice

1 tablespoon sunflower oil
1 teaspoon flax seeds
3 cups of water
2 cups beets, peeled

Directions:
Pour water in the Crock Pot and add beets. Cook them on High for 4 hours.   Then drain water, cool the beets and chop.   Put the chopped beets in the salad bowl.   Add capers, lettuce, walnuts, lemon juice, sunflower oil, and flax seeds. Carefully mix the salad.
Nutrition Info: Per Serving: 162 calories, 5.1g protein, 10.6g carbohydrates, 12.3g fat, 3g fiber, 0mg cholesterol, 115mg sodium, 365mg potassium.

---

754.   Aromatic Artichokes

Servings: 2   Cooking Time: 3 Hours
Ingredients:

4 artichokes, trimmed
2 tablespoons lemon juice
1 teaspoon minced garlic

4 teaspoons olive oil
1 teaspoon dried rosemary
1 cup of water

Directions:
Mix lemon juice with olive oil, minced garlic, and dried rosemary.   Then rub every artichoke with oil mixture and arrange it in the Crock Pot.   Add water and close the lid.   Cook the artichoke on High for 3 hours.
Nutrition Info: Per Serving: 240 calories, 10.8g protein, 35.2g carbohydrates, 10g fat, 17.9g fiber, 0mg cholesterol, 312mg sodium, 1230mg potassium.

---

755.   Potato Balls

Servings: 6   Cooking Time: 1.5 Hours
Ingredients:

2 cups mashed potato
1 tablespoon coconut cream
3 tablespoons breadcrumbs

1 teaspoon dried dill
2 oz scallions, diced
1 egg, beaten
2 tablespoons flour

½ cup of coconut milk

Directions:
In the mixing bowl mix mashed potato with coconut cream, breadcrumbs, dried dill, scallions, egg, and flour.   Make the potato balls and put them in the Crock Pot.   Add coconut milk and cook the meal on High for 1.5 hours.
Nutrition Info: Per Serving: 132 calories, 3.4g protein, 17.5g carbohydrates, 5.5g fat, 1.6g fiber, 28mg cholesterol, 273mg sodium, 287mg potassium.

---

756.   Shallot Saute

Servings: 2   Cooking Time: 2.5 Hours
Ingredients:

½ cup carrot, grated
1 cup shallot, sliced
1 teaspoon ground turmeric

½ teaspoon salt
1 teaspoon garlic, diced
½ cup milk

Directions:
Put all ingredients in the Crock Pot.   Close the lid and cook the saute on High for hours.   Then leave the cooked meal for   minutes to rest.
Nutrition Info: Per Serving: 105 calories, 4.4g protein, 20.3g carbohydrates, 1.5g fat, 0.9g fiber, 5mg cholesterol, 639mg sodium, 424mg potassium.

---

757.   Hot Sauce Oysters Mushrooms

Servings: 4   Cooking Time: 2 Hours
Ingredients:

2 tablespoons hot sauce
2 cups oysters mushrooms, sliced
½ cup of water

1 tablespoon avocado oil
1 teaspoon dried dill
1 teaspoon salt

Directions:
Mix sliced oysters with avocado oil, dried dill, and salt.   Put them in the Crock Pot.   Add water and cook the mushrooms on High for 2 hours. After this, drain the mushrooms and mix them with hot sauce.
Nutrition Info: Per Serving: 15 calories, 1.1g protein, 2.2g carbohydrates, 0.6g fat, 0.9g fiber, 0mg cholesterol, 778mg sodium, 149mg potassium.

---

758.   Pumpkin Bean Chili

Servings: 6   Cooking Time: 5 Hrs
Ingredients:

1 cup pumpkin puree
30 oz. canned kidney beans, drained
30 oz. canned roasted tomatoes, chopped
1 cup red lentils, dried
1 cup yellow onion, chopped

2 cups of water
1 tbsp chili powder
1 tbsp cocoa powder
½ tsp cinnamon powder
2 tsp cumin, ground
A pinch of cloves, ground
Salt and black pepper

1 jalapeno pepper,   to the taste
chopped   2 tomatoes, chopped

Directions:
Add pumpkin puree along with other ingredients except for tomatoes, to the Crock Pot.   Put the cooker's lid on and set the cooking time to 5 hours on High settings.   Serve with tomatoes on top. Enjoy.

Nutrition Info: Per Serving: Calories 266, Total Fat 6g, Fiber 4g, Total Carbs 12g, Protein 4g

759.   Eggplant Parmesan Casserole

Servings: 3   Cooking Time: 3 Hours

Ingredients:
1 medium eggplant,   1 large egg
sliced   1 cup almond flour
Salt and pepper to   1 cup parmesan
taste   cheese

Directions:
Place the eggplant slices in the crockpot.   Pour in the eggs and season with salt and pepper.   Stir in the almond flour and sprinkle with parmesan cheese.   Stir to combine everything.   Close the lid and cook on low for 3 hours or on high for 2 hours.

Nutrition Info: Calories per serving: 212; Carbohydrates: 17g; Protein: 15g; Fat:12.1 g; Sugar: 1.2g; Sodium: 231mg; Fiber:8.1 g

760.   Coconut Milk Lentils Bowl

Servings: 5   Cooking Time: 9 Hours

Ingredients:
2 cups brown lentils   1 teaspoon ground
3 cups of coconut   nutmeg
milk   1 teaspoon salt
3 cups of water

Directions:
Mix the brown lentils with salt and ground nutmeg and put in the Crock Pot.   Add coconut milk and water.   Close the lid and cook the lentils on Low for 9 hours.

Nutrition Info: Per Serving: 364 calories, 5.3g protein, 12.1g carbohydrates, 34.7g fat, 4.9g fiber, 0mg cholesterol, 491mg sodium, 382mg potassium.

761.Tarragon Pumpkin Bowl

Servings: 2   Cooking Time: 4 Hours

Ingredients:
2 cups pumpkin,   1 tablespoon coconut
chopped   oil
1 teaspoon dried   1 cup of water
tarragon   1 teaspoon salt

Directions:
Put all ingredients in the Crock Pot. Gently mix them.   Close the lid and cook pumpkin on High for 4 hours.

Nutrition Info: Per Serving: 143 calories, 2.8g protein, 20g carbohydrates, 7.5g fat, 7.1g fiber, 0mg cholesterol, 1179mg sodium, 515mg potassium.

762.   Chili Okra

Servings: 6   Cooking Time: 7 Hours

Ingredients:
6 cups okra, chopped   ½ teaspoon cayenne
1 cup tomato juice   pepper
1 teaspoon salt   1 tablespoon olive oil
½ teaspoon chili   1 cup vegetable stock
powder

Directions:
Put all ingredients from the list above in the Crock Pot.   Mix them gently and cook on Low for 7 hours.

Nutrition Info: Per Serving: 69 calories, 2.4g protein, 9.5g carbohydrates, 2.6g fat, 3.6g fiber, 0mg cholesterol, 514mg sodium, 399mg potassium.

763.   Pinto Beans Balls

Servings: 4   Cooking Time: 3 Hours

Ingredients:
½ cup pinto beans,   1 egg, beaten
cooked   2 tablespoons flour
1 teaspoon garam   1 teaspoon tomato
masala   paste
1 onion, diced,   1 tablespoon coconut
roasted   oil

Directions:
Mash the pinto beans with the help of the potato masher.   Then mix them with egg, garam masala, roasted onion, flour, and tomato paste.   Make the small balls from the mixture and put them in the Crock Pot.   Add coconut oil.   Cook the pinto beans balls for 3 hours on Low.

Nutrition Info: Per Serving: 155 calories, 7.3g protein, 21g carbohydrates, 4.9g fat, 4.5g fiber, 41mg cholesterol, 22mg sodium, 409mg potassium.

764.   Swedish Style Beets

Servings: 4   Cooking Time: 8 Hours

Ingredients:
¼ cup apple cider   1-pound beets
vinegar   1 teaspoon salt
1 tablespoon olive oil   ½ teaspoon sugar
                          3 cups of water

Directions:
Put beets in the Crock Pot.   Add water and cook the vegetables for 8 hours on Low.   Then drain water and peel the beets.   Chop the beets roughly and put in the big bowl.   Add all remaining ingredients and leave the beets for 2-3 hours to marinate.

Nutrition Info: Per Serving: 85 calories, 1.9g protein, 11.9g carbohydrates, 3.7g fat, 2.3g fiber, 0mg cholesterol, 675mg sodium, 359mg potassium.

765.   Crockpot Mediterranean Eggplant Salad

Servings: 2   Cooking Time: 4 Hours

Ingredients:
1 red onion, sliced   1 tablespoon smoked
2 bell peppers, sliced   paprika

3 extra virgin olive oil
1 eggplant, quartered
1 cup tomatoes, crushed

2 teaspoons cumin
Juice from 1 lemon, freshly squeezed
Salt and pepper to taste

Directions:
Place all ingredients in the CrockPot. Give a good stir. Close the lid and cook on high for hours or on low for 4 hours.
Nutrition Info: Calories per serving: 312; Carbohydrates: 30.2g; Protein: 5.6g; Fat: 22g; Sugar: 0.4g; Sodium: 519mg; Fiber: 27.1g

766. Masala Eggplants

Servings: 2   Cooking Time: 2 Hours
Ingredients:
½ cup coconut cream
1 teaspoon garam masala

½ cup of water
2 eggplants, chopped
1 teaspoon salt

Directions:
Sprinkle the eggplants with salt and leave for minutes. Then drain eggplant juice and transfer the vegetables in the Crock Pot. Add garam masala, water, and coconut cream. Cook the meal on High for 2 hours.
Nutrition Info: Per Serving: 275 calories, 6.8g protein, 35.5g carbohydrates, 15.3g fat, 20.7g fiber, 0mg cholesterol, 1186mg sodium, 1414mg potassium.

767. Crockpot Baked Tofu

Servings: 4   Cooking Time: 2 Hours
Ingredients:
1 small package extra firm tofu, sliced
3 tablespoons soy sauce
1 tablespoon sesame oil

2 teaspoons minced garlic
Juice from ½ lemon, freshly squeezed

Directions:
In a deep dish, mix together the soy sauce, sesame oil, garlic, and lemon. Add a few tablespoons of water if the sauce is too thick. Marinate the tofu slices for at least hours. Line the crockpot with foil and grease it with cooking spray. Place the slices of marinated tofu into the crockpot. Cook on low for 4 hours or on high for 2 hours. Make sure that the tofu slices have a crispy outer texture.
Nutrition Info: Calories per serving:145; Carbohydrates: 4.1g; Protein: 11.6g; Fat: 10.8g; Sugar: 0.6g; Sodium: 142mg; Fiber:1.5 g

768. Baby Kale, Mozzarella And Egg Bake

Servings: 6   Cooking Time: 4 Hours
Ingredients:
2 cups baby kale, chopped
2 teaspoons olive oil
1 ½ cup mozzarella

1 teaspoon garlic powder
1 teaspoon onion powder

cheese, grated
8 eggs, beaten

Salt and pepper to taste

Directions:
Place all ingredients in the CrockPot. Give a good stir. Close the lid and cook on high for hours or on low for 4 hours.
Nutrition Info: Calories per serving: 352; Carbohydrates:6.3 g; Protein: 32.1g; Fat: 21.6g; Sugar: 0.9g; Sodium: 841mg; Fiber: 3.7g

769. Sesame Asparagus

Servings: 4   Cooking Time: 3 Hours
Ingredients:
1-pound asparagus
½ cup of soy sauce
1 teaspoon sesame seeds

½ cup vegetable stock
1 tablespoon vegan butter

Directions:
Trim the asparagus and put it in the Crock Pot. Add soy sauce and vegetable stock. Then add sesame seeds and butter. Close the lid and cook the meal on High for 3 hours.
Nutrition Info: Per Serving: 71 calories, 4.7g protein, 7.1g carbohydrates, 3.5g fat, 2.7g fiber, 8mg cholesterol, 1915mg sodium, 304mg potassium.

770. Onion Balls

Servings: 4   Cooking Time: 2 Hours
Ingredients:
½ cup red lentils, cooked
½ cup onion, minced
1 teaspoon ground black pepper

¼ cup flax meal
1 teaspoon cornflour
½ teaspoon salt
½ cup of water
½ cup ketchup

Directions:
In the mixing bowl mix red lentils with minced onion, ground black pepper, flax meal, cornflour, and salt. Make the balls from the onion mixture and freeze them in the freezer for minutes. After this, mix water and ketchup in the Crock Pot. Add frozen balls and close the lid. Cook the meal on High for 2 hours.
Nutrition Info: Per Serving: 153 calories, 8.5g protein, 26.1g carbohydrates, 2.9g fat, 9.9g fiber, 0mg cholesterol, 628mg sodium, 430mg potassium.

771. Peach Tofu Crumble

Servings: 4   Cooking Time: 2 Hours
Ingredients:
4 peaches, pitted, halved
5 oz firm tofu, crumbled
½ cup coconut cream
1 teaspoon brown sugar

1 teaspoon vanilla extract
1 teaspoon vegan butter, melted
4 tablespoons bread crumbs

Directions:
Brush the ramekins with vegan butter. Then mix tofu with brown sugar and vanilla extract. Put ½ part of tofu in ramekins and top them with peaches. After this, add remaining tofu. Sprinkle it with coconut cream and breadcrumbs. Cover the ramekins with foil and transfer in the Crock Pot. Cook the meal on High for 2 hours.
Nutrition Info: Per Serving: 148 calories, 5.6g protein, 23.2g carbohydrates, 4.3g fat, 3g fiber, 6mg cholesterol, 69mg sodium, 364mg potassium.

772.	**Carrot Strips**

Servings: 2   Cooking Time: 1 Hour
Ingredients:

2 tablespoons sunflower oil	2 carrots, peeled
1 teaspoon dried thyme	½ teaspoon salt
	½ cup of water

Directions:
Cut the carrots into the strips. Then heat the sunflower oil in the skillet until hot. Put the carrot strips in the hot oil and roast for 2-minutes per side. Pour water in the Crock Pot. Add salt and dried thyme. Then add roasted carrot and cook the meal on High for 1 hour.
Nutrition Info: Per Serving: 150 calories, 0.6g protein, 6.3g carbohydrates, 14g fat, 1.7g fiber, 0mg cholesterol, 625mg sodium, 200mg potassium.

773.	**Oregano Cheese Pie**

Servings: 6   Cooking Time: 3.5 Hrs
Ingredients:

1 tsp baking soda	1 tsp salt
1 tbsp lemon juice	5 oz. Parmesan cheese, shredded
1 cup flour	
1 cup milk	2 eggs
5 oz. Cheddar cheese, shredded	½ tsp oregano
	1/3 tsp olive oil

Directions:
Sift flour with salt, oregano, baking soda and shredded cheese in a bowl. Beat eggs with lemon juice and milk in a separate bowl. Gradually stir in flour mixture and mix using a hand mixer until it forms a smooth dough. Layer the base of Crock Pot with olive oil and spread the dough in the cooker. Put the cooker's lid on and set the cooking time to 3 hours 30 minutes on High settings. Serve.
Nutrition Info: Per Serving: Calories 288, Total Fat 13.7g, Fiber 1g, Total Carbs 24.23g, Protein 16g

774.	**Quinoa Avocado Salad(2)**

Servings: 6   Cooking Time: 7 Hrs
Ingredients:

½ lemon, juiced	1 tsp canola oil
1 avocado, pitted, peeled and diced	½ cup fresh dill
1 red onion, diced	1 cup green peas, frozen
	1 tsp garlic powder

1 cup white quinoa
1 cup of water
Directions:
Add quinoa, green peas and water to the Crock Pot. Put the cooker's lid on and set the cooking time to 7 hours on Low settings. Transfer the cooked quinoa and peas to a salad bowl. Stir in the remaining ingredients for the salad and toss well. Serve fresh.
Nutrition Info: Per Serving: Calories 195, Total Fat 7.7g, Fiber 6g, Total Carbs 26.77g, Protein 6g

775.	**Split Pea Paste**

Servings: 4   Cooking Time: 2 Hours
Ingredients:

2 cups split peas	1 teaspoon salt
2 cups of water	1 teaspoon ground black pepper
1 tablespoon coconut oil	

Directions:
Pour water in the Crock Pot. Add split peas and close the lid. Cook them for 2 hours on high or until they are soft. Then drain water and transfer the split peas in the food processor. Add coconut oil, salt, and ground black pepper. Blend the mixture until smooth.
Nutrition Info: Per Serving: 367 calories, 24.2g protein, 59.8g carbohydrates, 4.6g fat, 25.3g fiber, 0mg cholesterol, 600mg sodium, 974mg potassium.

776.	**Sautéed Radish**

Servings: 4   Cooking Time: 2 Hours
Ingredients:

4 cups radish, halved	½ teaspoon salt
2 tablespoons sesame oil	1 tablespoon vegan butter
1 tablespoon dried dill	2 cups of water

Directions:
Put all ingredients except butter in the Crock Pot. Cook the mixture on High for hours. Then drain the liquid and transfer the cooked radish in the big bowl. Add butter and stir the radish well.
Nutrition Info: Per Serving: 106 calories, 1g protein, 4.4g carbohydrates, 9.8g fat, 2g fiber, 8mg cholesterol, 362mg sodium, 298mg potassium.

777.	**Mushroom Bourguignon**

Servings: 3   Cooking Time: 7 Hours
Ingredients:

½ cup mushrooms, chopped	¼ cup carrot, diced
¼ cup onion, chopped	1 teaspoon salt
½ cup green peas, frozen	2 tablespoons tomato paste
1 teaspoon dried thyme	3 cups vegetable stock

Directions:

Mix vegetable stock with tomato paste and pour liquid in the Crock Pot. Add all remaining ingredients and close the lid. Cook the meal on Low for 7 hours.
Nutrition Info: Per Serving: 45 calories, 2.8g protein, 8.8g carbohydrates, 0.3g fat, 2.9g fiber, 0mg cholesterol, 844mg sodium, 250mg potassium.

778.	**Squash Noodles**

Servings: 4   Cooking Time: 4 Hours
Ingredients:

1-pound butternut squash, seeded, halved	1 teaspoon salt
	½ teaspoon garlic powder
1 tablespoon vegan butter	3 cups of water

Directions:
Pour water in the Crock Pot. Add butternut squash and close the lid. Cook the vegetable on high for 4 hours. Then drain water and shred the squash flesh with the help of the fork and transfer in the bowl. Add garlic powder, salt, and butter. Mix the squash noodles.
Nutrition Info: Per Serving: 78 calories, 1.2g protein, 13.5g carbohydrates, 3g fat, 2.3g fiber, 8mg cholesterol, 612mg sodium, 406mg potassium

779.	**Okra Curry**

Servings: 4   Cooking Time: 2.5 Hours
Ingredients:

1 cup potatoes, chopped	1 teaspoon curry powder
1 cup okra, chopped	1 teaspoon dried dill
1 cup tomatoes, chopped	1 cup coconut cream
	1 cup of water

Directions:
Pour water in the Crock Pot. Add coconut cream, potatoes, tomatoes, curry powder, and dried dill. Cook the ingredients on High for 2 hours. Then add okra and carefully mix the meal. Cook it for 30 minutes on High.
Nutrition Info: Per Serving: 184 calories, 3g protein, 13.3g carbohydrates, 14.6g fat, 3.8g fiber, 0mg cholesterol, 18mg sodium, 508mg potassium.

780.	**Warming Butternut Squash Soup**

Servings: 9   Cooking Time: 8 Hrs
Ingredients:

2 lb. butternut squash, peeled and cubed	¼ tsp ground nutmeg
4 tsp minced garlic	1 tsp ground black pepper
½ cup onion, chopped	8 cups chicken stock
1 tsp salt	1 tbsp fresh parsley

Directions:
Spread the butternut squash in your Crock Pot. Add stock, garlic, and onion to the squash. Put the cooker's lid on and set the cooking time to 8 hours on Low settings. Add salt, black pepper, and nutmeg to the squash. Puree the cooked squash mixture using an immersion blender until smooth. Garnish with chopped parsley. Enjoy.
Nutrition Info: Per Serving: Calories 129, Total Fat 2.7g, Fiber 2g, Total Carbs 20.85g, Protein 7g

781.	**Vegetarian Red Coconut Curry**

Servings: 4   Cooking Time: 3 Hours
Ingredients:

1 cup broccoli florets	1 tablespoon red curry paste
1 large handful spinach, rinsed	1 teaspoon garlic, minced
1 cup coconut cream	

Directions:
Combine all ingredients in the crockpot. Close the lid and cook on low for 3 hours or on high for 1 hour.
Nutrition Info: Calories per serving: 226; Carbohydrates: 8g; Protein: 5.2g; Fat:21.4 g; Sugar: 0.4g; Sodium: 341mg; Fiber:4.3 g

782.	**Crockpot Eggplant Lasagna**

Servings: 4   Cooking Time: 4 Hours
Ingredients:

1 cup beefsteak tomatoes	1 cup chopped walnuts
½ cup basil leaves	2 large eggs, beaten
½ teaspoon thyme leaves	1 cup heavy cream
1 onion, diced	2 tablespoons olive oil
1 red bell pepper diced	1 eggplant, sliced using a mandolin
Salt and pepper to taste	1 cup mozzarella cheese

Directions:
In a blender or food processor, combine the tomatoes, basil leaves, thyme leaves, onion, and red bell pepper. Season with salt and pepper then pulse until smooth. Place in a bowl and add the chopped walnuts. In another bowl, combine the eggs and heavy cream. Set aside. Grease the bottom of the CrockPot with olive oil. Arrange the eggplant slices first and pour in a generous amount of the tomato sauce mixture. Pour the egg mixture and cheese on top. Repeat the layering until all ingredients are used up. Close the lid and cook on high for 3 hours or on low for 4 hours.
Nutrition Info: Calories per serving: 373; Carbohydrates: 19g; Protein: 23g; Fat: 14g; Sugar: 1.2g; Sodium: 963mg; Fiber: 13.8g!Follow

783.	**Sautéed Endives**

Servings: 4   Cooking Time: 40 Minutes
Ingredients:

1-pound endives, roughly chopped	1 teaspoon garlic, diced
½ cup of water	

1 tablespoon avocado oil	2 tablespoons coconut cream

Directions:
Pour water in the Crock Pot.   Add endives and garlic.   Close the lid and cook them on High for minutes.   Then add coconut cream and avocado oil.   Cook the endives for 10 minutes more.
Nutrition Info: Per Serving: 42 calories, 1.9g protein, 4.4g carbohydrates, 2.4g fat, 3.7g fiber, 6mg cholesterol, 41mg sodium, 376mg potassium.

784.   Light Chana Masala

Servings: 4   Cooking Time: 8 Hours
Ingredients:

1 teaspoon ginger, peeled, minced	1 jalapeno, chopped
1 teaspoon minced garlic	1 cup tomatoes, pureed
¼ cup fresh cilantro, chopped	1 cup chickpeas
	4 cups of water

Directions:
Put all ingredients in the Crock Pot and close the lid.   Cook the meal on Low for 8 hours.
Nutrition Info: Per Serving: 194 calories, 10.2g protein, 32.9g carbohydrates, 3.2g fat, 9.4g fiber, 0mg cholesterol, 22mg sodium, 568mg potassium.

785.   Creamy Garlic Potatoes

Servings: 6   Cooking Time: 7 Hrs
Ingredients:

2 lb. potatoes	½ tsp salt
1 cup heavy cream	1 tbsp fresh dill
1 tbsp minced garlic	1 tsp butter
1 tsp garlic powder	

Directions:
Liberally rub the potatoes with butter and place them in the Crock Pot.   Whisk cream with garlic powder, minced garlic fill, and salt in a bowl. Add cream mixture to the potatoes.   Put the cooker's lid on and set the cooking time to 7 hours on Low settings.   Serve warm.
Nutrition Info: Per Serving: Calories 198, Total Fat 8.3g, Fiber 4g, Total Carbs 28g, Protein 4g

786.   Curry Paneer

Servings: 2   Cooking Time: 2 Hours
Ingredients:

6 oz paneer, cubed	½ cup coconut cream
1 teaspoon garam masala	1 teaspoon olive oil
1 chili pepper, chopped	½ onion, diced
	1 teaspoon garlic paste

Directions:
In the mixing bowl mix diced onion, garlic paste, olive oil, chili pepper, coconut cream, and garam masala.   Then mix the mixture with cubed paneer and put in the Crock Pot.   Cook it on Low for 2 hours.

Nutrition Info: Per Serving: 309 calories, 7.1g protein, 22.5g carbohydrates, 22.4g fat, 3.5g fiber, 2mg cholesterol, 415mg sodium, 208mg potassium.

787.   Cauliflower Rice

Servings: 6   Cooking Time: 2 Hours
Ingredients:

4 cups cauliflower, shredded	1 tablespoon cream cheese
1 cup vegetable stock	1 teaspoon dried oregano
1 cup of water	

Directions:
Put all ingredients in the Crock Pot.   Close the lid and cook the cauliflower rice on High for hours.
Nutrition Info: Per Serving: 25 calories, 0.8g protein, 3.9g carbohydrates, 0.8g fat, 1.8g fiber, 2mg cholesterol, 153mg sodium, 211mg potassium

788.   Sweet Potato And Lentils Pate

Servings: 4   Cooking Time: 6 Hours
Ingredients:

1 cup sweet potato, chopped	1 tablespoon soy milk
½ cup red lentils	1 teaspoon cayenne pepper
2.5 cups water	½ teaspoon salt

Directions:
Put all ingredients in the Crock Pot.   Close the lid and cook the mixture on low for 6 hours.   When the ingredients are cooked, transfer them in the blender and blend until smooth.   Put the cooked pate in the bowl and store it in the fridge for up to days.
Nutrition Info: Per Serving: 140 calories, 7.4g protein, 25.1g carbohydrates, 1.3g fat, 9.1g fiber, 3mg cholesterol, 322mg sodium, 488mg potassium.

789.   Walnut Kale

Servings: 4   Cooking Time: 5 Hours
Ingredients:

5 cups kale, chopped	1 cup of coconut milk
2 oz walnuts, chopped	1 cup of water
1 teaspoon vegan butter	1 oz vegan Parmesan, grated

Directions:
Put all ingredients in the Crock Pot and gently stir. Then close the lid and cook the kale on Low for 5 hours.
Nutrition Info: Per Serving: 298 calories, 9.6g protein, 13.7g carbohydrates, 25.1g fat, 3.5g fiber, 8mg cholesterol, 120mg sodium, 644mg potassium.

790.   Eggplant Mini Wraps

Servings: 6   Cooking Time: 5 Hrs
Ingredients:

10 oz. eggplant, sliced into rounds	½ tsp ground black pepper
5 oz. halloumi cheese	1 tsp salt

1 tsp minced garlic   1 tsp paprika
3 oz. bacon, chopped   1 tomato

Directions:
Season the eggplant sliced with salt, paprika, and black pepper.   Add these slices to the Crock Pot and spread in a single layer.   Put the cooker's lid on and set the cooking time to 1 hour on High settings.   Allow the eggplant to cool then top them with tomato and cheese slices.   And top them with bacon and garlic.   Roll each slice and insert the toothpick to seal them.   Place these wrap in the Crock Pot carefully.   Put the cooker's lid on and set the cooking time to 4 hours on High settings.   Serve fresh.
Nutrition Info: Per Serving: Calories 131, Total Fat 9.4g, Fiber 2g, Total Carbs 7.25g, Protein 6g

791. Marinated Jalapeno Rings

Servings: 4   Cooking Time: 1 Hour

Ingredients:
1 cup of water   1 garlic clove, crushed
¼ cup apple cider vinegar   3 tablespoons sunflower oil
1 teaspoon peppercorns   5 oz jalapeno, sliced

Directions:
Put the sliced jalapeno in the plastic vessel (layer by layer).   Then put peppercorns in the Crock Pot. Add the garlic clove, sunflower oil, and apple cider vinegar.   Close the lid and cook the liquid on High for 1 hour.   After this, cool the liquid to the room temperature and pour it over the jalapenos. Close the plastic vessel and leave it in the fridge for 30-40 minutes before serving.
Nutrition Info: Per Serving: 109 calories, 0.6g protein, 2.8g carbohydrates, 10.7g fat, 1.2g fiber, 0mg cholesterol, 3mg sodium, 97mg potassium.

792. Mushroom Risotto

Servings: 4   Cooking Time: 6 Hours

Ingredients:
½ cup Arborio rice   1 teaspoon salt
2 cups brown mushrooms, chopped   1 teaspoon ground black pepper
1 yellow onion, diced   4 cups vegetable stock
2 tablespoons avocado oil

Directions:
Pour the vegetable stock in the Crock Pot.   Add ground black pepper and salt.   After this, add avocado oil, diced onion, mushrooms, and Arborio rice.   Close the lid and cook the risotto on Low for 6 hours.
Nutrition Info: Per Serving: 127 calories, 2.9g protein, 25.7g carbohydrates, 3.1g fat, 1.9g fiber, 0mg cholesterol, 1307mg sodium, 248mg potassium.

793. French Vegetable Stew

Servings: 6   Cooking Time: 9 Hrs

Ingredients:
2 yellow onions, chopped   4 zucchinis, sliced
1 eggplant, sliced   1 tsp oregano, dried
2 garlic cloves, minced   1 tsp sugar
2 green bell peppers, cut into medium strips   1 tsp basil, dried
6 oz. canned tomato paste   Salt and black pepper to the taste
2 tomatoes, cut into medium wedges   2 tbsp parsley, chopped
¼ cup olive oil

A pinch of red pepper flakes, crushed

Directions:
Add onions, zucchinis, eggplant, garlic, tomato paste, bell peppers, sugar, basil, salt, black pepper, and oregano to the Crock Pot.   Put the cooker's lid on and set the cooking time to 9 hours on Low settings.   Stir in parsley and pepper flakes. Serve warm.
Nutrition Info: Per Serving: Calories 269, Total Fat 7g, Fiber 6g, Total Carbs 17g, Protein 4g

794. Tri-bean Chili

Servings: 6   Cooking Time: 8 Hrs

Ingredients:
15 oz. canned kidney beans, drained   2 tbsp chili powder
30 oz. canned chili beans in sauce   2 yellow onions, chopped
15 oz. canned black beans, drained   2 garlic cloves, minced
2 green bell peppers, chopped   1 tsp oregano, dried
30 oz. canned tomatoes, crushed   1 tbsp cumin, ground
Salt and black pepper to the taste

Directions:
Add kidney beans, black beans, chili beans, and all the spices and veggies to the Crock Pot.   Put the cooker's lid on and set the cooking time to 8 hours on Low settings.   Serve warm.
Nutrition Info: Per Serving: Calories 314, Total Fat 6g, Fiber 5g, Total Carbs 14g, Protein 4g

795. Mung Beans Salad

Servings: 4   Cooking Time: 3 Hours

Ingredients:
½ avocado, chopped   3 cups of water
1 cup cherry tomatoes, halved   1 tablespoon lemon juice
½ cup corn kernels, cooked   1 tablespoon avocado oil
1 cup mung beans

Directions:
Put mung beans in the Crock Pot.   Add water and cook them on High for 3 hours.   Then drain water and transfer the mung beans in the salad bowl.   Add avocado, cherry tomatoes, corn kernels, and shake well.   Then sprinkle the salad with avocado oil and lemon juice.

Nutrition Info: Per Serving: 287 calories, 13.9g protein, 40g carbohydrates, 9.4g fat, 11.2g fiber, 0mg cholesterol, 20mg sodium, 932mg potassium.

796. Hot Tofu

Servings: 4   Cooking Time: 4 Hours
Ingredients:

1-pound firm tofu, cubed	1 tablespoon hot sauce
½ cup vegetable stock	1 teaspoon miso paste

Directions:
Mix vegetables tock with miso paste and pour in the Crock Pot.   Add hot sauce and tofu.   Close the lid and cook the meal on Low for 4 hours. Then transfer the tofu and liquid in the serving bowls.
Nutrition Info: Per Serving: 83 calories, 9.5g protein, 2.5g carbohydrates, 4.8g fat, 1.2g fiber, 0mg cholesterol, 168mg sodium, 176mg potassium.

797. Crockpot Cumin-roasted Vegetables

Servings: 2   Cooking Time: 4 Hours
Ingredients:

1 red bell pepper, chopped	6 cups kale leaves, chopped
1 yellow bell pepper, chopped	4 tablespoon olive oil
1 green bell pepper, chopped	1 teaspoon cumin
	1 teaspoon dried oregano
½ cup cherry tomatoes	¼ teaspoon salt
¼ cup pepita seeds	

Directions:
Place all ingredients in a mixing bowl. Toss to coat everything with oil.   Line the bottom of the CrockPot with foil.   Place the vegetables inside. Close the lid and cook on low for hours or on high for 6 hours until the vegetables are a bit brown on the edges.
Nutrition Info: Calories per serving:380; Carbohydrates: 13.8g; Protein: 8.6g; Fat:35.8g; Sugar:1.7 g; Sodium: 512mg; Fiber: 6.6g

798. Corn Fritters

Servings: 4   Cooking Time: 3 Hours
Ingredients:

1 cup mashed potato	1 teaspoon ground turmeric
1/3 cup corn kernels, cooked	½ teaspoon chili powder
1 egg, beaten	2 tablespoons coconut oil
2 tablespoons flour	
1 teaspoon salt	

Directions:
Put the coconut oil in the Crock Pot and melt it on low for   minutes.   Meanwhile, mix mashed potato with corn kernels, egg, flour, salt, ground turmeric, and chili powder.   Make the medium

size fritters and put them in the Crock Pot.   Cook them on Low for 3 hours.
Nutrition Info: Per Serving: 162 calories, 3.3g protein, 14.9g carbohydrates, 10.4g fat, 1.5g fiber, 41mg cholesterol, 777mg sodium, 246mg potassium.

799. Garam Masala Potato Bake

Servings: 2   Cooking Time: 6 Hours
Ingredients:

1 cup potatoes, chopped	3 eggs, beaten
1 teaspoon garam masala	1 tablespoon vegan butter
½ cup vegan mozzarella, shredded	2 tablespoons coconut cream

Directions:
Mix potatoes with garam masala.   Then put them in the Crock Pot.   Add vegan butter and mozzarella.   After this, mix coconut cream with eggs and pour the liquid over the mozzarella. Close the lid and cook the meal on Low for 6 hours.
Nutrition Info: Per Serving: 199 calories, 12.1g protein, 16.8g carbohydrates, 9.4g fat, 1.9g fiber, 252mg cholesterol, 156mg sodium, 398mg potassium.

800. Parmesan Scallops Potatoes

Servings: 5   Cooking Time: 7 Hours
Ingredients:

5 teaspoons vegan butter	5 potatoes
1 teaspoon ground black pepper	2 tablespoons flour
1 teaspoon garlic powder	3 cups of milk
	3 oz vegan Parmesan, grated

Directions:
Peel and slice the potatoes.   Then place the sliced potato in the Crock Pot in one layer.   Sprinkle the vegetables with ground black pepper, garlic powder, and butter.   After this, mix flour with milk and pour over the potatoes.   Then sprinkle the vegetables with Parmesan and close the lid. Cook the meal on Low for 7 hours.
Nutrition Info: Per Serving: 323 calories, 14.4g protein, 44.3g carbohydrates, 10.7g fat, 5.4g fiber, 34mg cholesterol, 267mg sodium, 967mg potassium.

801. Cauliflower Curry

Servings: 4   Cooking Time: 2 Hours
Ingredients:

4 cups cauliflower	2 cups of coconut milk
1 tablespoon curry paste	

Directions:
In the mixing bowl mix coconut milk with curry paste until smooth.   Put cauliflower in the Crock Pot.   Pour the curry liquid over the cauliflower and close the lid.   Cook the meal on High for 2 hours.

Nutrition Info: Per Serving: 236 calories, 4.9g protein, 13g carbohydrates, 30.9g fat, 5.1g fiber, 0mg cholesterol, 48mg sodium, 619mg potassium.

---

802. Tofu And Cauliflower Bowl

Servings: 3   Cooking Time: 2.15 Hours
Ingredients:

5 oz firm tofu, chopped	¼ cup of coconut milk
1 teaspoon curry paste	1 tablespoon sunflower oil
1 teaspoon dried basil	2 cups cauliflower, chopped
	1 cup of water

Directions:
Put cauliflower in the Crock Pot.   Add water and cook it on High for hours.   Meanwhile, mix curry paste with coconut milk, dried basil, and sunflower oil.   Then add tofu and carefully mix the mixture. Leave it for 30 minutes.   When the cauliflower is cooked, drain water.   Add tofu mixture and shake the meal well. Cook it on High for 15 minutes.
Nutrition Info: Per Serving: 148 calories, 5.7g protein, 5.9g carbohydrates, 12.5g fat, 2.5g fiber, 0mg cholesterol, 31mg sodium, 326mg potassium.

---

803. Braised Swiss Chard

Servings: 4   Cooking Time: 30 Minutes
Ingredients:

1-pound swiss chard, chopped	1 tablespoon sunflower oil
1 lemon	1 teaspoon salt
1 teaspoon garlic, diced	2 cups of water

Directions:
Put the swiss chard in the Crock Pot.   Cut the lemon into halves and squeeze it over the swiss chard.   After this, sprinkle the greens with diced garlic, sunflower oil, salt, and water.   Mix the mixture gently with the help of the spoon and close the lid.   Cook the greens on High for 30 minutes.
Nutrition Info: Per Serving: 58 calories, 2.2g protein, 5.8g carbohydrates, 3.9g fat, 2.3g fiber, 0mg cholesterol, 828mg sodium, 455mg potassium.

---

804. Curry Couscous

Servings: 4   Cooking Time: 20 Minutes
Ingredients:

1 cup of water	½ cup coconut cream
1 cup couscous	1 teaspoon salt

Directions:
Put all ingredients in the Crock Pot and close the lid.   Cook the couscous on High for   minutes.
Nutrition Info: Per Serving: 182 calories, 5.8g protein, 34.4g carbohydrates, 2g fat, 2.2g fiber, 6mg cholesterol, 597mg sodium, 84mg potassium.

---

805. Mediterranean Veggies

Servings: 8   Cooking Time: 7 Hrs
Ingredients:

1 zucchini, peeled and diced	2 tbsp olive oil
2 eggplants, peeled and diced	1 tsp ground black pepper
2 red onion, diced	1 tsp paprika
4 potatoes, peeled and diced	1 tsp salt
4 oz. asparagus, chopped	1 tbsp Mediterranean seasoning
	1 tsp minced garlic

Directions:
Mix Mediterranean seasoning with olive oil, paprika, salt, garlic, and black pepper in a large bowl.   Toss in all the veggies to this mixture and mix well.   Spread all the seasoned veggies in the Crock Pot.   Put the cooker's lid on and set the cooking time to 7 hours on Low settings.   Serve warm.
Nutrition Info: Per Serving: Calories 227, Total Fat 3.9g, Fiber 9g, Total Carbs 44.88g, Protein 6g

---

806. Marjoram Carrot Soup

Servings: 9   Cooking Time: 12 Hrs
Ingredients:

1 lb. carrot	1 tsp marjoram
1 tsp ground cardamom	5 cups chicken stock
¼ tsp nutmeg	½ cup yellow onion, chopped
1 tsp salt	1 tsp butter
3 tbsp fresh parsley	
1 tsp honey	

Directions:
Add butter and all the veggies to a suitable pan. Sauté these vegetables on low heat for 5 minutes then transfer to the Crock Pot.   Stir in cardamom, salt, chicken stock, marjoram, and nutmeg.   Put the cooker's lid on and set the cooking time to 12 hours on Low settings.   Puree the cooked veggie mixture using an immersion blender until smooth.   Garnish with honey and parsley.   Devour.
Nutrition Info: Per Serving: Calories 80, Total Fat 2.7g, Fiber 2g, Total Carbs 10.19g, Protein 4g

---

807. Fragrant Appetizer Peppers

Servings: 2   Cooking Time: 1.5 Hours
Ingredients:

4 sweet peppers, seeded	1 red onion, sliced
¼ cup apple cider vinegar	½ teaspoon sugar
1 teaspoon peppercorns	¼ cup of water
	1 tablespoon olive oil

Directions:
Slice the sweet peppers roughly and put in the Crock Pot.   Add all remaining ingredients and close the lid.   Cook the peppers on high for 1.5

hours.   Then cool the peppers well and store them in the fridge for up to 6 days.
Nutrition Info: Per Serving: 171 calories, 3.1g protein, 25.1g carbohydrates, 7.7g fat, 4.7g fiber, 0mg cholesterol, 11mg sodium, 564mg potassium.

808.	Minestrone Zucchini Soup

Servings: 8   Cooking Time: 4 Hrs
Ingredients:

2 zucchinis, chopped	3 carrots, chopped
1 yellow onion, chopped	1 lb. lentils, cooked
1 cup green beans, halved	4 cups veggie stock
	28 oz. canned tomatoes, chopped
3 celery stalks, chopped	1 tsp curry powder
4 garlic cloves, minced	½ tsp garam masala
10 oz. canned garbanzo beans	½ tsp cumin, ground
	Salt and black pepper to the taste

Directions:

Add carrots, zucchinis, and all other ingredients to the Crock Pot.   Put the cooker's lid on and set the cooking time to 4 hours on High settings.   Serve warm.
Nutrition Info: Per Serving: Calories 273, Total Fat 12g, Fiber 7g, Total Carbs 34g, Protein 10g

809.	Thyme Fennel Bulb

Servings: 4   Cooking Time: 3 Hours
Ingredients:

16 oz fennel bulb	1 teaspoon salt
1 tablespoon thyme	1 teaspoon peppercorns
1 cup of water	

Directions:

Chop the fennel bulb roughly and put it in the Crock Pot.   Add thyme, water, salt, and peppercorns.   Cook the fennel on High for hours. Then drain water, remove peppercorns, and transfer the fennel in the serving plates.
Nutrition Info: Per Serving: 38 calories, 1.5g protein, 9g carbohydrates, 0.3g fat, 3.9g fiber, 0mg cholesterol, 643mg sodium, 482mg potassium.

Side Dish Recipes

810.   Garlic Carrots Mix

Servings: 2   Cooking Time: 4 Hours

Ingredients:

1 pound carrots, sliced	½ cup tomato sauce
2 garlic cloves, minced	½ teaspoon oregano, dried
1 red onion, chopped	2 teaspoons lemon zest, grated
1 tablespoon olive oil	
A pinch of salt and black pepper	1 tablespoon lemon juice
	1 tablespoon chives, chopped

Directions:
In your Crock Pot, mix the carrots with the garlic, onion and the other ingredients, toss, put the lid on and cook on Low for 4 hours.   Divide the mix between plates and serve.
Nutrition Info:calories 219, fat 8, fiber 4, carbs 8, protein 17

811.Marjoram Rice Mix

Servings: 2   Cooking Time: 6 Hours

Ingredients:

1 cup wild rice	1 tablespoon olive oil
2 cups chicken stock	A pinch of salt and black pepper
1 carrot, peeled and grated	1 tablespoon green onions, chopped
2 tablespoons marjoram, chopped	

Directions:
In your Crock Pot, mix the rice with the stock and the other ingredients, toss, put the lid on and cook on Low for 6 hours.   Divide between plates and serve.
Nutrition Info:calories 200, fat 2, fiber 3, carbs 7, protein 5

812.   Green Beans And Mushrooms

Servings: 4   Cooking Time: 3 Hours

Ingredients:

1 pound fresh green beans, trimmed	1 cup chicken stock
1 small yellow onion, chopped	8 ounces mushrooms, sliced
6 ounces bacon, chopped	Salt and black pepper to the taste
1 garlic clove, minced	A splash of balsamic vinegar

Directions:
In your Crock Pot, mix beans with onion, bacon, garlic, stock, mushrooms, salt, pepper and vinegar, stir, cover and cook on Low for 3 hours.   Divide between plates and serve as a side dish.
Nutrition Info:calories 162, fat 4, fiber 5, carbs 8, protein 4

813.   Beans And Red Peppers

Servings: 2   Cooking Time: 2 Hrs.

Ingredients:

2 cups green beans, halved	Salt and black pepper to the taste
1 red bell pepper, cut into strips	1 and ½ tbsp honey mustard
1 tbsp olive oil	

Directions:
Add green beans, honey mustard, red bell pepper, oil, salt, and black to Crock Pot.   Put the cooker's lid on and set the cooking time to hours on High settings.   Serve warm.
Nutrition Info: Per Serving: Calories: 50, Total Fat: 0g, Fiber: 4g, Total Carbs: 8g, Protein: 2g

814.   Cabbage And Onion Mix

Servings: 2   Cooking Time: 2 Hours

Ingredients:

1 and ½ cups green cabbage, shredded	¼ cup veggie stock
1 cup red cabbage, shredded	2 tomatoes, chopped
	2 jalapenos, chopped
1 tablespoon olive oil	1 tablespoon chili powder
1 red onion, sliced	
2 spring onions, chopped	1 tablespoon chives, chopped
½ cup tomato paste	A pinch of salt and black pepper

Directions:
Grease your Crock Pot with the oil and mix the cabbage with the onion, spring onions and the other ingredients inside.   Toss, put the lid on and cook on High for hours.   Divide between plates and serve as a side dish.
Nutrition Info:calories 211, fat 3, fiber 3, carbs 6, protein 8

815.   Turmeric Potato Strips

Servings: 8   Cooking Time: 5 Hours

Ingredients:

3 lbs. potato, peeled and cut into strips	1 tbsp paprika
2 tomatoes, chopped	1 tsp salt
1 sweet pepper, chopped	½ tsp turmeric
	2 tbsp sesame oil

Directions:
Season the potato strips with salt, paprika, and turmeric.   Add oil and seasoned potatoes to the Crock Pot and toss them well.   Put the cooker's lid on and set the cooking time to hours on High settings.   Meanwhile, you can blend tomatoes with sweet pepper in a blender jug.   Pour this puree into the Crock Pot.   Put the cooker's lid on and set the cooking time to 2 hours on High settings.   Serve warm.

Nutrition Info: Per Serving: Calories: 176, Total Fat: 3.8g, Fiber: 5g, Total Carbs: 32.97g, Protein: 4g

816.   Nut Berry Salad

Servings: 4   Cooking Time: 1 Hour
Ingredients:

2 cups strawberries, halved	1 tbsp canola oil
2 tbsp mint, chopped	4 cups spinach, torn
1/3 cup raspberry vinegar	½ cup blueberries
2 tbsp honey	¼ cup walnuts, chopped
Salt and black pepper to the taste	1 oz. goat cheese, crumbled

Directions:
Toss strawberries with walnuts, spinach, honey, oil, salt, black pepper, blueberries, vinegar, and mint in the Crock Pot.   Put the cooker's lid on and set the cooking time to 1 hour on High settings.   Serve warm with cheese on top.
Nutrition Info: Per Serving: Calories: 200, Total Fat: 12g, Fiber: 4g, Total Carbs: 17g, Protein: 15g

817.   Hot Lentils

Servings: 2   Cooking Time: 6 Hours
Ingredients:

1 tablespoon thyme, chopped	½ cup veggie stock
½ tablespoon olive oil	1 tablespoon cider vinegar
1 cup canned lentils, drained	2 tablespoons tomato paste
2 garlic cloves, minced	1 tablespoon rosemary, chopped

Directions:
In your Crock Pot, mix the lentils with the thyme and the other ingredients, toss, put the lid on and cook on Low for 6 hours.   Divide between plates and serve as a side dish.
Nutrition Info:calories 200, fat 2, fiber 4, carbs 7, protein 8

818.   Slow-cooked White Onions

Servings: 5   Cooking Time: 9 Hours
Ingredients:

½ cup bread crumbs	1 tbsp salt
5 oz. Romano cheese, shredded	5 large white onions, peeled and wedges
¼ cup cream cheese	1 tsp ground black pepper
¼ cup half and half	
3 oz. butter	1 tsp garlic powder

Directions:
Add onion wedges to the insert of the Crock Pot. Mix breadcrumbs and shredded cheese in a suitable bowl.   Whisk the half and half cream with remaining ingredients.   Spread this mixture over the onion and then top it with breadcrumbs mixture.   Put the cooker's lid on and set the cooking time to 9 hours on Low settings.   Serve warm.

Nutrition Info: Per Serving: Calories: 349, Total Fat: 25.3g, Fiber: 3g, Total Carbs: 19.55g, Protein: 13g

819.   Cauliflower And Potatoes Mix

Servings: 2   Cooking Time: 4 Hours
Ingredients:

1 cup cauliflower florets	1 tablespoon chives, chopped
½ pound sweet potatoes, peeled and cubed	Salt and black pepper to the taste
1 cup veggie stock	1 teaspoon sweet paprika
½ cup tomato sauce	

Directions:
In your Crock Pot, mix the cauliflower with the potatoes, stock and the other ingredients, toss, put the lid on and cook on High for 4 hours.   Divide between plates and serve as a side dish.
Nutrition Info:calories 135, fat 5, fiber 1, carbs 7, protein 3

820.   Broccoli Mix

Servings: 10   Cooking Time: 2 Hours
Ingredients:

6 cups broccoli florets	¼ cup yellow onion, chopped
1 and ½ cups cheddar cheese, shredded	Salt and black pepper to the taste
10 ounces canned cream of celery soup	1 cup crackers, crushed
½ teaspoon Worcestershire sauce	2 tablespoons soft butter

Directions:
In a bowl, mix broccoli with cream of celery soup, cheese, salt, pepper, onion and Worcestershire sauce, toss and transfer to your Crock Pot.   Add butter, toss again, sprinkle crackers, cover and cook on High for hours.   Serve as a side dish.
Nutrition Info:calories 159, fat 11, fiber 1, carbs 11, protein 6

821.   Okra Side Dish(2)

Servings: 4   Cooking Time: 4 Hours
Ingredients:

1 pound okra, sliced	1 cup water
1 tomato, chopped	1 yellow onion, chopped
6 ounces tomato sauce	2 garlic cloves, minced
Salt and black pepper to the taste	

Directions:
In your Crock Pot, mix okra with tomato, tomato sauce, water, salt, pepper, onion and garlic, stir, cover and cook on Low for 4 hours.   Divide between plates and serve as a side dish.
Nutrition Info:calories 211, fat 4, fiber 6, carbs 17, protein 3

822.   Dill Mushroom Sauté

Servings: 2   Cooking Time: 3 Hours

Ingredients:

1 pound white mushrooms, halved

1 tablespoon olive oil

1 carrot, peeled and grated

2 green onions, chopped

1 red onion, sliced

1 garlic clove, minced

1 cup beef stock

½ cup tomato sauce

1 tablespoon dill, chopped

Directions:

Grease the Crock Pot with the oil and mix the mushrooms with the onion, carrot and the other ingredients inside.   Put the lid on, cook on Low for 3 hours, divide between plates and serve as a side dish.

Nutrition Info:calories 200, fat 6, fiber 4, carbs 28, protein 5

823.   Bacon Potatoes Mix

Servings: 2   Cooking Time: 6 Hours

Ingredients:

2 sweet potatoes, peeled and cut into wedges

1 tablespoon balsamic vinegar

A pinch of salt and black pepper

¼ teaspoon sage, dried

½ tablespoon sugar

A pinch of thyme, dried

1 tablespoon olive oil

½ cup veggie stock

2 bacon slices, cooked and crumbled

Directions:

In your Crock Pot, mix the potatoes with the vinegar, sugar and the other ingredients, toss, put the lid on and cook on Low for 6 hours   Divide between plates and serve as a side dish.

Nutrition Info:calories 209, fat 4, fiber 4, carbs 29, protein 4

824.   Garlic Risotto

Servings: 2   Cooking Time: 2 Hours

Ingredients:

1 small shallot, chopped

1 cup wild rice

1 cup chicken stock

1 tablespoons olive oil

2 garlic cloves, minced

Salt and black pepper to the taste

2 tablespoons cilantro, chopped

Directions:

In your Crock Pot, mix the rice with the stock, shallot and the other ingredients, toss, put the lid on and cook on High for 2 hours   Divide between plates and serve as a side dish.

Nutrition Info:calories 204, fat 7, fiber 3, carbs 17, protein 7

825.   Garlicky Black Beans

Servings: 8   Cooking Time: 7 Hours

Ingredients:

1 cup black beans, soaked overnight, drained and rinsed

1 cup of water

Salt and black pepper to the taste

1 spring onion, chopped

2 garlic cloves, minced

½ tsp cumin seeds

Directions:

Add beans, salt, black pepper, cumin seeds, garlic, and onion to the Crock Pot.   Put the cooker's lid on and set the cooking time to 7 hours on Low settings.   Serve warm.

Nutrition Info: Per Serving: Calories: 300, Total Fat: 4g, Fiber: 6g, Total Carbs: 20g, Protein: 15g

826.   Roasted Beets

Servings: 5   Cooking Time: 4 Hours

Ingredients:

10 small beets

5 teaspoons olive oil

A pinch of salt and black pepper

Directions:

Divide each beet on a tin foil piece, drizzle oil, season them with salt and pepper, rub well, wrap beets, place them in your Crock Pot, cover and cook on High for 4 hours.   Unwrap beets, cool them down a bit, peel, slice and serve them as a side dish.

Nutrition Info:calories 100, fat 2, fiber 2, carbs 4, protein 5

827.   Lemony Pumpkin Wedges

Servings: 4   Cooking Time: 6 Hours

Ingredients:

15 oz. pumpkin, peeled and cut into wedges

1 tbsp lemon juice

1 tsp salt

1 tsp honey

½ tsp ground cardamom

1 tsp lime juice

Directions:

Add pumpkin, lemon juice, honey, lime juice, cardamom, and salt to the Crock Pot.   Put the cooker's lid on and set the cooking time to 6 hours on Low settings.   Serve fresh.

Nutrition Info: Per Serving: Calories: 35, Total Fat: 0.1g, Fiber: 1g, Total Carbs: 8.91g, Protein: 1g

828.   Beans, Carrots And Spinach Salad

Servings: 6   Cooking Time: 7 Hours

Ingredients:

1 and ½ cups northern beans

1 yellow onion, chopped

2 garlic cloves, minced

½ teaspoon oregano, dried

Salt and black pepper to the taste

4 and ½ cups chicken stock

5 carrots, chopped

5 ounces baby spinach

2 teaspoons lemon peel, grated

1 avocado, peeled, pitted and chopped

3 tablespoons lemon juice

¾ cup feta cheese, crumbled

1/3 cup pistachios, chopped

Directions:
In your Crock Pot, mix beans with onion, carrots, garlic, oregano, salt, pepper and stock, stir, cover and cook on Low for 7 hours.   Drain beans and veggies, transfer them to a salad bowl, add baby spinach, lemon peel, avocado, lemon juice, pistachios and cheese, toss, divide between plates and serve as a side dish.
Nutrition Info: calories 300, fat 8, fiber 14, carbs 43, protein 16

829.	**Thai Side Salad**

Servings: 8   Cooking Time: 3 Hours
Ingredients:

8 ounces yellow summer squash, peeled and roughly chopped	2 tablespoons veggie stock
12 ounces zucchini, halved and sliced	2 garlic cloves, minced
2 cups button mushrooms, quartered	2 tablespoon Thai red curry paste
1 red sweet potatoes, chopped	1 tablespoon ginger, grated
2 leeks, sliced	1/3 cup coconut milk
	¼ cup basil, chopped

Directions:
In your Crock Pot, mix zucchini with summer squash, mushrooms, red pepper, leeks, garlic, stock, curry paste, ginger, coconut milk and basil, toss, cover and cook on Low for 3 hours.   Stir your Thai mix one more time, divide between plates and serve as a side dish.
Nutrition Info: calories 69, fat 2, fiber 2, carbs 8, protein 2

830.	**Eggplants With Mayo Sauce**

Servings: 8   Cooking Time: 5 Hours
Ingredients:

2 tbsp minced garlic	1 tsp salt
1 chili pepper, chopped	½ tsp ground black pepper
1 sweet pepper, chopped	18 oz. eggplants, peeled and diced
4 tbsp mayo	2 tbsp sour cream
1 tsp olive oil	

Directions:
Blend chili pepper, sweet peppers, salt, garlic, and black pepper in a blender until smooth.   Add eggplant and this chili mixture to the Crock Pot then toss them well.   Now mix mayo with sour cream and spread on top of eggplants.   Put the cooker's lid on and set the cooking time to 5 hours on High settings.   Serve warm
Nutrition Info: Per Serving: Calories: 40, Total Fat: 1.1g, Fiber: 3g, Total Carbs: 7.5g, Protein: 1g

831.	**Parmesan Rice**

Servings: 2   Cooking Time: 2 Hours And 30 Minutes
Ingredients:

1 cup rice	1 red onion, chopped
2 cups chicken stock	Salt and black pepper to the taste
1 tablespoon olive oil	
1 tablespoon lemon juice	1 tablespoon parmesan, grated

Directions:
In your Crock Pot, mix the rice with the stock, oil and the other ingredients, toss, put the lid on and cook on High for 2 hours and 30 minutes.   Divide between plates and serve as a side dish.
Nutrition Info: calories 162, fat 4, fiber 6, carbs 29, protein 6

832.	**Summer Squash Medley**

Servings: 4   Cooking Time: 2 Hrs
Ingredients:

¼ cup olive oil	2 tsp mustard
2 tbsp basil, chopped	Salt and black pepper to the taste
2 tbsp balsamic vinegar	3 summer squash, sliced
2 garlic cloves, minced	2 zucchinis, sliced

Directions:
Add squash, zucchinis, and all other ingredients to the Crock Pot.   Put the cooker's lid on and set the cooking time to hours on High settings.   Serve.
Nutrition Info: Per Serving: Calories: 179, Total Fat: 13g, Fiber: 2g, Total Carbs: 10g, Protein: 4g

833.	**Garlic Butter Green Beans**

Servings: 6   Cooking Time: 2 Hours
Ingredients:

22 ounces green beans	¼ cup butter, soft
2 garlic cloves, minced	2 tablespoons parmesan, grated

Directions:
In your Crock Pot, mix green beans with garlic, butter and parmesan, toss, cover and cook on High for 2 hours.   Divide between plates, sprinkle parmesan all over and serve as a side dish.
Nutrition Info: calories 60, fat 4, fiber 1, carbs 3, protein 1

834.	**Green Beans And Red Peppers**

Servings: 2   Cooking Time: 2 Hours
Ingredients:

2 cups green beans, halved	1 tablespoon olive oil
1 red bell pepper, cut into strips	1 and ½ tablespoon honey mustard
Salt and black pepper to the taste	

Directions:

In your Crock Pot, mix green beans with bell pepper, salt, pepper, oil and honey mustard, toss, cover and cook on High for 2 hours.   Divide between plates and serve as a side dish.
Nutrition Info:calories 50, fat 0, fiber 4, carbs 8, protein 2

835.	Veggies Rice Pilaf

Servings: 4   Cooking Time: 5 Hours
Ingredients:

2 cups basmati rice	2 tbsp butter
1 cup mixed carrots, peas, corn, and green beans	1 cinnamon stick
	1 tbsp cumin seeds
2 cups of water	2 bay leaves
½ tsp green chili, minced	3 whole cloves
	5 black peppercorns
½ tsp ginger, grated	2 whole cardamoms
3 garlic cloves, minced	1 tbsp sugar
	Salt to the taste

Directions:
Add water, rice, veggies and all other ingredients to the Crock Pot.   Put the cooker's lid on and set the cooking time to 5 hours on Low settings.   Discard the cinnamon and serve warm.
Nutrition Info: Per Serving: Calories: 300, Total Fat: 4g, Fiber: 3g, Total Carbs: 40g, Protein: 13g

836.	Sweet Potato And Cauliflower Mix

Servings: 2   Cooking Time: 4 Hours
Ingredients:

2 sweet potatoes, peeled and cubed	½ tablespoon sugar
1 cup cauliflower florets	1 tablespoon red curry paste
½ cup coconut milk	3 ounces white mushrooms, roughly chopped
1 teaspoons sriracha sauce	
A pinch of salt and black pepper	2 tablespoons cilantro, chopped

Directions:
In your Crock Pot, mix the sweet potatoes with the cauliflower and the other ingredients, toss, put the lid on and cook on Low for 4 hours.   Divide between plates and serve as a side dish.
Nutrition Info:calories 200, fat 3, fiber 5, carbs 15, protein 12

837.	Corn And Bacon

Servings: 20   Cooking Time: 4 Hours
Ingredients:

10 cups corn	A pinch of salt and black pepper
24 ounces cream cheese, cubed	4 bacon strips, cooked and crumbled
½ cup milk	
½ cup melted butter	2 tablespoons green onions, chopped
½ cup heavy cream	
¼ cup sugar	

Directions:

In your Crock Pot, mix corn with cream cheese, milk, butter, cream, sugar, salt, pepper, bacon and green onions, cover and cook on Low for 4 hours. Stir the corn, divide between plates and serve as a side dish.
Nutrition Info:calories 259, fat 20, fiber 2, carbs 18, protein 5

838.	Pumpkin Rice

Servings: 4   Cooking Time: 5 Hours
Ingredients:

2 ounces olive oil	4 cups chicken stock
1 small yellow onion, chopped	1 teaspoon thyme, chopped
2 garlic cloves, minced	½ teaspoon ginger, grated
12 ounces risotto rice	½ teaspoon cinnamon powder
6 ounces pumpkin puree	
½ teaspoon nutmeg, ground	½ teaspoon allspice, ground
	4 ounces heavy cream

Directions:
In your Crock Pot, mix oil with onion, garlic, rice, stock, pumpkin puree, nutmeg, thyme, ginger, cinnamon and allspice, stir, cover and cook on Low for 4 hours and 30 minutes.   Add cream, stir, cover, cook on Low for 30 minutes more, divide between plates and serve as a side dish.
Nutrition Info:calories 251, fat 4, fiber 3, carbs 30, protein 5

839.	Cauliflower Carrot Gratin

Servings: 12   Cooking Time: 7 Hours
Ingredients:

16 oz. baby carrots	6 tbsp butter, soft
1 cauliflower head, florets separated	1 tsp mustard powder
Salt and black pepper to the taste	1 and ½ cups of milk
1 yellow onion, chopped	6 oz. cheddar cheese, grated
	½ cup breadcrumbs

Directions:
Add carrots, cauliflower, and rest of the ingredients to the Crock Pot.   Put the cooker's lid on and set the cooking time to 7 hours on Low settings. Serve warm.
Nutrition Info: Per Serving: Calories: 182, Total Fat: 4g, Fiber: 7g, Total Carbs: 9g, Protein: 4g

840.	Buttery Spinach

Servings: 2   Cooking Time: 2 Hours
Ingredients:

1 pound baby spinach	1 cup heavy cream
½ teaspoon turmeric powder	½ teaspoon garam masala
A pinch of salt and black pepper	2 tablespoons butter, melted

Directions:

In your Crock Pot, mix the spinach with the cream and the other ingredients, toss, put the lid on and cook on Low for 2 hours.   Divide between plates and serve as a side dish.
Nutrition Info:calories 230, fat 12, fiber 2, carbs 9, protein 12

841.   Honey Glazed Vegetables

Servings: 12   Cooking Time: 6 Hrs.
Ingredients:

4 large carrots, peeled and chopped	½ cup brown sugar
3 red onions, chopped	1 tbsp salt
1 lb. potato, peeled and diced	1 tsp coriander
	1 tsp cilantro
3 sweet potatoes, peeled and diced	2 tbsp dried dill
	1 tbsp sesame oil
	3 oz. honey

Directions:
Toss onions, carrots, potato, and sweet potatoes with the rest of the ingredients in a Crock Pot.   Put the cooker's lid on and set the cooking time to 6 hours on Low settings.   Serve warm.
Nutrition Info: Per Serving: Calories: 148, Total Fat: 1.4g, Fiber: 3g, Total Carbs: 33g, Protein: 2g

842.   Minty Peas And Tomatoes

Servings: 2   Cooking Time: 3 Hours
Ingredients:

1 pound okra, sliced	Salt and black pepper to the taste
½ pound tomatoes, cut into wedges	1 tablespoon mint, chopped
1 tablespoon olive oil	3 green onions, chopped
½ cup veggie stock	
½ teaspoon chili powder	1 tablespoon chives, chopped

Directions:
Grease your Crock Pot with the oil, and mix the okra with the tomatoes and the other ingredients inside.   Put the lid on, cook on Low for 3 hours, divide between plates and serve as a side dish.
Nutrition Info:calories 70, fat 1, fiber 1, carbs 4, protein 6

843.   Italian Veggie Mix

Servings: 8   Cooking Time: 6 Hours
Ingredients:

38 ounces canned cannellini beans, drained	1 and ½ teaspoon Italian seasoning, dried and crushed
1 yellow onion, chopped	1 tomato, chopped
¼ cup basil pesto	15 ounces already cooked polenta, cut into medium pieces
19 ounces canned fava beans, drained	
4 garlic cloves, minced	2 cups spinach
	1 cup radicchio, torn

Directions:
In your Crock Pot, mix cannellini beans with fava beans, basil pesto, onion, garlic, Italian seasoning,

polenta, tomato, spinach and radicchio, toss, cover and cook on Low for 6 hours.   Divide between plates and serve as a side dish.
Nutrition Info:calories 364, fat 12, fiber 10, carbs 45, protein 21

844.   Pink Salt Rice

Servings: 8   Cooking Time: 5 Hours
Ingredients:

1 tsp salt	2 cups pink rice
2 and ½ cups of water	

Directions:
Add rice, salt, and water to the Crock Pot.   Put the cooker's lid on and set the cooking time to 5 hours on Low settings.   Serve warm.
Nutrition Info: Per Serving: Calories: 120, Total Fat: 3g, Fiber: 3g, Total Carbs: 16g, Protein: 4g

845.   Cinnamon Applesauce

Servings: 5   Cooking Time: 6 Hrs.
Ingredients:

1 lb. red apples, peeled and chopped	1 tsp ground cinnamon
2 oz. cinnamon stick	4 oz. water
1 tsp ground ginger	½ tsp salt
½ tsp nutmeg	1 tbsp lime juice

Directions:
Add red apples, cinnamon stick, salt, cinnamon ground, water, lime juice, nutmeg, and ginger to the Crock Pot.   Put the cooker's lid on and set the cooking time to 6 hours on High settings.   Discard the cinnamon sticks from the apples.   Serve fresh.   Transfer the dish to the serving bowls and serve it or keep in the fridge for not more than 3 days. Enjoy!
Nutrition Info: Per Serving: Calories: 86, Total Fat: 0.4g, Fiber: 9g, Total Carbs: 22.93g, Protein: 1g

846.   Dill Cauliflower Mash

Servings: 6   Cooking Time: 5 Hours
Ingredients:

1 cauliflower head, florets separated	2 tablespoons butter, melted
1/3 cup dill, chopped	A pinch of salt and black pepper
6 garlic cloves	

Directions:
Put cauliflower in your Crock Pot, add dill, garlic and water to cover cauliflower, cover and cook on High for 5 hours.   Drain cauliflower and dill, add salt, pepper and butter, mash using a potato masher, whisk well and serve as a side dish.
Nutrition Info:calories 187, fat 4, fiber 5, carbs 12, protein 3

847.   Maple Sweet Potatoes

Servings: 10   Cooking Time: 5 Hours
Ingredients:

8 sweet potatoes, halved and sliced
1 cup walnuts, chopped
½ cup maple syrup
½ cup cherries, dried and chopped
¼ cup apple juice
A pinch of salt

Directions:
Arrange sweet potatoes in your Crock Pot, add walnuts, dried cherries, maple syrup, apple juice and a pinch of salt, toss a bit, cover and cook on Low for 5 hours. Divide between plates and serve as a side dish.
Nutrition Info:calories 271, fat 6, fiber 4, carbs 26, protein 6

848. Lemon Artichokes

Servings: 2   Cooking Time: 3 Hours
Ingredients:
2 medium artichokes, trimmed
1 tablespoon lemon juice
1 cup veggie stock
1 tablespoon lemon zest, grated
Salt to the taste

Directions:
In your Crock Pot, mix the artichokes with the stock and the other ingredients, toss, put the lid on and cook on Low for 3 hours. Divide artichokes between plates and serve as a side dish.
Nutrition Info:calories 100, fat 2, fiber 5, carbs 10, protein 4

849. Maple Brussels Sprouts

Servings: 12   Cooking Time: 3 Hours
Ingredients:
1 cup red onion, chopped
2 pounds Brussels sprouts, trimmed and halved
Salt and black pepper to the taste
¼ cup apple juice
3 tablespoons olive oil
¼ cup maple syrup
1 tablespoon thyme, chopped

Directions:
In your Crock Pot, mix Brussels sprouts with onion, salt, pepper and apple juice, toss, cover and cook on Low for 3 hours. In a bowl, mix maple syrup with oil and thyme, whisk really well, add over Brussels sprouts, toss well, divide between plates and serve as a side dish.
Nutrition Info:calories 100, fat 4, fiber 4, carbs 14, protein 3

850. Mashed Potatoes(2)

Servings: 2   Cooking Time: 6 Hours
Ingredients:
1 pound gold potatoes, peeled and cubed
2 garlic cloves, chopped
1 cup milk
1 cup water
2 tablespoons butter
A pinch of salt and white pepper

Directions:
In your Crock Pot, mix the potatoes with the water, salt and pepper, put the lid on and cook on Low for 6 hours. Mash the potatoes, add the rest of the ingredients, whisk and serve.
Nutrition Info:calories 135, fat 4, fiber 2, carbs 10, protein 4

851. Jalapeno Meal

Servings: 6   Cooking Time: 6 Hrs.
Ingredients:
12 oz. jalapeno pepper, cut in half and deseeded
2 tbsp olive oil
1 tbsp balsamic vinegar
1 onion, sliced
1 garlic clove, sliced
1 tsp ground coriander
4 tbsp water

Directions:
Place the jalapeno peppers in the Crock Pot. Top the pepper with olive oil, balsamic vinegar, onion, garlic, coriander, and water. Put the cooker's lid on and set the cooking time to 6 hours on Low settings. Serve warm.
Nutrition Info: Per Serving: Calories: 67, Total Fat: 4.7g, Fiber: 2g, Total Carbs: 6.02g, Protein: 1g

852. Tomato And Corn Mix

Servings: 2   Cooking Time: 4 Hours
Ingredients:
1 red onion, sliced
2 spring onions, chopped
1 cup corn
1 cup tomatoes, cubed
1 tablespoon olive oil
½ red bell pepper, chopped
½ cup tomato sauce
¼ teaspoon sweet paprika
½ teaspoon cumin, ground
1 tablespoon chives, chopped
Salt and black pepper to the taste

Directions:
Heat up a pan with the oil over medium-high heat, add the onion , spring onions and bell pepper and cook for   minutes. Transfer the mix to the Crock Pot, add the corn and the other ingredients, toss, put the lid on and cook on Low for 4 hours. Divide the mix between plates and serve as a side dish.
Nutrition Info:calories 312, fat 4, fiber 6, carbs 12, protein 6

853. Spinach And Squash Side Salad

Servings: 12   Cooking Time: 4 Hours
Ingredients:
3 pounds butternut squash, peeled and cubed
1 yellow onion, chopped
2 teaspoons thyme, chopped
3 garlic cloves, minced
A pinch of salt and black pepper
10 ounces veggie stock
6 ounces baby spinach

Directions:

In your Crock Pot, mix squash cubes with onion, thyme, salt, pepper and stock, stir, cover and cook on Low for 4 hours.   Transfer squash mix to a bowl, add spinach, toss, divide between plates and serve as a side dish.
Nutrition Info:calories 100, fat 1, fiber 4, carbs 18, protein 4

854.   Blueberry Spinach Salad

Servings: 3   Cooking Time: 1 Hour
Ingredients:

¼ cup pecans, chopped	1 tbsp olive oil
½ tsp sugar	4 cups spinach
2 tsp maple syrup	2 oranges, peeled and
1 tbsp white vinegar	cut into segments
2 tbsp orange juice	1 cup blueberries

Directions:
Add pecans, maple syrup, and rest of the ingredients to the Crock Pot.   Put the cooker's lid on and set the cooking time to 1 hour on High settings.   Serve warm.
Nutrition Info: Per Serving: Calories: 140, Total Fat: 4g, Fiber: 3g, Total Carbs: 10g, Protein: 3g

855.   Butter Glazed Yams

Servings: 7   Cooking Time: 4 Hrs.
Ingredients:

2 lb. yams, peeled and diced	4 oz. white sugar
5 tbsp butter, melted	½ tsp salt
5 oz. brown sugar	1 tsp vanilla extract
	2 tbsp cornstarch

Directions:
Add melted butter, brown sugar, yams, white sugar, salt, and vanilla extract to the Crock Pot.   Put the cooker's lid on and set the cooking time to 4 hours on High settings.   Toss well, then stir in cornstarch, continue cooking for 10 minutes on High.   Mix well and serve.
Nutrition Info: Per Serving: Calories: 404, Total Fat: 16.4g, Fiber: 6g, Total Carbs: 63.33g, Protein: 3g

856.   Mustard Brussels Sprouts(2)

Servings: 2   Cooking Time: 3 Hours
Ingredients:

½ pounds Brussels sprouts, trimmed and halved	1 tablespoons olive oil
	2 tablespoons maple syrup
A pinch of salt and black pepper	1 tablespoon thyme, chopped
2 tablespoons mustard	
½ cup veggie stock	

Directions:
In your Crock Pot, mix the sprouts with the mustard and the other ingredients, toss, put the lid on and cook on Low for 3 hours.   Divide between plates and serve as a side dish.

Nutrition Info:calories 170, fat 4, fiber 4, carbs 14, protein 6

857.   Rice And Farro Pilaf

Servings: 12   Cooking Time: 5 Hours
Ingredients:

1 shallot, chopped	6 cups chicken stock
1 teaspoon garlic, minced	Salt and black pepper to the taste
A drizzle of olive oil	1 tablespoon parsley and sage, chopped
1 and ½ cups whole grain farro	½ cup hazelnuts, toasted and chopped
¾ cup wild rice	¾ cup cherries, dried

Directions:
In your Crock Pot, mix oil with garlic, shallot, farro, rice, stock, salt, pepper, sage and parsley, hazelnuts and cherries, toss, cover and cook on Low for 5 hours.   Divide between plates and serve as a side dish.
Nutrition Info:calories 120, fat 2, fiber 7, carbs 20, protein 3

858.   Italian Squash And Peppers Mix

Servings: 4   Cooking Time: 1 Hour And 30 Minutes
Ingredients:

2 red bell peppers, cut into wedges	12 small squash, peeled and cut into wedges
2 green bell peppers, cut into wedges	Salt and black pepper to the taste
1/3 cup Italian dressing	1 tablespoon parsley, chopped
1 red onion, cut into wedges	

Directions:
In your Crock Pot, mix squash with red bell peppers, green bell peppers, salt, pepper and Italian dressing, cover and cook on High for hour and 30 minutes.   Add parsley, toss, divide between plates and serve as a side dish.
Nutrition Info:calories 80, fat 2, fiber 3, carbs 11, protein 2

859.   Red Curry Veggie Mix

Servings: 2   Cooking Time: 3 Hours
Ingredients:

2 zucchinis, cubed	¼ tablespoon Thai red curry paste
1 eggplant, cubed	
½ cup button mushrooms, quartered	¼ tablespoon ginger, grated
1 small red sweet potatoes, chopped	Salt and black pepper to the taste
½ cup veggie stock	2 tablespoons coconut milk
1 garlic cloves, minced	

Directions:

In your Crock Pot, mix the zucchinis with the eggplant and the other ingredients, toss, put the lid on and cook on Low for 3 hours.   Divide between plates and serve as a side dish.
Nutrition Info:calories 169, fat 2, fiber 2, carbs 15, protein 6

860.	Dill Mixed Fennel

Servings: 7   Cooking Time: 3 Hour
Ingredients:

10 oz. fennel bulbs, diced	1 tsp oregano
2 tbsp olive oil	1 tsp basil
1 tsp ground black pepper	3 tbsp white wine
1 tsp paprika	1 tsp salt
1 tsp cilantro	2 garlic cloves
	1 tsp dried dill

Directions:
Add fennel bulbs and all other ingredients to the Crock Pot.   Put the cooker's lid on and set the cooking time to 3.5 hours on High settings. Serve warm.
Nutrition Info: Per Serving: Calories: 53, Total Fat: 4.1g, Fiber: 2g, Total Carbs: 4g, Protein: 1g

861.	Nut And Berry Side Salad

Servings: 4   Cooking Time: 1 Hour
Ingredients:

2 cups strawberries, halved	Salt and black pepper to the taste
2 tablespoons mint, chopped	4 cups spinach, torn
1/3 cup raspberry vinegar	½ cup blueberries
2 tablespoons honey	¼ cup walnuts, chopped
1 tablespoon canola oil	1 ounce goat cheese, crumbled

Directions:
In your Crock Pot, mix strawberries with mint, vinegar, honey, oil, salt, pepper, spinach, blueberries and walnuts, cover and cook on High for hour.   Divide salad on plates, sprinkle cheese on top and serve as a side dish.
Nutrition Info:calories 200, fat 12, fiber 4, carbs 17, protein 15

862.	Turmeric Buckwheat

Servings: 6   Cooking Time: 4 Hrs
Ingredients:

4 tbsp milk powder	4 cups chicken stock
2 tbsp butter	1 tbsp salt
1 carrot	1 tbsp turmeric
4 cup buckwheat	1 tsp paprika

Directions:
Whisk milk powder with buckwheat, stock, salt, turmeric, and paprika in the Crock Pot.   Stir in carrot strips and mix gently.   Put the cooker's lid on and set the cooking time to 4 hours on High settings.   Stir in butter then serve warm.

Nutrition Info: Per Serving: Calories: 238, Total Fat: 6.6g, Fiber: 4g, Total Carbs: 37.85g, Protein: 9g

863.	Okra And Corn

Servings: 4   Cooking Time: 8 Hours
Ingredients:

3 garlic cloves, minced	28 ounces canned tomatoes, crushed
1 small green bell pepper, chopped	1 teaspoon oregano, dried
1 small yellow onion, chopped	1 teaspoon thyme, dried
1 cup water	1 teaspoon marjoram, dried
16 ounces okra, sliced	A pinch of cayenne pepper
2 cups corn	Salt and black pepper to the taste
1 and ½ teaspoon smoked paprika	

Directions:
In your Crock Pot, mix garlic with bell pepper, onion, water, okra, corn, paprika, tomatoes, oregano, thyme, marjoram, cayenne, salt and pepper, cover, cook on Low for 8 hours, divide between plates and serve as a side dish.
Nutrition Info:calories 182, fat 3, fiber 6, carbs 8, protein 5

864.	Creamy Coconut Potatoes

Servings: 2   Cooking Time: 4 Hours
Ingredients:

½ pound gold potatoes, halved and sliced	2 ounces coconut milk
2 scallions, chopped	¼ cup veggie stock
1 tablespoon avocado oil	Salt and black pepper to the taste
	1 tablespoons parsley, chopped

Directions:
In your Crock Pot, mix the potatoes with the scallions and the other ingredients, toss, put the lid on and cook on High for 4 hours.   Divide the mix between plates and serve.
Nutrition Info:calories 306, fat 14, fiber 4, carbs 15, protein 12

865.	Rice And Veggies

Servings: 4   Cooking Time: 5 Hours
Ingredients:

2 cups basmati rice	2 tablespoons butter
1 cup mixed carrots, peas, corn and green beans	1 cinnamon stick
2 cups water	1 tablespoon cumin seeds
½ teaspoon green chili, minced	2 bay leaves
½ teaspoon ginger, grated	3 whole cloves
3 garlic cloves, minced	5 black peppercorns
	2 whole cardamoms
	1 tablespoon sugar
	Salt to the taste

Directions:
Put the water in your Crock Pot, add rice, mixed veggies, green chili, grated ginger, garlic, cinnamon stick, whole cloves, butter, cumin seeds, bay leaves, cardamoms, black peppercorns, salt and sugar, stir, cover and cook on Low for 5 hours.   Discard cinnamon, divide between plates and serve as a side dish.
Nutrition Info:calories 300, fat 4, fiber 3, carbs 40, protein 13

866.   Sage Peas

Servings: 2   Cooking Time: 2 Hours
Ingredients:

1 pound peas	¼ teaspoon sage, dried
1 red onion, sliced	
½ cup veggie stock	Salt and black pepper to the taste
½ cup tomato sauce	
2 garlic cloves, minced	1 tablespoon dill, chopped

Directions:
In your Crock Pot, combine the peas with the onion, stock and the other ingredients, toss, put the lid on and cook on Low for 2 hours.   Divide between plates and serve as a side dish.
Nutrition Info:calories 100, fat 4, fiber 3, carbs 15, protein 4

867.   Mac Cream Cups

Servings: 6   Cooking Time: 8 Hours
Ingredients:

6 oz. puff pastry	1 tbsp flour
1 cup fresh basil	1 tbsp cornstarch
7 oz. elbow macaroni, cooked	1 tsp salt
1 egg	1 tbsp turmeric
¼ cup heavy cream	1 tsp olive oil

Directions:
Roll the puff pastry and cut it into 6 squares. Layer a muffin tray with olive oil and place one square into each muffin cup.   Press the puff pastry square into the muffin cup.   Beat egg with cream, flour, salt, cornstarch, and turmeric in a suitable bowl.   Stir in macaroni then divide this mixture into the muffin cups.   Place this muffin tray in the Crock Pot.   Put the cooker's lid on and set the cooking time to 8 hours on Low settings. Serve warm.
Nutrition Info: Per Serving: Calories: 270, Total Fat: 15.4g, Fiber: 2g, Total Carbs: 26.67g, Protein: 6g

868.   Savoy Cabbage Mix

Servings: 2   Cooking Time: 2 Hours
Ingredients:

1 pound Savoy cabbage, shredded	½ cup veggie stock
1 red onion, sliced	1 carrot, grated
1 tablespoon olive oil	½ cup tomatoes, cubed

A pinch of salt and black pepper	½ teaspoon sweet paprika
	½ inch ginger, grated

Directions:
In your Crock Pot, mix the cabbage with the onion, oil and the other ingredients, toss, put the lid on and cook on High for 2 hours.   Divide the mix between plates and serve as a side dish.
Nutrition Info:calories 100, fat 3, fiber 4, carbs 5, protein 2

869.   Balsamic-glazed Beets

Servings: 6   Cooking Time: 2 Hours
Ingredients:

1 lb. beets, sliced	3 tbsp almonds
5 oz. orange juice	6 oz. goat cheese
3 oz. balsamic vinegar	1 tsp minced garlic
	1 tsp olive oil

Directions:
Toss the beets with balsamic vinegar, orange juice, and olive oil in the insert of Crock Pot.   Put the cooker's lid on and set the cooking time to 7 hours on Low settings.   Toss goat cheese with minced garlic and almonds in a bowl.   Spread this cheese garlic mixture over the beets.   Put the cooker's lid on and set the cooking time to 10 minutes on High settings.   Serve warm.
Nutrition Info: Per Serving: Calories: 189, Total Fat: 11.3g, Fiber: 2g, Total Carbs: 12g, Protein: 10g

870.   Creamy Chipotle Sweet Potatoes

Servings: 10   Cooking Time: 4 Hours
Ingredients:

1 sweet onion, chopped	4 big sweet potatoes, shredded
2 tablespoons olive oil	8 ounces coconut cream
¼ cup parsley, chopped	16 ounces bacon, cooked and chopped
2 shallots, chopped	
2 teaspoons chipotle pepper, crushed	½ teaspoon sweet paprika
Salt and black pepper	Cooking spray

Directions:
Heat up a pan with the oil over medium-high heat, add shallots and onion, stir, cook for 6 minutes and transfer to a bowl.   Add parsley, chipotle pepper, salt, pepper, sweet potatoes, coconut cream, paprika and bacon, stir, pour everything in your Crock Pot after you've greased it with some cooking spray, cover, cook on Low for 4 hours, leave aside to cool down a bit, divide between plates and serve as a side dish.
Nutrition Info:calories 260, fat 14, fiber 6, carbs 20, protein 15

871.   Herbed Balsamic Beets

Servings: 4   Cooking Time: 7 Hours

Ingredients:

6 medium assorted-color beets, peeled and cut into wedges	2 tbsp olive oil
	1 tbsp tarragon, chopped
2 tbsp balsamic vinegar	Salt and black pepper to the taste
2 tbsp chives, chopped	1 tsp orange peel, grated

Directions:
Add beets, tarragon, and rest of the ingredients to the Crock Pot.   Put the cooker's lid on and set the cooking time to 7 hours on Low settings.   Serve warm.
Nutrition Info: Per Serving: Calories: 144, Total Fat: 3g, Fiber: 1g, Total Carbs: 17g, Protein: 3g

872.   Cauliflower Rice And Spinach

Servings: 8   Cooking Time: 3 Hours
Ingredients:

2 garlic cloves, minced	20 ounces spinach, chopped
2 tablespoons butter, melted	6 ounces coconut cream
1 yellow onion, chopped	Salt and black pepper to the taste
¼ teaspoon thyme, dried	2 cups cauliflower rice
3 cups veggie stock	

Directions:
Heat up a pan with the butter over medium heat, add onion, stir and cook for 4 minutes.   Add garlic, thyme and stock, stir, cook for 1 minute more and transfer to your Crock Pot.   Add spinach, coconut cream, cauliflower rice, salt and pepper, stir a bit, cover and cook on High for hours. Divide between plates and serve as a side dish.
Nutrition Info:calories 200, fat 4, fiber 4, carbs 8, protein 2

873.   Cumin Quinoa Pilaf

Servings: 2   Cooking Time: 2 Hours
Ingredients:

1 cup quinoa	1 teaspoon turmeric powder
2 teaspoons butter, melted	2 cups chicken stock
Salt and black pepper to the taste	1 teaspoon cumin, ground

Directions:
Grease your Crock Pot with the butter, add the quinoa and the other ingredients, toss, put the lid on and cook on High for 2 hours   Divide between plates and serve as a side dish.
Nutrition Info:calories 152, fat 3, fiber 6, carbs 8, protein 4

874.   Beans Risotto

Servings: 6   Cooking Time: 5 Hours
Ingredients:

1 lb. red kidney beans, soaked overnight and	4 garlic cloves, chopped
	1 green bell pepper,

drained	chopped
Salt to the taste	1 tsp thyme, dried
1 tsp olive oil	2 bay leaves
1 lb. smoked sausage, roughly chopped	5 cups of water
1 yellow onion, chopped	2 green onions, minced
1 celery stalk, chopped	2 tbsp parsley, minced

Directions:
Add red beans, oil, sausage, and rest of the ingredients to the Crock Pot.   Put the cooker's lid on and set the cooking time to 5 hours on Low settings.   Serve warm.
Nutrition Info: Per Serving: Calories: 200, Total Fat: 5g, Fiber: 6g, Total Carbs: 20g, Protein: 5g

875.   Balsamic Okra Mix

Servings: 4   Cooking Time: 2 Hours
Ingredients:

1 cup cherry tomatoes, halved	2 cups okra, sliced
1 tablespoon olive oil	2 tablespoons balsamic vinegar
½ teaspoon turmeric powder	2 tablespoons basil, chopped
½ cup canned tomatoes, crushed	1 tablespoon thyme, chopped

Directions:
In your Crock Pot, mix the okra with the tomatoes, crushed tomatoes and the other ingredients, toss, put the lid on and cook on High for 2 hours. Divide between plates and serve as a side dish.
Nutrition Info:calories 233, fat 12, fiber 4, carbs 8, protein 4

876.   Asparagus Mix(2)

Servings: 4   Cooking Time: 6 Hours
Ingredients:

10 ounces cream of celery	2 eggs, hard-boiled, peeled and sliced
12 ounces asparagus, chopped	1 cup cheddar cheese, shredded
1 teaspoon olive oil	

Directions:
Grease your Crock Pot with the oil, add cream of celery and cheese to the Crock Pot and stir.   Add asparagus and eggs, cover and cook on Low for 6 hours.   Divide between plates and serve as a side dish.
Nutrition Info:calories 241, fat 5, fiber 4, carbs 5, protein 12

877.   Tarragon Sweet Potatoes

Servings: 4   Cooking Time: 3 Hours
Ingredients:

1 pound sweet potatoes, peeled and cut into wedges	Salt and black pepper to the taste
	1 tablespoon olive oil
1 cup veggie stock	1 tablespoon tarragon, dried
½ teaspoon chili powder	

½ teaspoon cumin, ground   2 tablespoons balsamic vinegar

Directions:
In your Crock Pot, mix the sweet potatoes with the stock, chili powder and the other ingredients, toss, put the lid on and cook on High for 3 hours. Divide the mix between plates and serve as a side dish.
Nutrition Info:calories 80, fat 4, fiber 4, carbs 8, protein 4

878. Rice With Artichokes

Servings: 4   Cooking Time: 4 Hrs
Ingredients:

1 tbsp olive oil
5 oz. Arborio rice
2 garlic cloves, minced
1 and ¼ cups chicken stock
1 tbsp white wine
6 oz. graham crackers, crumbled
1 and ¼ cups of water

15 oz. canned artichoke hearts, chopped
16 oz. cream cheese
1 tbsp parmesan, grated
1 and ½ tbsp thyme, chopped
Salt and black pepper to the taste

Directions:
Add oil, rice, artichokes, garlic, water, wine, crackers, and stock to the Crock Pot.   Put the cooker's lid on and set the cooking time to 4 hours on Low settings.   Stir in cream cheese, salt, parmesan, thyme, and black pepper.   Mix well and serve warm.
Nutrition Info: Per Serving: Calories: 230, Total Fat: 3g, Fiber: 5g, Total Carbs: 30g, Protein: 4g

879. Butternut Squash And Eggplant Mix

Servings: 2   Cooking Time: 4 Hours
Ingredients:

1 butternut squash, peeled and roughly cubed
1 eggplant, roughly cubed
1 red onion, chopped
Cooking spray
½ cup veggie stock

¼ cup tomato paste
½ tablespoon parsley, chopped
Salt and black pepper to the taste
2 garlic cloves, minced

Directions:
Grease the Crock Pot with the cooking spray and mix the squash with the eggplant, onion and the other ingredients inside.   Put the lid on and cook on Low for 4 hours.   Divide between plates and serve as a side dish.
Nutrition Info:calories 114, fat 4, fiber 4, carbs 18, protein 4

880. Lemon Kale Mix

Servings: 2   Cooking Time: 2 Hours
Ingredients:

1 yellow bell pepper, chopped

1 tablespoon lemon juice

1 red bell pepper, chopped
1 tablespoon olive oil
1 red onion, sliced
4 cups baby kale
1 teaspoon lemon zest, grated

½ cup veggie stock
1 garlic clove, minced
A pinch of salt and black pepper
1 tablespoon basil, chopped

Directions:
In your Crock Pot, mix the kale with the oil, onion, bell peppers and the other ingredients, toss, put the lid on and cook on Low for 2 hours.   Divide the mix between plates and serve as a side dish.
Nutrition Info:calories 251, fat 9, fiber 6, carbs 7, protein 8

881. Apples And Potatoes

Servings: 10   Cooking Time: 7 Hours
Ingredients:

2 green apples, cored and cut into wedges
3 pounds sweet potatoes, peeled and cut into medium wedges

1 cup coconut cream
½ cup dried cherries
1 cup apple butter
1 and ½ teaspoon pumpkin pie spice

Directions:
In your Crock Pot, mix sweet potatoes with green apples, cream, cherries, apple butter and spice, toss, cover and cook on Low for 7 hours.   Toss, divide between plates and serve as a side dish.
Nutrition Info:calories 351, fat 8, fiber 5, carbs 48, protein 2

882. Carrot Beet Salad

Servings: 6   Cooking Time: 7 Hours
Ingredients:

½ cup walnuts, chopped
¼ cup lemon juice
½ cup olive oil
1 shallot, chopped
1 tsp Dijon mustard
Salt and black pepper to the taste

1 tbsp brown sugar
2 beets, peeled and cut into wedges
2 carrots, peeled and sliced
1 cup parsley
5 oz. arugula

Directions:
Add beets, carrots, and rest of the ingredients to the Crock Pot.   Put the cooker's lid on and set the cooking time to 7 hours on Low settings.   Serve warm.
Nutrition Info: Per Serving: Calories: 100, Total Fat: 3g, Fiber: 3g, Total Carbs: 7g, Protein: 3g

883. Farro Mix

Servings: 2   Cooking Time: 4 Hours
Ingredients:

2 scallions, chopped
2 garlic cloves, minced
1 tablespoon olive oil
1 cup whole grain farro

2 cups chicken stock
Salt and black pepper to the taste
½ tablespoon parsley, chopped

1 tablespoon cherries, dried

Directions:
In your Crock Pot, mix the farro with the scallions, garlic and the other ingredients, toss, put the lid on and cook on Low for 4 hours.   Divide between plates and serve as a side dish.
Nutrition Info:calories 152, fat 4, fiber 5, carbs 20, protein 4

884.   Classic Veggies Mix

Servings: 4   Cooking Time: 3 Hours
Ingredients:

1 and ½ cups red onion, cut into medium chunks
1 cup cherry tomatoes, halved
2 and ½ cups zucchini, sliced
2 cups yellow bell pepper, chopped
1 cup mushrooms, sliced
2 tablespoons basil, chopped
1 tablespoon thyme, chopped
½ cup olive oil
½ cup balsamic vinegar

Directions:
In your Crock Pot, mix onion pieces with tomatoes, zucchini, bell pepper, mushrooms, basil, thyme, oil and vinegar, toss to coat everything, cover and cook on High for 3 hours.   Divide between plates and serve as a side dish.
Nutrition Info:calories 150, fat 2, fiber 2, carbs 6, protein 5

885.   Mashed Potatoes(1)

Servings: 12   Cooking Time: 4 Hours
Ingredients:

3 pounds gold potatoes, peeled and cubed
1 bay leaf
6 garlic cloves, minced
28 ounces chicken stock
1 cup milk
¼ cup butter
Salt and black pepper to the taste

Directions:
In your Crock Pot, mix potatoes with bay leaf, garlic, salt, pepper and stock, cover and cook on Low for 4 hours.   Drain potatoes, mash them, mix with butter and milk, blend really, divide between plates and serve as a side dish.
Nutrition Info:calories 135, fat 4, fiber 2, carbs 22, protein 4

886.   Zucchini Casserole

Servings: 10   Cooking Time: 2 Hours
Ingredients:

7 cups zucchini, sliced
2 cups crackers, crushed
2 tablespoons melted butter
1/3 cup yellow onion,
1 cup cheddar cheese, shredded
1/3 cup sour cream
Salt and black pepper to the taste
1 tablespoon parsley,

chopped
1 cup chicken stock
chopped
Cooking spray

Directions:
Grease your Crock Pot with cooking spray and arrange zucchini and onion in the pot.   Add melted butter, stock, sour cream, salt and pepper and toss.   Add cheese mixed with crackers, cover and cook on High for 2 hours.   Divide zucchini casserole on plates, sprinkle parsley all over and serve as a side dish.
Nutrition Info:calories 180, fat 6, fiber 1, carbs 14, protein 4

887.   Cornbread Cream Pudding

Servings: 8   Cooking Time: 8 Hours
Ingredients:

11 oz. cornbread mix
1 cup corn kernels
3 cups heavy cream
1 cup sour cream
3 eggs
1 chili pepper
1 tsp salt
1 tsp ground black pepper
2 oz. pickled jalapeno
¼ tbsp sugar
1 tsp butter

Directions:
Whisk eggs in a suitable bowl and add cream and cornbread mix.   Mix it well then add salt, chili pepper, sour cream, sugar, butter, and black pepper.   Add corn kernels and pickled jalapeno then mix well to make a smooth dough.   Spread this dough in the insert of a Crock Pot.   Put the cooker's lid on and set the cooking time to 8 hours on Low settings.   Slice and serve.
Nutrition Info: Per Serving: Calories: 398, Total Fat: 27.9g, Fiber: 2g, Total Carbs: 29.74g, Protein: 9g

888.   Ramen Noodles

Servings: 5   Cooking Time: 25 Minutes
Ingredients:

1 tbsp ramen seasoning
10 oz. ramen noodles
4 cups chicken stock
1 tsp salt
3 tbsp soy sauce
1 tsp paprika
1 tbsp butter

Directions:
Add chicken stock, butter, ramen, paprika, noodles and all other ingredients to the Crock Pot.   Put the cooker's lid on and set the cooking time to minutes on High settings.   Serve warm.
Nutrition Info: Per Serving: Calories: 405, Total Fat: 19.2g, Fiber: 6g, Total Carbs: 49.93g, Protein: 15g

889.   Butter Green Beans

Servings: 2   Cooking Time: 2 Hours
Ingredients:

1 pound green beans, trimmed and halved
2 tablespoons butter, melted
1 teaspoon rosemary, dried
½ cup veggie stock
1 tablespoon chives, chopped
Salt and black pepper to the taste

¼ teaspoon soy sauce

Directions:
In your Crock Pot, combine the green beans with the melted butter, stock and the other ingredients, toss, put the lid on and cook on Low for 2 hours. Divide between plates and serve as a side dish.
Nutrition Info:calories 236, fat 6, fiber 8, carbs 10, protein 6

890.   Mexican Rice

Servings: 8   Cooking Time: 4 Hours
Ingredients:

1 cup long grain rice
1 and ¼ cups veggie stock
½ cup cilantro, chopped

½ avocado, pitted, peeled and chopped
Salt and black pepper to the taste
¼ cup green hot sauce

Directions:
Put the rice in your Crock Pot, add stock, stir, cover, cook on Low for 4 hours, fluff with a fork and transfer to a bowl.   In your food processor, mix avocado with hot sauce and cilantro, blend well, pour over rice, toss well, add salt and pepper, divide between plates and serve as a side dish.
Nutrition Info:calories 100, fat 3, fiber 6, carbs 18, protein 4

891.   Mint Farro Pilaf

Servings: 2   Cooking Time: 4 Hours
Ingredients:

½ tablespoon balsamic vinegar
½ cup whole grain farro
A pinch of salt and black pepper
1 cup chicken stock

½ tablespoon olive oil
1 tablespoon green onions, chopped
1 tablespoon mint, chopped

Directions:
In your Crock Pot, mix the farro with the vinegar and the other ingredients, toss, put the lid on and cook on Low for 4 hours.   Divide between plates and serve.
Nutrition Info:calories 162, fat 3, fiber 6, carbs 9, protein 4

892.   Cider Dipped Farro

Servings: 6   Cooking Time: 5 Hours
Ingredients:

1 tbsp apple cider vinegar
1 cup whole-grain farro
1 tsp lemon juice
Salt to the taste
3 cups of water
1 tbsp olive oil

½ cup cherries, dried and chopped
¼ cup green onions, chopped
10 mint leaves, chopped
2 cups cherries, pitted and halved

Directions:
Add water and farro to the Crock Pot.   Put the cooker's lid on and set the cooking time to 5 hours on Low settings.   Toss the cooker farro with salt, cherries, mint, green onion, lemon juice, and oil in a bowl.   Serve fresh.
Nutrition Info: Per Serving: Calories: 162, Total Fat: 3g, Fiber: 6g, Total Carbs: 12g, Protein: 4g

893.   Glazed Baby Carrots

Servings: 6   Cooking Time: 6 Hours
Ingredients:

½ cup peach preserves
½ cup butter, melted
2 pounds baby carrots
1 teaspoon vanilla extract
A pinch of salt and black pepper

2 tablespoon sugar
A pinch of nutmeg, ground
½ teaspoon cinnamon powder
2 tablespoons water

Directions:
Put baby carrots in your Crock Pot, add butter, peach preserves, sugar, vanilla, salt, pepper, nutmeg, cinnamon and water, toss well, cover and cook on Low for 6 hours.   Divide between plates and serve as a side dish.
Nutrition Info:calories 283, fat 14, fiber 4, carbs 28, protein 3

894.   Squash Side Salad

Servings: 8   Cooking Time: 4 Hours
Ingredients:

1 tablespoon olive oil
1 cup carrots, chopped
1 yellow onion, chopped
1 teaspoon sugar
1 and ½ teaspoons curry powder
1 garlic clove, minced

1 big butternut squash, peeled and cubed
A pinch of sea salt and black pepper
¼ teaspoon ginger, grated
½ teaspoon cinnamon powder
3 cups coconut milk

Directions:
In your Crock Pot, mix oil with carrots, onion, sugar, curry powder, garlic, squash, salt, pepper, ginger, cinnamon and coconut milk, stir well, cover and cook on Low for 4 hours.   Stir, divide between plates and serve as a side dish.
Nutrition Info:calories 200, fat 4, fiber 4, carbs 17, protein 4

895.   Lemony Beets

Servings: 6   Cooking Time: 8 Hours
Ingredients:

6 beets, peeled and cut into medium wedges
2 tablespoons olive oil

2 tablespoons honey
Salt and black pepper to the taste
1 tablespoon white vinegar

2 tablespoons lemon juice
½ teaspoon lemon peel, grated

Directions:
In your Crock Pot, mix beets with honey, oil, lemon juice, salt, pepper, vinegar and lemon peel, cover and cook on Low for 8 hours.   Divide between plates and serve as a side dish.
Nutrition Info: calories 80, fat 3, fiber 4, carbs 8, protein 4

| 896. | Baby Carrots And Parsnips Mix |

Servings: 2   Cooking Time: 6 Hours
Ingredients:

1 tablespoon avocado oil
1 pound baby carrots, peeled
½ pound parsnips, peeled and cut into sticks
1 teaspoon sweet paprika
½ cup tomato paste
½ cup veggie stock
½ teaspoon chili powder
A pinch of salt and black pepper
2 garlic cloves, minced
1 tablespoon dill, chopped

Directions:
Grease the Crock Pot with the oil and mix the carrots with the parsnips, paprika and the other ingredients inside.   Toss, put the lid on and cook on Low for 6 hours.   Divide everything between plates and serve as a side dish.
Nutrition Info: calories 273, fat 7, fiber 5, carbs 8, protein 12

| 897. | Potatoes And Leeks Mix |

Servings: 2   Cooking Time: 4 Hours
Ingredients:

2 leeks, sliced
½ pound sweet potatoes, cut into medium wedges
½ tablespoon balsamic vinegar
½ cup veggie stock
1 tablespoon chives, chopped
½ teaspoon pumpkin pie spice

Directions:
In your Crock Pot, mix the leeks with the potatoes and the other ingredients, toss, put the lid on and cook on High for 4 hours.   Divide between plates and serve as a side dish.
Nutrition Info: calories 351, fat 8, fiber 5, carbs 48, protein 7

| 898. | Chorizo And Cauliflower Mix |

Servings: 4   Cooking Time: 5 Hours
Ingredients:

1 pound chorizo, chopped
1 yellow onion, chopped
½ teaspoon garlic powder
12 ounces canned green chilies, chopped
1 cauliflower head, riced
2 tablespoons green onions, chopped

Salt and black pepper to the taste
Directions:
Heat up a pan over medium heat, add chorizo and onion, stir, brown for a few minutes and transfer to your Crock Pot.   Add chilies, garlic powder, salt, pepper, cauliflower and green onions, toss, cover and cook on Low for 5 hours.   Divide between plates and serve as a side dish.
Nutrition Info: calories 350, fat 12, fiber 4, carbs 6, protein 20

| 899. | Cauliflower Mash |

Servings: 2   Cooking Time: 5 Hours
Ingredients:

1 pound cauliflower florets
1 tablespoon dill, chopped
2 garlic cloves, minced
½ cup heavy cream
1 tablespoons butter, melted
A pinch of salt and black pepper

Directions:
In your Crock Pot, mix the cauliflower with the cream and the other ingredients, toss, put the lid on and cook on High for 5 hours.   Mash the mix, whisk, divide between plates and serve.
Nutrition Info: calories 187, fat 4, fiber 5, carbs 7, protein 3

| 900. | Herbed Eggplant Cubes |

Servings: 8   Cooking Time: 4 Hrs
Ingredients:

17 oz. eggplants, peeled and cubed
1 tbsp salt
1 tsp ground black pepper
1 tsp cilantro
4 cups of water
7 tbsp mayo
1 tsp onion powder
1 tsp garlic powder
1 tbsp nutmeg
3 tbsp butter

Directions:
Add eggplant, salt, and water to the Crock Pot.   Put the cooker's lid on and set the cooking time to 1 hour on High settings.   Meanwhile, mix remaining spices, butter, and mayo in a bowl.   Drain the cooked eggplants and return them to the Crock Pot.   Now add the butter-mayo mixture to the eggplants.   Put the cooker's lid on and set the cooking time to 3 hours on Low settings.   Serve warm.
Nutrition Info: Per Serving: Calories: 67, Total Fat: 4.8g, Fiber: 2g, Total Carbs: 6.09g, Protein: 1g

| 901. | Creamy Butter Parsnips |

Servings: 5   Cooking Time: 7 Hours
Ingredients:

1 cup cream
2 tsp butter
1 lb. parsnip, peeled and chopped
1 yellow onion, chopped
1 carrot, chopped
1 tsp salt
1 tsp ground white pepper
½ tsp paprika

1 tbsp chives, chopped   1 tbsp salt

¼ tsp sugar

Directions:
Add parsnips, carrot, and rest of the ingredients to the Crock Pot. Put the cooker's lid on and set the cooking time to 7 hours on Low settings. Serve warm.

Nutrition Info: Per Serving: Calories: 190, Total Fat: 11.2g, Fiber: 4g, Total Carbs: 22g, Protein: 3g

902. Mexican Avocado Rice

Servings: 8   Cooking Time: 4 Hrs

Ingredients:

1 cup long-grain rice
1 and ¼ cups veggie stock
½ cup cilantro, chopped

½ avocado, pitted, peeled and chopped
Salt and black pepper to the taste
¼ cup green hot sauce

Directions:
Add rice and stock to the Crock Pot. Put the cooker's lid on and set the cooking time to 4 hours on Low settings. Meanwhile, blend avocado flesh with hot sauce, cilantro, salt, and black pepper. Serve the cooked rice with avocado sauce on top.

Nutrition Info: Per Serving: Calories: 100, Total Fat: 3g, Fiber: 6g, Total Carbs: 18g, Protein: 4g

903. Goat Cheese Rice

Servings: 6   Cooking Time: 4 Hours

Ingredients:

2 garlic cloves, minced
2 tablespoons olive oil
¾ cup yellow onion, chopped
1 and ½ cups Arborio rice
½ cup white wine
12 ounces spinach, chopped

3 and ½ cups hot veggie stock
Salt and black pepper to the taste
4 ounces goat cheese, soft and crumbled
2 tablespoons lemon juice
1/3 cup pecans, toasted and chopped

Directions:
In your Crock Pot, mix oil with garlic, onion, rice, wine, salt, pepper and stock, stir, cover and cook on Low for 4 hours. Add spinach, toss and leave aside for a few minutes Add lemon juice and goat cheese, stir, divide between plates and serve with pecans on top as a side dish.

Nutrition Info: calories 300, fat 12, fiber 4, carbs 20, protein 15

904. Creamy Red Cabbage

Servings: 9   Cooking Time: 8 Hours

Ingredients:

17 oz. red cabbage, sliced
1 cup fresh cilantro, chopped

1 tsp salt
1 tbsp tomato paste
1 tsp ground black pepper

3 red onions, diced
1 tbsp sliced almonds
1 cup sour cream
½ cup chicken stock

1 tsp cumin
½ tsp thyme
2 tbsp butter
1 cup green peas

Directions:
Add cabbage, onion and all other ingredients to the Crock Pot. Put the cooker's lid on and set the cooking time to 8 hours on Low settings. Serve warm.

Nutrition Info: Per Serving: Calories: 112, Total Fat: 5.9g, Fiber: 3g, Total Carbs: 12.88g, Protein: 4g

905. Baked Potato

Servings: 6   Cooking Time: 8 Hours

Ingredients:

6 large potatoes, peeled and cubed
3 oz. mushrooms, chopped
1 onion, chopped
1 tsp butter

½ tsp salt
½ tsp minced garlic
1 tsp sour cream
½ tsp turmeric
1 tsp olive oil

Directions:
Grease the insert of the Crock Pot with olive oil. Toss in potatoes, onion, mushrooms, and rest of the ingredients. Put the cooker's lid on and set the cooking time to 8 hours on Low settings. Serve warm.

Nutrition Info: Per Serving: Calories: 309, Total Fat: 1.9g, Fiber: 9g, Total Carbs: 66.94g, Protein: 8g

906. Cauliflower And Broccoli Mix

Servings: 10   Cooking Time: 7 Hours

Ingredients:

4 cups broccoli florets
4 cups cauliflower florets
7 ounces Swiss cheese, torn
14 ounces Alfredo sauce

1 yellow onion, chopped
Salt and black pepper to the taste
1 teaspoon thyme, dried
½ cup almonds, sliced

Directions:
In your Crock Pot, mix broccoli with cauliflower, cheese, sauce, onion, salt, pepper and thyme, stir, cover and cook on Low for 7 hours. Add almonds, divide between plates and serve as a side dish.

Nutrition Info: calories 177, fat 7, fiber 2, carbs 10, protein 7

907. Buttery Artichokes

Servings: 5   Cooking Time: 6 Hrs.

Ingredients:

13 oz. artichoke heart halved
1 tsp salt

1 garlic clove, peeled
4 tbsp butter
4 oz. Parmesan, shredded

4 cups chicken stock
1 tsp turmeric
Directions:
Add artichoke, stock, salt, and turmeric to the Crock Pot.   Put the cooker's lid on and set the cooking time to 6 hours on Low settings.   Drain and transfer the cooked artichoke to the serving plates.   Drizzle, cheese, and butter over the artichoke.   Serve warm.
Nutrition Info: Per Serving: Calories: 272, Total Fat: 12.8g, Fiber: 4g, Total Carbs: 24.21g, Protein: 17g

908.	Buttery Mushrooms

Servings: 6   Cooking Time: 4 Hours
Ingredients:

1 yellow onion, chopped
1 pounds mushrooms, halved
1 teaspoon Italian seasoning

½ cup butter, melted
Salt and black pepper to the taste
1 teaspoon sweet paprika

Directions:
In your Crock Pot, mix mushrooms with onion, butter, Italian seasoning, salt, pepper and paprika,
toss, cover and cook on Low for 4 hours.   Divide between plates and serve as a side dish.
Nutrition Info:calories 120, fat 6, fiber 1, carbs 8, protein 4

909.	Zucchini Onion Pate

Servings: 6   Cooking Time: 6 Hours
Ingredients:

3 medium zucchinis, peeled and chopped
2 red onions, grated
6 tbsp tomato paste
½ cup fresh dill
1 tsp salt

1 tsp butter
1 tbsp brown sugar
½ tsp ground black pepper
1 tsp paprika
¼ chili pepper

Directions:
Add zucchini to the food processor and blend for 3 minutes until smooth.   Transfer the zucchini blend to the Crock Pot.   Stir in onions and all other ingredients.   Put the cooker's lid on and set the cooking time to 6 hours on Low settings.   Serve warm.
Nutrition Info: Per Serving: Calories: 45, Total Fat: 0.8g, Fiber: 2g, Total Carbs: 9.04g, Protein: 1g

910. Sweet Potato Dip

Servings: 2   Cooking Time: 4 Hours

Ingredients:

- 2 sweet potatoes, peeled and cubed
- ½ cup coconut cream
- ½ teaspoon turmeric powder
- ½ teaspoon garam masala
- 2 garlic cloves, minced
- ½ cup veggie stock
- 1 cup basil leaves
- 2 tablespoons olive oil
- 1 tablespoon lemon juice
- A pinch of salt and black pepper

Directions:

In your Crock Pot, mix the sweet potatoes with the cream, turmeric and the other ingredients, toss, put the lid on and cook on High for 4 hours.   Blend using an immersion blender, divide into bowls and serve as a party dip.

Nutrition Info: calories 253, fat 5, fiber 6, carbs 13, protein 4

911. Basic Pepper Salsa

Servings: 6   Cooking Time: 5 Hours

Ingredients:

- 7 cups tomatoes, chopped
- 1 green bell pepper, chopped
- 1 red bell pepper, chopped
- 2 yellow onions, chopped
- 4 jalapenos, chopped
- ¼ cup apple cider vinegar
- 1 tsp coriander, ground
- 1 tbsp cilantro, chopped
- 3 tbsp basil, chopped
- Salt and black pepper to the taste

Directions:

Add jalapenos, tomatoes and all other ingredients to the Crock Pot.   Put the cooker's lid on and set the cooking time to 5 hours on Low settings.   Mix gently and serve.

Nutrition Info: Per Serving: Calories: 172, Total Fat: 3g, Fiber: 5g, Total Carbs: 8g, Protein: 4g

912. Crab Dip(1)

Servings: 2   Cooking Time: 1 Hour

Ingredients:

- 1 tablespoon lime zest, grated
- ½ tablespoon lime juice
- 2 tablespoons mayonnaise
- 2 ounces crabmeat
- 2 green onions, chopped
- 2 ounces cream cheese, cubed
- Cooking spray

Directions:

Grease your Crock Pot with the cooking spray, and mix the crabmeat with the lime zest, juice and the other ingredients inside.   Put the lid on, cook on Low for 1 hour, divide into bowls and serve as a party dip.

Nutrition Info: calories 100, fat 3, fiber 2, carbs 9, protein 4

913. Bulgur And Beans Salsa

Servings: 2   Cooking Time: 8 Hours

Ingredients:

- 1 cup veggie stock
- 1 small yellow onion, chopped
- 1 red bell pepper, chopped
- 1 garlic clove, minced
- 5 ounces canned kidney beans, drained
- ½ cup bulgur
- ½ cup salsa
- 1 tablespoon chili powder
- ¼ teaspoon oregano, dried
- Salt and black pepper to the taste

Directions:

In your Crock Pot, mix the bulgur with the stock and the other ingredients, toss, put the lid on and cook on Low for 8 hours.   Divide into bowls and serve cold as an appetizer.

Nutrition Info: calories 351, fat 4, fiber 6, carbs 12, protein 4

914. Eggplant Salad

Servings: 2   Cooking Time: 8 Hours

Ingredients:

- 2 eggplants, cubed
- 2 scallions, chopped
- 1 red bell pepper, chopped
- ½ teaspoon coriander, ground
- ½ cup mild salsa
- 1 teaspoon cumin, ground
- A pinch of salt and black pepper
- 1 tablespoon lemon juice

Directions:

In your Crock Pot, combine the eggplants with the scallions, pepper and the other ingredients, toss, put the lid on, cook on Low for 8 hours, divide into bowls and serve cold as an appetizer salad.

Nutrition Info: calories 203, fat 2, fiber 3, carbs 7, protein 8

915. Apple And Carrot Dip

Servings: 2   Cooking Time: 6 Hours

Ingredients:

- 1 cup carrots, peeled and grated
- ¼ teaspoon cloves, ground
- ¼ teaspoon ginger powder
- 1 tablespoon lemon juice
- 2 cups apples, peeled, cored and chopped
- ½ tablespoon lemon zest, grated
- ½ cup coconut cream
- ¼ teaspoon nutmeg, ground

Directions:

In your Crock Pot, mix the apples with the carrots, cloves and the other ingredients, toss, put the lid on

and cook on Low for 6 hours. Bend using an immersion blender, divide into bowls and serve.
Nutrition Info:calories 212, fat 4, fiber 6, carbs 12, protein 3

916. Italian Mussels Salad

Servings: 4   Cooking Time: 1 Hour
Ingredients:

28 ounces canned tomatoes, crushed	2 pounds mussels, cleaned and scrubbed
½ cup white onion, chopped	2 tablespoons red pepper flakes
2 jalapeno peppers, chopped	2 garlic cloves, minced
¼ cup dry white wine	Salt to the taste
¼ cup extra virgin olive oil	½ cup basil, chopped
¼ cup balsamic vinegar	Lemon wedges for serving

Directions:
In your Crock Pot, mix tomatoes with onion, jalapenos, wine, oil, vinegar, garlic, pepper flakes, salt, basil and mussels, cover and cook on High for hour. Discard unopened mussels, divide everything into bowls and serve with lemon wedges.
Nutrition Info:calories 100, fat 1, fiber 1, carbs 7, protein 2

917.Ginger Chili Peppers

Servings: 7   Cooking Time: 3 Hours
Ingredients:

2 tbsp balsamic vinegar	3 tbsp water
10 oz. red chili pepper, chopped	1 tsp oregano
	1 tsp ground black pepper
4 garlic cloves, peeled and sliced	4 tbsp olive oil
1 white onion, chopped	1 tsp ground nutmeg
	½ tsp ground ginger

Directions:
Spread the red chili peppers in the Crock Pot. Mix onion and garlic with remaining ingredients and spread on top of chili peppers. Put the cooker's lid on and set the cooking time to hours on High settings. Serve.
Nutrition Info: Per Serving: Calories: 96, Total Fat: 8g, Fiber: 1g, Total Carbs: 5.87g, Protein: 1g

918. Corn Dip(1)

Servings: 12   Cooking Time: 3 Hours
Ingredients:

9 cups corn, rice and wheat cereal	1 cup peanuts
1 cup cheerios	1 tablespoon salt
2 cups pretzels	¼ cup
6 tablespoons hot, melted butter	Worcestershire sauce
	1 teaspoon garlic powder

Directions:

In your Crock Pot, mix cereal with cheerios, pretzels, peanuts, butter, salt, Worcestershire sauce and garlic powder, toss well, cover and cook on Low for 3 hours. Divide into bowls and serve as a snack.
Nutrition Info:calories 182, fat 4, fiber 5, carbs 8, protein 8

919. Carrot Broccoli Fritters

Servings: 12   Cooking Time: 4 Hrs
Ingredients:

2 large carrots, grated	1 tsp salt
4 oz. broccoli, chopped	1 tsp paprika
	1 tsp butter
1 tbsp cream cheese	4 tbsp fresh cilantro, chopped
¼ cup flour	1 egg
1 tsp ground black pepper	3 oz. celery stalk

Directions:
Whisk egg with cream cheese, salt, flour, cilantro, black pepper, and paprika in a bowl. Stir in celery stalk, carrots and broccoli, and mix to well to form a dough. Divide the broccoli dough into 2 or 4 pieces and roll them into fritters. Grease the base of Crock Pot with butter and these fritters inside. Put the cooker's lid on and set the cooking time to 3 hours on High settings. Flip the Crock Pot fritters and again cover to cook for another 1 hour. Serve fresh,
Nutrition Info: Per Serving: Calories: 37, Total Fat: 1.6g, Fiber: 1g, Total Carbs: 4.22g, Protein: 2g

920. Beef Dip(1)

Servings: 2   Cooking Time: 4 Hours
Ingredients:

1 pound beef meat, ground	1 tablespoon sriracha sauce
1 carrot, peeled and grated	3 tablespoons beef stock
2 spring onions, chopped	1 teaspoon hot sauce
	3 ounces heavy cream

Directions:
In your Crock Pot, mix the beef meat with the stock, hot sauce and the other ingredients, whisk, put the lid on and cook on Low for 4 hours. Divide the mix into bowls and serve as a party dip.
Nutrition Info:calories 301, fat 3, fiber 6, carbs 11, protein 5

921. Apple Sausage Snack

Servings: 15   Cooking Time: 2 Hrs
Ingredients:

2 lbs. sausages, sliced	18 oz. apple jelly
	9 oz. Dijon mustard

Directions:
Add sausage slices, apple jelly, and mustard to the Crock Pot. Put the cooker's lid on and set the cooking time to hours on Low settings. Serve fresh.
Nutrition Info: Per Serving: Calories: 200, Total Fat: 3g, Fiber: 1g, Total Carbs: 9g, Protein: 10g

922. White Cheese & Green Chilies Dip

Servings: 8 (4 Ounces Per Serving)   Cooking Time: 55 Minutes

Ingredients:

- 1 lb. white cheddar, cut into cubes
- 2 tablespoons butter, salted
- 1 can (11 oz.) green chilies, drained
- 1 cup cream cheese
- 1 tablespoons pepper flakes, (optional)
- 3 tablespoons milk
- 3 tablespoons water

Directions:

Cut chilies into quarters.   Place all the ingredients (except milk and water) in Crock-Pot.   Close the lid and cook on HIGH for 30 minutes.   Stir the mixture until it is well combined and then add water and milk; continue to stir until it reaches desired consistency.   Close lid and cook for another 20 minutes.   Let cool and serve.

Nutrition Info: Calories: 173.76, Total Fat: 15.16 g, Saturated Fat: 7.53 g, Cholesterol: 37.71 g, Sodium: 394.08 mg, Potassium: 309.15 mg, Total Carbohydrates: 6.67 g, Fiber: 0.52 g, Sugar: 2.13 g, Protein: 2.88 g

923. Spinach, Walnuts And Calamari Salad

Servings: 2   Cooking Time: 4 Hours And 30 Minutes

Ingredients:

- 2 cups baby spinach
- ½ cup walnuts, chopped
- ½ cup mild salsa
- 1 cup calamari rings
- ½ cup kalamata olives, pitted and halved
- ½ teaspoons thyme, chopped
- 2 garlic cloves, minced
- 1 cup tomatoes, cubed
- A pinch of salt and black pepper
- ¼ cup veggie stock

Directions:

In your Crock Pot, mix the salsa with the calamari rings and the other ingredients except the spinach, toss, put the lid on and cook on High for 4 hours. Add the spinach, toss, put the lid on, cook on High for 30 minutes more, divide into bowls and serve.

Nutrition Info:calories 160, fat 1, fiber 4, carbs 18, protein 4

924. Spinach And Walnuts Dip

Servings: 2   Cooking Time: 2 Hours

Ingredients:

- ½ cup heavy cream
- ½ cup walnuts, chopped
- 1 garlic clove, chopped
- 1 cup baby spinach
- 1 tablespoon mayonnaise
- Salt and black pepper to the taste

Directions:

In your Crock Pot, mix the spinach with the walnuts and the other ingredients, toss, put the lid on and cook on High for 2 hours.   Blend using an immersion blender, divide into bowls and serve as a party dip.

Nutrition Info:calories 260, fat 4, fiber 2, carbs 12, protein 5

925. Lentils Hummus

Servings: 2   Cooking Time: 4 Hours

Ingredients:

- 1 cup chicken stock
- 1 cup canned lentils, drained
- 2 tablespoons tahini paste
- ¼ teaspoon onion powder
- ¼ cup heavy cream
- A pinch of salt and black pepper
- ¼ teaspoon turmeric powder
- 1 teaspoon lemon juice

Directions:

In your Crock Pot, mix the lentils with the stock, onion powder, salt and pepper, toss, put the lid on and cook on High for 4 hours.   Drain the lentils, transfer to your blender, add the rest of the ingredients, pulse well, divide into bowls and serve.

Nutrition Info:calories 192, fat 7, fiber 7, carbs 12, protein 4

926. Cheeseburger Dip

Servings: 10   Cooking Time: 3 Hours

Ingredients:

- 1 pound beef, ground
- 1 teaspoon garlic powder
- Salt and black pepper to the taste
- 2 tablespoons Worcestershire sauce
- 8 bacon strips, chopped
- 3 garlic cloves, minced
- 1 yellow onion, chopped
- 12 ounces cream cheese, soft
- 1 cup sour cream
- 2 tablespoons ketchup
- 2 tablespoons mustard
- 10 ounces canned tomatoes and chilies, chopped
- 1 and ½ cup cheddar cheese, shredded
- 1 cup mozzarella, shredded

Directions:

In your Crock Pot, mix beef with garlic, salt, pepper, Worcestershire sauce, bacon, garlic, onion, cream cheese, sour cream, ketchup, mustard, tomatoes and chilies, cheddar and mozzarella, stir, cover and cook on Low for 3 hours.   Divide into bowls and serve.

Nutrition Info:calories 251, fat 5, fiber 8, carbs 16, protein 4

927. Paprika Cod Sticks

Servings: 2   Cooking Time: 2 Hours

Ingredients:

- 1 eggs whisked
- ½ pound cod fillets, cut into medium
- ½ cup almond flour
- ½ teaspoon turmeric

strips
½ teaspoon cumin, ground
½ teaspoon coriander, ground

powder
A pinch of salt and black pepper
¼ teaspoon sweet paprika
Cooking spray

Directions:
In a bowl, mix the flour with cumin, coriander and the other ingredients except the fish, eggs and cooking spray.   Put the egg in another bowl and whisk it.   Dip the fish sticks in the egg and then dredge them in the flour mix.   Grease the Crock Pot with cooking spray, add fish sticks, put the lid on, cook on High for 2 hours, arrange on a platter and serve.
Nutrition Info:calories 200, fat 2, fiber 4, carbs 13, protein 12

928.   Walnuts And Almond Muffins

Servings: 8 (2.5 Ounces Per Serving)   Cooking Time: 1 Hour And 10 Minutes
Ingredients:

½ cup flaxseed	2 teaspoon vanilla extract
1 cup almond flour	
¾ cup walnuts, chopped	½ teaspoon baking soda
2 eggs	
½ cup coconut oil	¼ teaspoon liquid Stevia
¼ cup sweetener	

Directions:
Add all ingredients to a mixing bowl and beat until well mixed.   Spoon batter into silicone muffin pans.   Sprinkle with finely chopped walnuts.   Place inside the Crock-Pot, right on the ceramic bottom.   Close the lid and cook for about hour on HIGH.   Serve hot or cold.
Nutrition Info: Calories: 384, Total Fat: 35.03 g, Saturated Fat: 13.9 g, Cholesterol: 46.5 mg, Sodium: 100.16 mg, Potassium: 269.16 mg, Total Carbohydrates: 12.88 g, Fiber: 5.26 g, Sugar: 5.72 g, Protein: 8.76 g

929.   Beans Spread

Servings: 2   Cooking Time: 6 Hours
Ingredients:

1 cup canned black beans, drained	½ teaspoon balsamic vinegar
2 tablespoons tahini paste	½ tablespoon olive oil
¼ cup veggie stock	

Directions:
In your Crock Pot, mix the beans with the tahini paste and the other ingredients, toss, put the lid on and cook on Low for 6 hours.   Transfer to your food processor, blend well, divide into bowls and serve.
Nutrition Info:calories 221, fat 6, fiber 5, carbs 19, protein 3

930.   Piquant Mushrooms

Servings: 3 (13.2 Ounces Per Serving)   Cooking Time: Low Setting-4 Hours Or High-2 Hours
Ingredients:

2 tablespoons ghee/butter	1 teaspoon chili powder
1 lb. mushrooms, fresh	Basil, oregano, parsley, and thyme, to taste
Ginger, grated	2 cups water
1 onion, chopped	Salt and pepper to taste
2 cloves garlic, chopped	
1 tablespoon olive oil	1 tablespoon fresh lemon juice

Directions:
Rinse and slice mushrooms.   Peel and grate ginger.   Place mushrooms and all remaining ingredients in Crock-Pot.   Stir in the water.   Cover with lid and cook on LOW for 3-4 hours or on HIGH for 2 hours.   Just before serving, sprinkle with fresh lemon juice and parsley.   Serve with steak bites.
Nutrition Info: Calories: 95.01 , Total Fat: 5.17 g,
Saturated Fat: 0.75 g, Cholesterol: 0 mg ,
Sodium: 21.7 mg, Potassium: 563.92 mg, Total Carbohydrates: 7.97 g, Fiber: 2.42 g, Sugar: 4.9 g, Protein: 5.33 g

931.   Cheese Stuffed Meat Balls

Servings: 9   Cooking Time: 9 Hours
Ingredients:

10 oz. ground pork	1 tsp oregano
1 tbsp minced garlic	1 cup panko bread crumbs
1 tsp ground black pepper	1 tsp chili flakes
1 tsp salt	1 egg
1 tsp paprika	2 tsp milk
6 oz. Romano cheese, cut into cubes	1 tsp olive oil

Directions:
Mix ground pork with oregano, chili flakes, paprika, salt, garlic, and black pepper in a bowl. Stir in beaten egg and milk, then mix well with your hands.   Make golf ball-sized meatballs out of this beef mixture and insert one cheese cubes into each ball.   Roll each meatball in the bread crumbs to coat well.   Place these cheese-stuffed meatballs in the Crock Pot.   Put the cooker's lid on and set the cooking time to 9 hours on Low settings.   Serve warm.
Nutrition Info: Per Serving: Calories: 167, Total Fat: 9.2g, Fiber: 0g, Total Carbs: 3.92g, Protein: 17g

932.   Almond Spread

Servings: 2   Cooking Time: 8 Hours
Ingredients:

¼ cup almonds	1 cup heavy cream
½ teaspoon nutritional yeast flakes	A pinch of salt and black pepper

Directions:
In your Crock Pot, mix the almonds with the cream and the other ingredients, toss, put the lid on and cook on Low for 8 hours.   Transfer to a blender, pulse well, divide into bowls and serve.
Nutrition Info:calories 270, fat 4, fiber 4, carbs 8, protein 10

933.	Black Bean Salsa Salad

Servings: 6   Cooking Time: 4 Hours
Ingredients:

1 tablespoon soy sauce	1 cup salsa
½ teaspoon cumin, ground	6 cups romaine lettuce leaves
1 cup canned black beans	½ cup avocado, peeled, pitted and mashed

Directions:
In your Crock Pot, mix black beans with salsa, cumin and soy sauce, stir, cover and cook on Low for 4 hours.   In a salad bowl, mix lettuce leaves with black beans mix and mashed avocado, toss and serve.
Nutrition Info:calories 221, fat 4, fiber 7, carbs 12, protein 3

934.	Mushroom Dip(1)

Servings: 2   Cooking Time: 5 Hours
Ingredients:

4 ounces white mushrooms, chopped	A pinch of salt and black pepper
1 eggplant, cubed	1 tablespoon balsamic vinegar
½ cup heavy cream	
½ tablespoon tahini paste	½ tablespoon basil, chopped
2 garlic cloves, minced	½ tablespoon oregano, chopped

Directions:
In your Crock Pot, mix the mushrooms with the eggplant, cream and the other ingredients, toss, put the lid on and cook on High for 5 hours.   Divide the mushroom mix into bowls and serve as a dip.
Nutrition Info:calories 261, fat 7, fiber 6, carbs 10, protein 6

935.	Roasted Parmesan Green Beans

Servings: 8 (4.4 Ounces Per Serving)   Cooking Time: 4 Hours And 5 Minutes
Ingredients:

2 lbs. green beans, fresh, trimmed	1 teaspoon salt and black pepper
2 tablespoons olive oil	½ cup Parmesan cheese, grated

Directions:
Rinse and pat dry green beans with paper towel. Drizzle with olive oil and sprinkle with salt and pepper. Using your fingers coat the beans evenly with olive oil and spread them out do not overlap them.   Place green beans in greased Crock-Pot. Sprinkle with Parmesan cheese. Cover and cook on HIGH for 3-4 hours.   Serve.
Nutrition Info: Calories: 91.93, Total Fat: 5.41 g, Saturated Fat: 1.6 g, Cholesterol: 5.5 mg, Sodium: 337.43 mg, Potassium: 247.12 mg, Total Carbohydrates: 6.16 g, Fiber: 3.06 g, Sugar: 3.75 g, Protein: 4.48 g

936.	Cashew Dip

Servings: 10   Cooking Time: 3 Hours
Ingredients:

1 cup water	A pinch of salt and black pepper
1 cup cashews	
10 ounces hummus	¼ teaspoon mustard powder
¼ teaspoon garlic powder	
¼ teaspoon onion powder	1 teaspoon apple cider vinegar

Directions:
In your Crock Pot, mix water with cashews, salt and pepper, stir, cover and cook on High for 3 hours. Transfer to your blender, add hummus, garlic powder, onion powder, mustard powder and vinegar, pulse well, divide into bowls and serve.
Nutrition Info:calories 192, fat 7, fiber 7, carbs 12, protein 4

937.	Mushroom Salsa

Servings: 4   Cooking Time: 5 Hours
Ingredients:

2 cups white mushrooms, sliced	½ teaspoon oregano, dried
1 cup cherry tomatoes halved	½ cup black olives, pitted and sliced
1 cup spring onions, chopped	3 garlic cloves, minced
½ teaspoon chili powder	1 cup mild salsa
½ teaspoon rosemary, dried	Salt and black pepper to the taste

Directions:
In your Crock Pot, mix the mushrooms with the cherry tomatoes and the other ingredients, toss, put the lid on and cook on Low for 5 hours.   Divide into bowls and serve as a snack.
Nutrition Info:calories 205, fat 4, fiber 7, carbs 9, protein 3

938.	Apple Jelly Sausage Snack

Servings: 15   Cooking Time: 2 Hours
Ingredients:

2 pounds sausages, sliced	9 ounces Dijon mustard
18 ounces apple jelly	

Directions:
Place sausage slices in your Crock Pot, add apple jelly and mustard, toss to coat well, cover and cook on Low for 2 hours.   Divide into bowls and serve as a snack.

172

Nutrition Info:calories 200, fat 3, fiber 1, carbs 9, protein 10

939.   Apple Chutney

Servings: 10   Cooking Time: 9 Hours
Ingredients:

1 cup wine vinegar	1 jalapeno pepper
4 oz. brown sugar	1 tsp ground
2 lbs. apples, chopped	cardamom
4 oz. onion, chopped	½ tsp ground cinnamon
	1 tsp chili flakes

Directions:
Mix brown sugar with wine vinegar in the Crock Pot.   Put the cooker's lid on and set the cooking time to 1 hour on High settings.   Add chopped apples and all other ingredients to the cooker. Put the cooker's lid on and set the cooking time to 8 hours on Low settings.   Mix well and mash the mixture with a fork.   Serve.
Nutrition Info: Per Serving: Calories: 101, Total Fat: 0.2g, Fiber: 3g, Total Carbs: 25.04g, Protein: 0g

940.   Salmon Bites

Servings: 2   Cooking Time: 2 Hours
Ingredients:

1 pound salmon fillets, boneless	½ teaspoon turmeric powder
¼ cup chili sauce	2 tablespoons grape jelly
A pinch of salt and black pepper	

Directions:
In your Crock Pot, mix the salmon with the chili sauce and the other ingredients, toss gently, put the lid on and cook on High for 2 hours.   Serve as an appetizer.
Nutrition Info:calories 200, fat 6, fiber 3, carbs 15, protein 12

941.   Chicken Taco Nachos

Servings: 10   Cooking Time: 4 Hrs
Ingredients:

1 tbsp taco seasoning	1 tsp minced garlic
16 oz. chicken breast, boneless, diced	4 tbsp tomato sauce
1 tsp salt	1 tsp thyme
1 tsp paprika	1 tbsp chives, chopped
1 onion, chopped	6 oz. Cheddar cheese, shredded
1 chili pepper, chopped	7 oz. tortilla chips
2 tbsp salsa	1 avocado, pitted, peeled and diced

Directions:
Mix taco seasoning, salt, thyme, and paprika in a shallow bowl.   Set the chicken in the Crock Pot and drizzle the taco mixture over it.   Add tomato sauce, salsa, garlic, chili pepper, and onion to the cooker.   Put the cooker's lid on and set the cooking time to 2 hours on High settings.   Use

two forks and shred the slow-cooked chicken. Spread the tortilla chip on the serving plate and top Place the tortilla chips on the serving plate and top them with shredded chicken.   Add chives, cheese, and avocado pieces.   Serve.
Nutrition Info: Per Serving: Calories: 249, Total Fat: 11.8g, Fiber: 3g, Total Carbs: 21.56g, Protein: 14g

942.   Spicy Mussels

Servings: 4   Cooking Time: 1 Hour
Ingredients:

2 tablespoons olive oil	2 pounds mussels, scrubbed and debearded
1 yellow onion, chopped	2 teaspoons garlic, minced
½ teaspoon red pepper flakes	½ cup chicken stock
14 ounces tomatoes, chopped	2 teaspoons oregano, dried

Directions:
In your Crock Pot, mix oil with onions, pepper flakes, garlic, stock, oregano, tomatoes and mussels, stir, cover and cook on High for hour Divide between bowls and serve.
Nutrition Info:calories 83, fat 2, fiber 2, carbs 8, protein 3

943.   Garlic Parmesan Dip

Servings: 7   Cooking Time: 6 Hours
Ingredients:

10 oz. garlic cloves, peeled	1 tsp cayenne pepper
5 oz. Parmesan	1 tbsp dried dill
1 cup cream cheese	1 tsp turmeric
	½ tsp butter

Directions:
Add garlic cloves, cream cheese and all other ingredients to the Crock Pot.   Put the cooker's lid on and set the cooking time to 6 hours on Low settings.   Mix well and blend the dip with a hand blender.   Serve.
Nutrition Info: Per Serving: Calories: 244, Total Fat: 11.5g, Fiber: 1g, Total Carbs: 23.65g, Protein: 13g

944.   Beef Tomato Meatballs

Servings: 8   Cooking Time: 8 Hrs
Ingredients:

1 and ½ lbs. beef, ground	1 egg, whisked
16 oz. canned tomatoes, crushed	2 garlic cloves, minced
14 oz. canned tomato puree	1 yellow onion, chopped
¼ cup parsley, chopped	Salt and black pepper to the taste

Directions:
Mix beef with parsley, egg, garlic, onion, and black pepper in a bowl.   Make 16 small meatballs out of this beef mixture.   Add tomato puree, tomatoes,

and meatballs to the Crock Pot.   Put the cooker's lid on and set the cooking time to 8 hours on Low settings.   Serve warm.

Nutrition Info: Per Serving: Calories: 160, Total Fat: 5g, Fiber: 3g, Total Carbs: 10g, Protein: 7g

945.   Macadamia Nuts Snack

Servings: 2   Cooking Time: 2 Hours

Ingredients:

½ pound macadamia nuts	¼ cup water
1 tablespoon avocado oil	½ teaspoon oregano, dried
½ tablespoon chili powder	½ teaspoon onion powder

Directions:

In your Crock Pot, mix the macadamia nuts with the oil and the other ingredients, toss, put the lid on, cook on Low for 2 hours, divide into bowls and serve as a snack.

Nutrition Info:calories 108, fat 3, fiber 2, carbs 9, protein 2

946.   Stuffed Peppers Platter

Servings: 2   Cooking Time: 4 Hours

Ingredients:

1 red onion, chopped	1 teaspoons olive oil
½ teaspoon sweet paprika	½ cup corn
½ tablespoon chili powder	A pinch of salt and black pepper
1 garlic clove, minced	2 colored bell peppers, tops and insides scooped out
1 cup white rice, cooked	½ cup tomato sauce

Directions:

In a bowl, mix the onion with the oil, paprika and the other ingredients except the peppers and tomato sauce, stir well and stuff the peppers the with this mix.   Put the peppers in the Crock Pot, add the sauce, put the lid on and cook on Low for 4 hours.   Transfer the peppers on a platter and serve as an appetizer.

Nutrition Info:calories 253, fat 5, fiber 4, carbs 12, protein 3

947.   Cajun Almonds And Shrimp Bowls

Servings: 2   Cooking Time: 2 Hours

Ingredients:

1 cup almonds	½ cup black olives, pitted and halved
1 pound shrimp, peeled and deveined	
½ cup kalamata olives, pitted and halved	½ cup mild salsa
	½ tablespoon Cajun seasoning

Directions:

In your Crock Pot, mix the shrimp with the almonds, olives and the other ingredients, toss, put

the lid on and cook on High for 2 hours.   Divide between small plates and serve as an appetizer.

Nutrition Info:calories 100, fat 2, fiber 3, carbs 7, protein 3

948.   Beef Meatballs

Servings: 8   Cooking Time: 8 Hours

Ingredients:

1 and ½ pounds beef, ground	1 egg, whisked
16 ounces canned tomatoes, crushed	2 garlic cloves, minced
14 ounces canned tomato puree	1 yellow onion, chopped
¼ cup parsley, chopped	Salt and black pepper to the taste

Directions:

In a bowl, mix beef with egg, parsley, garlic, black pepper and onion, stir well and shape   meatballs. Place them in your Crock Pot, add tomato puree and crushed tomatoes on top, cover and cook on Low for 8 hours.   Arrange them on a platter and serve.

Nutrition Info:calories 160, fat 5, fiber 3, carbs 10, protein 7

949.   Apple Wedges With Peanuts

Servings: 5   Cooking Time: 2 Hours

Ingredients:

1 tbsp peanut butter	½ tsp cinnamon
3 tbsp peanut, crushed	1 tbsp butter
6 green apples, cut into wedges	2 tsp water
	1 tsp lemon zest
	1 tsp lemon juice

Directions:

Toss the peanuts with peanut butter, butter, lemon zest, cinnamon, and lemon juice in a bowl.   Stir in apple wedges and mix well to coat them. Transfer the apple to the Crock Pot along with 2 tsp water.   Put the cooker's lid on and set the cooking time to 2 hours on High settings.   Serve.

Nutrition Info: Per Serving: Calories: 20, Total Fat: 6.9g, Fiber: 6g, Total Carbs: 35.16g, Protein: 4g

950.   Cauliflower Spread

Servings: 2   Cooking Time: 7 Hours

Ingredients:

1 cup cauliflower florets	½ cup heavy cream
1 tablespoon mayonnaise	¼ teaspoon smoked paprika
1 tablespoon lemon juice	¼ teaspoon mustard powder
½ teaspoon garlic powder	A pinch of salt and black pepper

Directions:

In your Crock Pot, combine the cauliflower with the cream, mayonnaise and the other ingredients, toss, put the lid on and cook on Low for 7 hours.

Transfer to a blender, pulse well, into bowls and serve as a spread.

Nutrition Info: calories 152, fat 13.8, fiber 1.5, carbs 6.2, protein 2

951. Caramel Corn

Servings: 13   Cooking Time: 2 Hours

Ingredients:

½ cup butter
1 teaspoon vanilla extract
¼ cup corn syrup
1 cup brown sugar
1 teaspoon baking soda
12 cups plain popcorn
1 cup mixed nuts
Cooking spray

Directions:

Grease your Crock Pot with cooking spray, add butter, vanilla, corn syrup, brown sugar and baking soda, cover and cook on High for hour, stirring after 30 minutes.   Add popcorn, toss, cover and cook on Low for 1 hour more.   Add nuts, toss, divide into bowls and serve as a snack.

Nutrition Info: calories 250, fat 14, fiber 1, carbs 20, protein 2

952. Caramel Milk Dip

Servings: 4   Cooking Time: 2 Hours

Ingredients:

1 cup butter
12 oz. condensed milk
2 cups brown sugar
1 cup of corn syrup

Directions:

Add butter, milk, corn syrup, and sugar to the Crock Pot.   Put the cooker's lid on and set the cooking time to hours on High settings.   Serve warm.

Nutrition Info: Per Serving: Calories: 172, Total Fat: 2g, Fiber: 6g, Total Carbs: 12g, Protein: 4g

953. Wild Rice Pilaf

Servings: 8 (6.8 Ounces Per Serving)   Cooking Time: 3 Hours And 10 Minutes

Ingredients:

2 green onion, chopped
2 cups long grain wild rice
1 cup whole tomatoes, sliced
1 teaspoon seasonings, thyme, basil, rosemary
4 cups water
1 lemon rind, finely grated
4 tablespoons olive oil
Sea salt and fresh cracked pepper to taste

Directions:

Place all the ingredients in Crock-Pot except the seasonings and lemon rind, and give it a good stir.   Close the lid and cook on HIGH for ½ hours or on LOW for 3 hours. After done cooking add seasoning to taste.   Sprinkle with lemon rind and serve hot.

Nutrition Info: Calories: 209.81, Total Fat: 7.31 g, Saturated Fat: 1.01 g, Cholesterol: 0 mg, Sodium: 8.69 mg, Potassium: 237.85 mg, Fiber: 2.87 g, Sugar: 1.75 g, Protein: 6.22 g

954. Zucchini Spread

Servings: 2   Cooking Time: 6 Hours

Ingredients:

1 tablespoon walnuts, chopped
2 zucchinis, grated
1 teaspoon balsamic vinegar
1 cup heavy cream
1 tablespoon tahini paste
1 tablespoon chives, chopped

Directions:

In your Crock Pot, combine the zucchinis with the cream, walnuts and the other ingredients, whisk, put the lid on and cook on Low for 6 hours. Blend using an immersion blender, divide into bowls and serve as a party spread.

Nutrition Info: calories 221, fat 6, fiber 5, carbs 9, protein 3

955. Beer And Cheese Dip

Servings: 10   Cooking Time: 1 Hour

Ingredients:

12 ounces cream cheese
4 cups cheddar cheese, shredded
6 ounces beer
1 tablespoon chives, chopped

Directions:

In your Crock Pot, mix cream cheese with beer and cheddar, stir, cover and cook on Low for hour. Stir your dip, add chives, divide into bowls and serve.

Nutrition Info: calories 212, fat 4, fiber 7, carbs 16, protein 5

956. Buffalo Meatballs

Servings: 36   Cooking Time: 3 Hours And 10 Minutes

Ingredients:

1 cup breadcrumbs
2 pounds chicken, ground
¾ cup buffalo wings sauce
½ cup yellow onion, chopped
3 garlic cloves, minced
2 eggs
Salt and black pepper to the taste
2 tablespoons olive oil
¼ cup butter, melted
1 cup blue cheese dressing

Directions:

In a bowl, mix chicken with breadcrumbs, eggs, onion, garlic, salt and pepper, stir and shape small meatballs out of this mix.   Heat up a pan with the oil over medium-high heat, add meatballs, brown them for a few minutes on each side and transfer them to your Crock Pot.   Add melted butter and buffalo wings sauce, cover and cook on Low for hours.   Arrange meatballs on a platter and serve them with the blue cheese dressing on the side.

Nutrition Info: calories 100, fat 7, fiber 1, carbs 4, protein 4

957. Peanut Bombs

Servings: 9   Cooking Time: 6 Hours

Ingredients:

1 cup peanut	1 tsp salt
½ cup flour	1 tsp turmeric
1 egg	4 tbsp milk
1 tsp butter, melted	¼ tsp nutmeg

Directions:
First, blend the peanuts in a blender then stir in flour. Beat egg with milk, nutmeg, turmeric, and salt in a bowl. Stir in the peanut-flour mixture and mix well to form a dough. Grease the base of the Crock Pot with melted butter. Divide the dough into golf ball-sized balls and place them the cooker. Put the cooker's lid on and set the cooking time to hours on Low settings. Serve.
Nutrition Info: Per Serving: Calories: 215, Total Fat: 12.7g, Fiber: 2g, Total Carbs: 17.4g, Protein: 10g

958. Walnuts Bowls

Servings: 2 Cooking Time: 2 Hours
Ingredients:

Cooking spray	½ tablespoon lemon zest, grated
1 cup walnuts, chopped	
2 tablespoons balsamic vinegar	½ tablespoons olive oil
1 tablespoon smoked paprika	1 teaspoon rosemary, dried

Directions:
Grease your Crock Pot with the cooking spray, add walnuts and the other ingredients inside, toss, put the lid on and cook on Low for 2 hours. Divide into bowls and serve them as a snack.
Nutrition Info:calories 100, fat 2, fiber 2, carbs 3, protein 2

959. Cinnamon Pecans Snack

Servings: 2 Cooking Time: 3 Hours
Ingredients:

½ tablespoon cinnamon powder	¼ cup water
½ tablespoon avocado oil	½ teaspoon chili powder
	2 cups pecans

Directions:
In your Crock Pot, mix the pecans with the cinnamon and the other ingredients, toss, put the lid on and cook on Low for 3 hours. Divide the pecans into bowls and serve as a snack.
Nutrition Info:calories 172, fat 3, fiber 5, carbs 8, protein 2

960. Marsala Cheese Mushrooms

Servings: 6 Cooking Time: 8 Hours 20 Minutes
Ingredients:

4 oz. marsala	5 oz. cream, whipped
8 oz. button mushrooms	1 oz. corn starch
½ cup fresh dill	3 garlic cloves, chopped
	3 oz. Cheddar cheese

2 oz. shallot, chopped	1 tsp salt
3 oz. chicken stock	½ tsp paprika

Directions:
Add mushrooms to the base of the Crock Pot. Mix Marsala wine with chicken stock and pour over the mushrooms. Now add shallot, salt, and paprika to the cooker. Put the cooker's lid on and set the cooking time to 8 hours on Low settings. Whisk cream with dill, cornstarch, and cheese. Add this cream-cheese mixture to the cooked mushrooms. Put the cooker's lid on and set the cooking time to 20 minutes on High settings. Serve.
Nutrition Info: Per Serving: Calories: 254, Total Fat: 10.3g, Fiber: 5g, Total Carbs: 35.7g, Protein: 9g

961. Mozzarella Basil Tomatoes

Servings: 8 Cooking Time: 30 Minutes
Ingredients:

3 tbsp fresh basil	1 tsp chili flakes
5 oz. Mozzarella, sliced	1 tbsp olive oil
	1 tsp minced garlic
4 large tomatoes, sliced	½ tsp onion powder
	½ tsp cilantro

Directions:
Whisk olive oil with onion powder, cilantro, garlic, and chili flakes in a bowl. Rub all the tomato slices with this cilantro mixture. Top each tomato slice with cheese slice and then place another tomato slice on top to make a sandwich. Insert a toothpick into each tomato sandwich to seal it. Place them in the base of the Crock Pot. Put the cooker's lid on and set the cooking time to 20 minutes on High settings. Garnish with basil. Enjoy.
Nutrition Info: Per Serving: Calories: 59, Total Fat: 1.9g, Fiber: 2g, Total Carbs: 4.59g, Protein: 7g

962. Cordon Bleu Dip

Servings: 6 Cooking Time: 1 Hour 30 Minutes
Ingredients:

16 oz. cream cheese	3 garlic cloves, minced
2 chicken breasts, baked and shredded	6 oz. ham, chopped
1 cup cheddar cheese, shredded	2 tbsp green onions
1 cup Swiss cheese, shredded	Salt and black pepper to the taste

Directions:
Add cream cheese, chicken and all other ingredients to the Crock Pot. Put the cooker's lid on and set the cooking time to 1.5 hours on Low settings. Serve warm.
Nutrition Info: Per Serving: Calories: 243, Total Fat: 5g, Fiber: 8g, Total Carbs: 15g, Protein: 3g

963. Eggplant Salsa(1)

Servings: 2 Cooking Time: 7 Hours
Ingredients:

2 cups eggplant, chopped
1 teaspoon capers, drained
1 cup black olives, pitted and halved
2 garlic cloves, minced
½ cup mild salsa
½ tablespoon basil, chopped
1 teaspoon balsamic vinegar
A pinch of salt and black pepper

Directions:
In your Crock Pot, mix the eggplant with the capers and the other ingredients, toss, put the lid on and cook on Low for 7 hours.   Divide into bowls and serve as an appetizer.
Nutrition Info:calories 170, fat 3, fiber 5, carbs 10, protein 5

964.   Chickpea Hummus

Servings: 10   Cooking Time: 8 Hrs
Ingredients:
1 cup chickpeas, dried
2 tbsp olive oil
A pinch of salt and black pepper
3 cup of water
1 garlic clove, minced
1 tbsp lemon juice

Directions:
Add chickpeas, salt, water, and black pepper to the Crock Pot.   Put the cooker's lid on and set the cooking time to 8 hours on Low settings.   Drain and transfer the chickpeas to a blender jug.   Add salt, black pepper, lemon juice, garlic, and olive oil. Blend the chickpeas dip until smooth.   Serve.
Nutrition Info: Per Serving: Calories: 211, Total Fat: 6g, Fiber: 7g, Total Carbs: 8g, Protein: 4g

965.   Fava Bean Onion Dip

Servings: 6   Cooking Time: 5 Hours
Ingredients:
1 lb. fava bean, rinsed
1 cup yellow onion, chopped
4 and ½ cups of water
1 bay leaf
¼ cup olive oil
1 garlic clove, minced
2 tbsp lemon juice
Salt to the taste

Directions:
Add 4 cups water, bay leaf, salt, and fava beans to the Crock Pot.   Put the cooker's lid on and set the cooking time to 3 hours on low settings.   Drain the Crock Pot beans and discard the bay leaf. Return the cooked beans to the cooker and add onion, garlic, and ½ cup water.   Put the cooker's lid on and set the cooking time to 2 hours on Low settings.   Blend the slow-cooked beans with lemon juice and olive oil.   Serve.
Nutrition Info: Per Serving: Calories: 300, Total Fat: 3g, Fiber: 1g, Total Carbs: 20g, Protein: 6g

966.   Chickpeas Salsa

Servings: 2   Cooking Time: 6 Hours
Ingredients:
1 cup canned chickpeas, drained
½ cup black olives,
1 cup veggie stock
¼ tablespoons

pitted and halved
1 small yellow onion, chopped
¼ tablespoon ginger, grated
4 garlic cloves, minced
coriander, ground
¼ tablespoons red chili powder
¼ tablespoons garam masala
1 tablespoon lemon juice

Directions:
In your Crock Pot, mix the chickpeas with the stock, olives and the other ingredients, toss, put the lid on and cook on Low for 6 hours.   Divide into bowls and serve as an appetizer.
Nutrition Info:calories 355, fat 5, fiber 14, carbs 16, protein 11

967.   Cheesy Mushroom Dip

Servings: 6   Cooking Time: 4 Hrs
Ingredients:
2 cups green bell peppers, chopped
1 cup yellow onion, chopped
3 garlic cloves, minced
28 oz. tomato sauce
1 lb. mushrooms, chopped
½ cup goat cheese, crumbled
Salt and black pepper to the taste

Directions:
Add mushrooms, bell peppers and all other ingredients to the Crock Pot.   Put the cooker's lid on and set the cooking time to 4 hours on Low settings.   Serve.
Nutrition Info: Per Serving: Calories: 255, Total Fat: 4g, Fiber: 7g, Total Carbs: 9g, Protein: 3g

968.   Lemon Peel Snack

Servings: 80 Pieces   Cooking Time: 4 Hours
Ingredients:
5 big lemons, sliced halves, pulp removed and peel cut into strips
2 and ¼ cups white sugar
5 cups water

Directions:
Put strips in your instant Crock Pot, add water and sugar, stir cover and cook on Low for 4 hours. Drain lemon peel and keep in jars until serving.
Nutrition Info:calories 7, fat 1, fiber 1, carbs 2, protein 1

969.   Blue Cheese Parsley Dip

Servings: 7   Cooking Time: 7 Hours
Ingredients:
1 cup parsley, chopped
8 oz. celery stalk, chopped
6 oz. Blue cheese, chopped
1 tbsp apple cider vinegar
6 oz. cream
1 tsp minced garlic
1 tsp paprika
¼ tsp ground red pepper
1 onion, peeled and grated

Directions:

Whisk the cream with cream cheese in a bowl and add to the Crock Pot. Toss in parsley, celery stalk, garlic, onion, apple cider vinegar, and red pepper ground. Put the cooker's lid on and set the cooking time to 7 hours on Low settings. Mix the dip after hours of cooking then resume cooked. Serve.

Nutrition Info: Per Serving: Calories: 151, Total Fat: 11.9g, Fiber: 1g, Total Carbs: 5.14g, Protein: 7g

970. Cauliflower Dip

Servings: 2   Cooking Time: 5 Hours
Ingredients:

1 cup cauliflower florets	2 tablespoons lemon juice
½ cup heavy cream	1 tablespoon basil, chopped
1 tablespoon tahini paste	1 teaspoon rosemary, dried
½ cup white mushrooms, chopped	A pinch of salt and black pepper
2 garlic cloves, minced	

Directions:
In your Crock Pot, mix the cauliflower with the cream, tahini paste and the other ingredients, toss, put the lid on and cook on Low for 5 hours. Transfer to a blender, pulse well, divide into bowls and serve as a party dip.

Nutrition Info:calories 301, fat 7, fiber 6, carbs 10, protein 6

971.Eggplant Zucchini Dip

Servings: 4   Cooking Time: 4 Hrs 10 Minutes
Ingredients:

1 eggplant	1 celery stick, chopped
1 zucchini, chopped	
2 tbsp olive oil	1 tomato, chopped
2 tbsp balsamic vinegar	2 tbsp tomato paste
1 tbsp parsley, chopped	1 and ½ tsp garlic, minced
1 yellow onion, chopped	A pinch of sea salt
	Black pepper to the taste

Directions:
Rub the eggplant with cooking oil and grill it for 5 minutes per side on a preheated grill. Chop the grilled eggplant and transfer it to the Crock Pot. Add tomato, parsley and all other ingredients to the cooker. Put the cooker's lid on and set the cooking time to hours on High settings. Serve.

Nutrition Info: Per Serving: Calories: 110, Total Fat: 1g, Fiber: 2g, Total Carbs: 7g, Protein: 5g

972. Onion Dip(2)

Servings: 6   Cooking Time: 4 Hours
Ingredients:

7 cups tomatoes, chopped	¼ cup apple cider vinegar
1 yellow onion, chopped	1 tablespoon cilantro, chopped
1 red onion, chopped	1 tablespoon sage, chopped
3 jalapenos, chopped	
1 red bell pepper, chopped	3 tablespoons basil, chopped
1 green bell pepper, chopped	Salt to the taste

Directions:
In your Crock Pot, mix tomatoes with onion, jalapenos, red bell pepper, green bell pepper, vinegar, sage, cilantro and basil, stir, cover and cook on Low for 4 hours. Transfer to your food processor, add salt, pulse well, divide into bowls and serve.

Nutrition Info:calories 162, fat 7, fiber 4, carbs 7, protein 3

973. Corn Dip(2)

Servings: 2   Cooking Time: 2 Hours
Ingredients:

1 cup corn	2 ounces cream cheese, cubed
1 tablespoon chives, chopped	¼ teaspoon chili powder
½ cup heavy cream	

Directions:
In your Crock Pot, mix the corn with the chives and the other ingredients, whisk, put the lid on and cook on Low for 2 hours. Divide into bowls and serve as a dip.

Nutrition Info:calories 272, fat 5, fiber 10, carbs 12, protein 4

974. Thyme Pepper Shrimp

Servings: 5   Cooking Time: 25 Minutes
Ingredients:

1 tsp sage	2 tbsp heavy cream
1 tbsp Piri Piri sauce	1 tsp salt
1 tsp thyme	¼ cup butter
1 tbsp cayenne pepper	1 lb. shrimp, peeled
	½ cup fresh parsley

Directions:
Blend butter with Piri Piri, thyme, sage, cayenne pepper, salt, and cream in a blender until smooth. Add this buttercream mixture to the Crock Pot. Put the cooker's lid on and set the cooking time to 10 minutes on High settings. Now add the shrimp to the Crock Pot and cover again to cook for another 15 minutes. Serve warm.

Nutrition Info: Per Serving: Calories: 199, Total Fat: 12.9g, Fiber: 1g, Total Carbs: 1.28g, Protein: 19g

975. Maple Glazed Turkey Strips

Servings: 8   Cooking Time: 3.5 Hours
Ingredients:

15 oz. turkey fillets, cut into strips	1 tbsp butter
2 tbsp honey	1 tsp paprika
1 tbsp maple syrup	1 tsp oregano
1 tsp cayenne pepper	1 tsp dried dill
	2 tbsp mayo

Directions:

Place the turkey strips in the Crock Pot. Add all other spices, herbs, and mayo on top of the turkey. Put the cooker's lid on and set the cooking time to hours on High settings. During this time, mix honey with maples syrup and melted butter in a bowl. Pour this honey glaze over the turkey evenly. Put the cooker's lid on and set the cooking time to 30 minutes on High settings. Serve warm.

Nutrition Info: Per Serving: Calories: 295, Total Fat: 25.2g, Fiber: 0g, Total Carbs: 6.82g, Protein: 10g

---

976. Cheesy Pork Rolls

Servings: 8   Cooking Time: 7 Hours

Ingredients:

3 oz. Monterey cheese, sliced	1 tsp ground pepper
6 oz. ground pork	5 oz. Cheddar cheese, sliced
2 oz. onion, chopped	1 tbsp pesto sauce
1 tbsp sliced garlic	8 flour tortilla
1 tsp salt	1 tsp olive oil

Directions:

Grease the base of your Crock Pot with olive oil. Add ground pepper with onion, pesto sauce, ground pork, and onion to the Crock Pot. Put the cooker's lid on and set the cooking time to 5 hours on High settings. Mix well, then divide this beef mixture into each tortilla. Drizzle chopped cheese over the tortilla filling. Roll all the tortilla and place them in the Crock Pot. Put the cooker's lid on and set the cooking time to 2 hours on High settings. Serve.

Nutrition Info: Per Serving: Calories: 270, Total Fat: 10.8g, Fiber: 1g, Total Carbs: 27.52g, Protein: 16g

---

977. Eggplant Salsa(2)

Servings: 4   Cooking Time: 7 Hours

Ingredients:

1 and ½ cups tomatoes, chopped	4 garlic cloves, minced
3 cups eggplant, cubed	2 teaspoons balsamic vinegar
2 teaspoons capers	1 tablespoon basil, chopped
6 ounces green olives, pitted and sliced	Salt and black pepper to the taste

Directions:

In your Crock Pot, mix tomatoes with eggplant cubes, capers, green olives, garlic, vinegar, basil, salt and pepper, toss, cover and cook on Low for 7 hours. Divide salsa into bowls and serve.

Nutrition Info:calories 200, fat 6, fiber 5, carbs 9, protein 2

---

978. Chicken Cordon Bleu Dip

Servings: 6   Cooking Time: 1 Hour And 30 Minutes

Ingredients:

16 ounces cream cheese	3 garlic cloves, minced
2 chicken breasts, baked and shredded	6 ounces ham, chopped
1 cup cheddar cheese, shredded	2 tablespoons green onions
1 cup Swiss cheese, shredded	Salt and black pepper to the taste

Directions:

In your Crock Pot, mix cream cheese with chicken, cheddar cheese, Swiss cheese, garlic, ham, green onions, salt and pepper, stir, cover and cook on Low for hour and 30 minutes. Divide into bowls and serve as a snack.

Nutrition Info:calories 243, fat 5, fiber 8, carbs 15, protein 3

---

979. Almond Buns

Servings: 6 (1.9 Ounces Per Serving)   Cooking Time: 20 Minutes

Ingredients:

3 cups almond flour	5 tablespoons butter
1 ½ teaspoons sweetener of your choice (optional)	2 eggs
	1 ½ teaspoons baking powder

Directions:

In a mixing bowl, combine the dry ingredients. In another bowl, whisk the eggs. Add melted butter to mixture and mix well. Divide almond mixture equally into 6 parts. Grease the bottom of Crock-Pot and place in 6 almond buns. Cover and cook on HIGH for 2 to 2 ½ hours or LOW for 4 to 4 ½ hours. Serve hot.

Nutrition Info: Calories: 219.35, Total Fat: 20.7 g, Saturated Fat: 7.32 g, Cholesterol: 87.44 mg, Sodium: 150.31 mg, Potassium: 145.55 mg, Total Carbohydrates: 4.59 g, Fiber: 1.8 g, Sugar: 1.6 g, Protein: 6.09 g

---

980. Eggplant Dip

Servings: 4   Cooking Time: 4 Hours And 10 Minutes

Ingredients:

1 eggplant	1 celery stick, chopped
1 zucchini, chopped	1 tomato, chopped
2 tablespoons olive oil	2 tablespoons tomato paste
2 tablespoons balsamic vinegar	1 and ½ teaspoons garlic, minced
1 tablespoon parsley, chopped	A pinch of sea salt
1 yellow onion, chopped	Black pepper to the taste

Directions:

Brush eggplant with the oil, place on preheated grill and cook over medium-high heat for 5 minutes on each side. Leave aside to cool down, chop it and put in your Crock Pot. Also add, zucchini, vinegar, onion, celery, tomato, parsley, tomato paste, garlic, salt and pepper and stir everything.

Cover and cook on High for hours. Stir your spread again very well, divide into bowls and serve.
Nutrition Info:calories 110, fat 1, fiber 2, carbs 7, protein 5

981. Slow-cooked Lemon Peel

Servings: 80 Pieces   Cooking Time: 4 Hrs
Ingredients:

- 5 big lemons, peel cut into strips
- 5 cups of water
- 2 and ¼ cups white sugar

Directions:
Spread the lemon peel in the Crock Pot and top it with sugar and water.   Put the cooker's lid on and set the cooking time to 4 hours on Low settings. Drain the cooked peel and serve.
Nutrition Info: Per Serving: Calories: 7, Total Fat: 1g, Fiber: 1g, Total Carbs: 2g, Protein: 1g

982. Apple Dip

Servings: 8   Cooking Time: 1 Hour And 30 Minutes
Ingredients:

- 5 apples, peeled and chopped
- ½ teaspoon cinnamon powder
- 12 ounces jarred caramel sauce
- A pinch of nutmeg, ground

Directions:
In your Crock Pot, mix apples with cinnamon, caramel sauce and nutmeg, stir, cover and cook on High for hour and 30 minutes.   Divide into bowls and serve.
Nutrition Info:calories 200, fat 3, fiber 6, carbs 10, protein 5

983. Cheeseburger Cream Dip

Servings: 10   Cooking Time: 3 Hours
Ingredients:

- 1 lb. beef, ground
- 1 tsp garlic powder
- Salt and black pepper to the taste
- 2 tbsp Worcestershire sauce
- 8 bacon strips, chopped
- 3 garlic cloves, minced
- 1 yellow onion, chopped
- 12 oz. cream cheese, soft
- 1 cup sour cream
- 2 tbsp ketchup
- 2 tbsp mustard
- 10 oz. canned tomatoes and chilies, chopped
- 1 and ½ cup cheddar cheese, shredded
- 1 cup mozzarella, shredded

Directions:
Add beef, Worcestershire sauce and all other ingredients to the Crock Pot.   Put the cooker's lid on and set the cooking time to 3 hours on Low settings.   Serve fresh.
Nutrition Info: Per Serving: Calories: 251, Total Fat: 5g, Fiber: 8g, Total Carbs: 16g, Protein: 4g

984. Cheeseburger Meatballs

Servings: 12   Cooking Time: 3 Hours
Ingredients:

- 2 bacon slices, chopped
- 1 pound beef, ground
- ¼ cup milk
- ½ cup yellow onion, chopped
- ½ cup breadcrumbs
- 1 egg, whisked
- 1 tablespoon honey
- Salt and black pepper to the taste
- 3 ounces cheddar cheese, cubed
- 18 ounces bbq sauce
- 24 dill pickle slices

Directions:
In a bowl, mix beef with bacon, milk, onion, breadcrumbs, egg, honey, salt and pepper, stir well and shape medium meatballs out of this mix. Place a cheddar cube in each meatball, seal them well, put them in your Crock Pot, add bbq sauce, cover and cook on Low for 3 hours.   Thread dill pickles on cocktail picks and serve them with your cheeseburger meatballs.
Nutrition Info:calories 200, fat 8, fiber 1, carbs 24, protein 10

985. Caramel Dip

Servings: 4   Cooking Time: 2 Hours
Ingredients:

- 1 cup butter
- 12 ounces condensed milk
- 2 cups brown sugar
- 1 cup corn syrup

Directions:
In your Crock Pot, mix butter with condensed milk, sugar and corn syrup, cover and cook on High for 2 hours stirring often.   Divide into bowls and serve.
Nutrition Info:calories 172, fat 2, fiber 6, carbs 12, protein 4

986. Glazed Sausages

Servings: 24   Cooking Time: 4 Hours
Ingredients:

- 10 ounces jarred red pepper jelly
- 1/3 cup bbq sauce
- ½ cup brown sugar
- 24 ounces cocktail-size sausages
- 16 ounces pineapple chunks and juice
- 1 tablespoons cornstarch
- 2 tablespoons water
- Cooking spray

Directions:
Grease your Crock Pot with cooking spray, add pepper jelly, bbq sauce, brown sugar, pineapple and sausages, stir, cover and cook on Low for 3 hours.   Add cornstarch mixed with the water, whisk everything and cook on High for 1 more hour.   Arrange sausages on a platter and serve them as a snack.
Nutrition Info:calories 170, fat 10, fiber 1, carbs 17, protein 4

987. Tamale Dip

Servings: 8   Cooking Time: 2 Hours
Ingredients:

1 jalapeno, chopped
8 ounces cream cheese, cubed
¾ cup cheddar cheese, shredded
½ cup Monterey jack cheese, shredded
2 garlic cloves, minced
15 ounces enchilada sauce

1 cup canned corn, drained
1 cup rotisserie chicken, shredded
1 tablespoon chili powder
Salt and black pepper to the taste
1 tablespoon cilantro, chopped

Directions:
In your Crock Pot, mix jalapeno with cream cheese, cheddar cheese, Monterey cheese, garlic, enchilada sauce, corn, chicken, chili powder, salt and pepper, stir, cover and cook on Low for 2 hours.　Add cilantro, stir, divide into bowls and serve as a snack.
Nutrition Info:calories 200, fat 4, fiber 7, carbs 20, protein 4

988.　Candied Pecans

Servings: 4　Cooking Time: 3 Hours
Ingredients:
1 cup white sugar
1 and ½ tablespoons cinnamon powder
½ cup brown sugar
1 egg white, whisked

4 cups pecans
2 teaspoons vanilla extract
¼ cup water

Directions:
In a bowl, mix white sugar with cinnamon, brown sugar and vanilla and stir.　Dip pecans in egg white, then in sugar mix and put them in your Crock Pot, also add the water, cover and cook on Low for 3 hours.　Divide into bowls and serve as a snack.
Nutrition Info:calories 152, fat 4, fiber 7, carbs 16, protein 6

989.　Carrots Spread

Servings: 4　Cooking Time: 7 Hours
Ingredients:
2 cups carrots, peeled and grated
½ cup heavy cream
1 teaspoon turmeric powder
1 teaspoon sweet paprika

1 cup coconut milk
1 teaspoon garlic powder
¼ teaspoon mustard powder
A pinch of salt and black pepper

Directions:
In your Crock Pot, mix the carrots with the cream, turmeric and the other ingredients, whisk, put the lid on and cook on Low for 7 hours.　Divide the mix into bowls and serve as a party spread.
Nutrition Info:calories 291, fat 7, fiber 4, carbs 14, protein 3

990.　Pineapple And Tofu Salsa

Servings: 2　Cooking Time: 6 Hours
Ingredients:

½ cup firm tofu, cubed
1 cup pineapple, peeled and cubed
1 cup cherry tomatoes, halved
½ tablespoons sesame oil

1 tablespoon soy sauce
½ cup pineapple juice
½ tablespoon ginger, grated
1 garlic clove, minced

Directions:
In your Crock Pot, mix the tofu with the pineapple and the other ingredients, toss, put the lid on and cook on Low for 6 hours.　Divide into bowls and serve as an appetizer.
Nutrition Info:calories 201, fat 5, fiber 7, carbs 15, protein 4

991.　Rice Snack Bowls

Servings: 2　Cooking Time: 6 Hours
Ingredients:
½ cup wild rice
1 red onion, sliced
½ cup brown rice
2 cups veggie stock
½ cup baby spinach
½ cup cherry tomatoes, halved
2 tablespoons pine nuts, toasted

1 tablespoon raisins
1 tablespoon chives, chopped
1 tablespoon dill, chopped
½ tablespoon olive oil
A pinch of salt and black pepper

Directions:
In your Crock Pot, mix the rice with the onion, stock and the other ingredients, toss, put the lid on and cook on Low for 6 hours.　Divide in to bowls and serve as a snack.
Nutrition Info:calories 301, fat 6, fiber 6, carbs 12, protein 3

992.　Potato Salsa

Servings: 6　Cooking Time: 8 Hours
Ingredients:
1 sweet onion, chopped
¼ cup white vinegar
2 tablespoons mustard
Salt and black pepper to the taste

1 and ½ pounds gold potatoes, cut into medium cubes
¼ cup dill, chopped
1 cup celery, chopped
Cooking spray

Directions:
Spray your Crock Pot with cooking spray, add onion, vinegar, mustard, salt and pepper and whisk well.　Add celery and potatoes, toss them well, cover and cook on Low for 8 hours.　Divide salad into small bowls, sprinkle dill on top and serve.
Nutrition Info:calories 251, fat 6, fiber 7, carbs 12, protein 7

993.　Creamy Mushroom Bites

Servings: 10　Cooking Time: 5 Hours
Ingredients:
7 oz. shiitake mushroom, chopped

1 tsp salt
½ tsp chili flakes

2 eggs
1 tbsp cream cheese
3 tbsp panko bread crumbs
2 tbsp flour
1 tsp minced garlic

1 tsp olive oil
1 tsp ground coriander
½ tsp nutmeg
1 tbsp almond flour
1 tsp butter, melted

Directions:
Toss the mushrooms with salt, chili flakes, olive oil, ground coriander, garlic, and nutmeg in a skillet. Stir cook for 5 minutes approximately on medium heat.   Whisk eggs with flour, cream cheese, and bread crumbs in a suitable bowl.   Stir in sauteed mushrooms and butter then mix well.   Knead this mushroom dough and divide it into golf ball-sized balls.   Pour the oil from the skillet in the Crock Pot.   Add the mushroom dough balls to the cooker.   Put the cooker's lid on and set the cooking time to 3 hours on High settings.   Flip the balls and cook for another 2 hours on high heat. Serve.

Nutrition Info: Per Serving: Calories: 65, Total Fat: 3.5g, Fiber: 1g, Total Carbs: 6.01g, Protein: 3g

994.   Artichoke Dip(1)

Servings: 2   Cooking Time: 2 Hours
Ingredients:

2 ounces canned artichoke hearts, drained and chopped
2 tablespoons mayonnaise
¼ cup mozzarella, shredded

2 ounces heavy cream
2 green onions, chopped
½ teaspoon garam masala
Cooking spray

Directions:
Grease your Crock Pot with the cooking spray, and mix the artichokes with the cream, mayo and the other ingredients inside.   Stir, cover, cook on Low for hours, divide into bowls and serve as a party dip.

Nutrition Info:calories 100, fat 3, fiber 2, carbs 7, protein 3

995.   Mushroom Dip(2)

Servings: 6   Cooking Time: 4 Hours
Ingredients:

2 cups green bell peppers, chopped
1 cup yellow onion, chopped
3 garlic cloves, minced
1 pound mushrooms, chopped

28 ounces tomato sauce
½ cup goat cheese, crumbled
Salt and black pepper to the taste

Directions:
In your Crock Pot, mix bell peppers with onion, garlic, mushrooms, tomato sauce, cheese, salt and pepper, stir, cover and cook on Low for 4 hours. Divide into bowls and serve.

Nutrition Info:calories 255, fat 4, fiber 7, carbs 9, protein 3

996.   Spinach Mussels Salad

Servings: 4   Cooking Time: 1 Hour
Ingredients:

2 lbs. mussels, cleaned and scrubbed
1 radicchio, cut into thin strips
1 white onion, chopped
1 lb. baby spinach

½ cup dry white wine
1 garlic clove, crushed
½ cup of water
A drizzle of olive oil

Directions:
Add mussels, onion, water, oil, garlic, and wine to the Crock Pot.   Put the cooker's lid on and set the cooking time to 1 hour on High settings.   Spread the radicchio and spinach in the serving plates. Divide the cooked mussels over the spinach leaves. Serve.

Nutrition Info: Per Serving: Calories: 59, Total Fat: 4g, Fiber: 1g, Total Carbs: 1g, Protein: 1g

997.   Tomato And Mushroom Salsa

Servings: 2   Cooking Time: 4 Hours
Ingredients:

1 cup cherry tomatoes, halved
1 cup mushrooms, sliced
1 small yellow onion, chopped
1 garlic clove, minced

12 ounces tomato sauce
¼ cup cream cheese, cubed
1 tablespoon chives, chopped
Salt and black pepper to the taste

Directions:
In your Crock Pot, mix the tomatoes with the mushrooms and the other ingredients, toss, put the lid on and cook on Low for 4 hours.   Divide into bowls and serve as a party salsa

Nutrition Info:calories 285, fat 4, fiber 7, carbs 12, protein 4

998.   Beef Dip(2)

Servings: 2   Cooking Time: 7 Hours And 10 Minutes
Ingredients:

½ pounds beef, minced
3 spring onions, minced
1 tablespoon olive oil
1 cup mild salsa
2 ounces white mushrooms, chopped
¼ cup pine nuts, toasted

2 garlic cloves, minced
1 tablespoon hives, chopped
½ teaspoon coriander, ground
½ teaspoon rosemary, dried
A pinch of salt and black pepper

Directions:
Heat up a pan with the oil over medium heat, add the spring onions, mushrooms, garlic and the meat, stir, brown for   minutes and transfer to your Crock Pot.   Add the rest of the ingredients, toss, put the

lid on and cook on Low for 7 hours.   Divide the dip into bowls and serve.
Nutrition Info:calories 361, fat 6, fiber 6, carbs 12, protein 3

999.   Tacos

Servings: 2   Cooking Time: 4 Hours
Ingredients:

13 ounces canned pinto beans, drained
¼ cup chili sauce
2 ounces chipotle pepper in adobo sauce, chopped
½ tablespoon cocoa powder
¼ teaspoon cinnamon powder
4 taco shells

Directions:
In your Crock Pot, mix the beans with the chili sauce and the other ingredients except the taco shells, toss, put the lid on and cook on Low for 4 hours.   Divide the mix into the taco shells and serve them as an appetizer.
Nutrition Info:calories 352, fat 3, fiber 6, carbs 12, protein 10

1000.   Simple Salsa

Servings: 6   Cooking Time: 5 Hours
Ingredients:

7 cups tomatoes, chopped
1 green bell pepper, chopped
1 red bell pepper, chopped
2 yellow onions,
4 jalapenos, chopped
1 teaspoon coriander, ground
1 tablespoon cilantro, chopped
3 tablespoons basil, chopped
chopped
¼ cup apple cider vinegar
Salt and black pepper to the taste

Directions:
In your Crock Pot, mix tomatoes with green and red peppers, onions, jalapenos, vinegar, coriander, salt and pepper, stir, cover and cook on Low for 5 hours.   Add basil and cilantro, stir, divide into bowls and serve.
Nutrition Info:calories 172, fat 3, fiber 5, carbs 8, protein 4

1001.   Bbq Chicken Dip

Servings: 10   Cooking Time: 1 Hour And 30 Minutes
Ingredients:

1 and ½ cups bbq sauce
1 small red onion, chopped
24 ounces cream cheese, cubed
2 cups rotisserie chicken, shredded
3 bacon slices, cooked and crumbled
1 plum tomato, chopped
½ cup cheddar cheese, shredded
1 tablespoon green onions, chopped

Directions:
In your Crock Pot, mix bbq sauce with onion, cream cheese, rotisserie chicken, bacon, tomato, cheddar and green onions, stir, cover and cook on Low for hour and 30 minutes.   Divide into bowls and serve.
Nutrition Info:calories 251, fat 4, fiber 6, carbs 10, protein 4

3-Week Meal Plan

Week 1
Monday
Breakfast: 1. Mushroom Quiche
Lunch: 135. Chicken And Peppers Mix
Dinner: 100. Bbq Tofu

Tuesday
Breakfast: 2. "baked" Creamy Brussels Sprouts
Lunch: 138. Beef Bolognese Sauce
Dinner: 102. Dinner Millet Bowl

Wednesday
Breakfast: 3. Eggs With Brussel Sprouts
Lunch: 103. Beef Broccoli Sauté
Dinner: 118. White Bean Chard Stew

Thursday
Breakfast: 4. Egg Bake
Lunch: 104. Buffalo Chicken Drumsticks
Dinner: 141. Vegetarian Coconut Curry

Friday
Breakfast: 5. Quinoa And Chia Pudding
Lunch: 144. Creamy Chicken And Mushroom Pot Pie
Dinner: 105. Quinoa Tofu Veggie Stew

Saturday
Breakfast: 6. Apple Breakfast Rice
Lunch: 106. Black Bean Pork Stew
Dinner: 145. Marinated Mushrooms

Sunday
Breakfast: 7. Greek Mushrooms Casserole
Lunch: 107. Chicken Shrimp Jambalaya
Dinner: 142. Broccoli With Peanuts

Week 2
Monday
Breakfast: 8. Pumpkin And Quinoa Mix
Lunch: 148. Hungarian Beef Goulash
Dinner: 108. Spinach Bean Casserole

Tuesday
Breakfast: 9. Creamy Strawberries Oatmeal
Lunch: 146. Chicken Dip
Dinner: 109. Mustard Pork Chops And Carrots

Wednesday
Breakfast: 10. Apple And Chia Mix
Lunch: 147. Miso Braised Pork
Dinner: 110. Boston Baked Beans

Thursday
Breakfast: 11. Vanilla Maple Oats
Lunch: 112. Intense Mustard Pork Chops

Dinner: 149. Cauliflower Mashed Potatoes

Friday
Breakfast: 12. Scrambled Spinach Eggs
Lunch: 113. Creamy Salsa Verde Chicken
Dinner: 154. Chunky Beef Pasta Sauce

Saturday
Breakfast: 13. Breakfast Spinach Pie
Lunch: 158. Texas Style Braised Beef
Dinner: 114. Beans And Mushroom Stew

Sunday
Breakfast: 14. Chicken Frittata
Lunch: 160. Mexican Shredded Chicken
Dinner: 115. Asiago Chickpea Stew

Week 3
Monday
Breakfast: 15. Peach, Vanilla And Oats Mix
Lunch: 163. Teriyaki Pork
Dinner: 116. African Sweet Potato Stew

Tuesday
Breakfast: 16. Eggplant Pate
Lunch: 164. Turkey And Mushrooms
Dinner: 117. Garlic Roasted Pork Belly

Wednesday
Breakfast: 17. Baguette Boats
Lunch: 121. Spicy Swiss Steak
Dinner: 123. Veggie Soup

Thursday
Breakfast: 18. Squash Bowls
Lunch: 125. Honey Sesame Glazed Chicken
Dinner: 165. Bbq Pork Ribs

Friday
Breakfast: 19. Jalapeno Muffins
Lunch: 126. Red Chile Pulled Pork
Dinner: 166. Bavarian Beef Roast

Saturday
Breakfast: 20. Cheesy Eggs
Lunch: 127. Summer Squash Lasagna
Dinner: 167. Lime Cilantro Chicken

Sunday
Breakfast: 21. Ham Stuffed Pockets
Lunch: 129. Onion Pork Tenderloin
Dinner: 171. Spinach Lentil Stew

CPSIA information can be obtained
at www.ICGtesting.com
Printed in the USA
LVHW020254050323
740942LV00005B/751